Hugh Selsick

Editor

Sleep Disorders in Psychiatric Patients

A Practical Guide

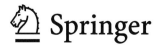 Springer

Editor
Hugh Selsick
Insomnia Clinic
Royal London Hospital for Integrated Medicine
London
United Kingdom

ISBN 978-3-642-54835-2   ISBN 978-3-642-54836-9   (eBook)
https://doi.org/10.1007/978-3-642-54836-9

Library of Congress Control Number: 2018940536

Printed on acid-free paper

This Springer imprint is published by the registered company Springer-Verlag GmbH, DE part of Springer Nature
The registered company address is: Heidelberger Platz 3, 14197 Berlin, Germany

To:

My parents Ica and Resa who made everything possible.

My wife Ella, without whom nothing would ever get done.

My children Joey, Miri and Leila who make everything worthwhile.

Acknowledgments

This book would not have been possible without the input and support of many people. I am immensely grateful to the authors who have given so freely of their time and expertise; Wilma McHugh and all at Springer for their phenomenal forbearance; my patients who have inspired me to persist with this project; my sister Aiden Selsick whose proof-reading of this book took it from distant dream to solid reality; my sister Ricki Outis and colleagues Adam Birdseye, Iain Duncan, Sakina Dastagir and Sara Stevens for their help with the graphics and my friends for all their support and humour. Finally, I am most grateful to my wife Ella and my children Joey, Leila and Miri. Pursuing this project has inevitably meant I have not spent as much time with you as I wanted to. Thank you for your support, love and patience.

Introduction

Sleep is ubiquitous and occupies a third of our lives. Whilst we still do not fully understand the functions of sleep, the fact that we spend so much time in this vulnerable state testifies to its importance. Furthermore, given how much time we devote to sleep itis not surprising that there is a lot that can go wrong with this vital biological function. Sleep has long fascinated people but the scientific study of sleep and its disorders is a very new endeavour. It is not an exaggeration to say that we are still only scraping the surface of this vast field.

One could make the same argument with regard to our understanding of the human mind and its disorders. The mind is surely the most individual and variable aspect of the human organism. This makes it incredibly difficult to find universal principles that apply to all minds and therefore all disorders of the mind.

Given the enormous variability of the human mind and psychiatric disorders and our still rudimentary understanding of sleep, the problem of applying sleep medicine research to patients with psychiatric disorders seems an impossible task. Indeed if one asks a specific question about the interactions between sleep and psychiatric disorders or how to treat a sleep disorder in a specific patient with a psychiatric condition one would be very fortunate to find research that specifically addresses that question.

This complexity makes the field of sleep and psychiatry challenging but it is also what makes it so fascinating. When approaching patients with co-morbid sleep and psychiatric disorders one can bring to bear three sources of knowledge. The first is the existing research. Incomplete as it is, there is still a wealth of useful information in the growing body of research. The second is the application of basic principles to specific clinical situations. Understanding the underlying science of sleep, the nature of sleep and psychiatric disorders, and the mechanisms of medication and other treatments allows one to make informed and decisions about how to treat each individual patient. Finally, as with all aspects of medicine, there is a wealth of knowledge in the accumulated clinical experience of those who work in the field.

The book is divided into three sections: *Foundations* contains a basic introduction to normal sleep, taking a sleep history, the classification of sleep disorders, the various sleep investigations and the impact of psychiatric drugs on sleep. *Insomnia* has a section of its own; it was felt that insomnia required a more detailed treatment as it is the sleep disorder most likely to present to psychiatric clinics and is often the disorder that sleep specialists feel the least confident in managing. The final section,

Other Sleep Disorders addresses the broad categories of sleep disorders with the exception of insomnia. Each chapter describes the aetiology, symptoms, assessment and treatment of these disorders. One can read the book all the way through but one can also refer to individual chapters as needed.

Sleep medicine is a truly multidisciplinary branch of medicine and one that is growing and evolving all the time. I sincerely hope that this book will be useful to all clinicians who encounter sleep disorders and psychiatric disorders. But ultimately, it is my greatest hope that this book will benefit the patients that we treat. Sleep is often thought of as the "Cinderella" of medicine. The importance of sleep is too often forgotten by medical professionals, but rarely forgotten by patients. My experience as a psychiatrist is that we often have a complex relationship with our patients. Unlike other branches of medicine where doctors and patients usually agree on the nature of the illness and the best treatment plan, in psychiatry we often have very different explanations for symptoms from our patients and there is not infrequently conflict about the treatment. But even when doctor and patient are unable to reach agreement on the nature of the patient's symptoms or the importance of their psychiatric treatment, they can find common ground on the importance of good sleep and can strengthen the therapeutic relationship by working together to help the patient to sleep well. The successful treatment of their sleep problems will be immensely satisfying to the clinician, and positively life changing for the patient.

Contents

Part 1
Foundations

Normal Sleep

Rexford Muza

1.1   Introduction—Definition of Sleep

The Oxford dictionary defines sleep as 'a condition of body and mind which typically recurs for several hours every night, in which the nervous system is inactive, the eyes closed, the postural muscles relaxed, and consciousness practically suspended'. Sleep is episodic and, unlike unconsciousness, is promptly reversible. Sleep is a brain state, a physiological process and a behavioural process. The familiar behavioural characteristics of sleep include recumbence, quiescence and eye closure. While asleep, there is reduced awareness and reduced responsiveness to external stimuli. In addition to the diminution of sensory awareness, an active initiating mechanism of sleep is also believed to be at play. Sleep is also associated with relative motor inhibition. The external observable behaviour of an asleep individual suggests relative inactivity; this masks the intense neurological and physiological activity which goes on in sleep. Sleep is also tightly controlled by a complex neuronal circuitry.

Sleep is universal and is a requirement which cannot be resisted. We spend a third of our lives sleeping. Sleep touches nearly every aspect of our physiology and psychology; the amount and quality of sleep we have impacts on our daytime functioning, yet the purpose of sleep is still something of a mystery. Some have found it useful to look at sleep as a drive state such as hunger or thirst. Although the real reason for sleep remains poorly defined, it is known that sleep deprivation has deleterious consequences (Banks and Dinger 2007; Cirelli and Tononi 2008; Durmer and Dinges 2005; Knutson et al. 2007; Oliver et al. 2009; Gangwisch et al. 2006; Thomas et al. 2003; Thorne et al. 1999; Welsh et al. 1998). It has been postulated that sleep is needed for restoration, conservation of energy and memory

R. Muza
Sleep Disorders Centre, Guy's and St Thomas' Hospital, London, UK
e-mail: Rexford.Muza@gstt.nhs.uk

© Springer-Verlag GmbH Germany, part of Springer Nature 2018
H. Selsick (ed.), *Sleep Disorders in Psychiatric Patients*,
https://doi.org/10.1007/978-3-642-54836-9_1

consolidation (Genzel et al. 2014; Maquet 2001; Sejnowski and Destexhe 2000; Siegel 2005). Whatever the functions of sleep are, it is quite clear that sleep is essential for all animals, particularly during periods of growth. A growing brain needs more sleep than an adult brain; daily sleep amount is highest during periods when the nervous system is developing. Some have indeed regarded sleep as being 'of the brain, by the brain and for the brain'.

1.2   Sleep Architecture

Sleep architecture describes the pattern or structure of sleep. Sleep is broadly divided into NREM sleep and REM sleep (Carskadon and Dement 1994). The first description of non-rapid-eye movement (NREM) sleep was by Loomis back in 1937 (Loomis et al. 1938). Aserinsky and Kleitman then went on to describe rapid-eye-movement (REM) sleep in the early 1950s (Aserinsky and Kleitman 1953; Dement and Kleitman 1957). This was followed in 1968 by the publication of the standards for sleep staging using electroencephalography (EEG), electromyography (EMG) and electro-oculography (EOG) by Rechtschaffen and Rales (Rechtschaffen and Kales 1968). This has evolved over the past few decades and has culminated in the current American Academy of Sleep Medicine (AASM) scoring manual (Iber et al. 2007).

NREM sleep is further divided into stage N1, stage N2 and stage N3. In a healthy adult, sleep is entered through NREM sleep. The normal sleep cycle in a healthy adult starts with stage N1 (drowsiness), followed by the intermediate stage N2 and then stage N3 which is also known as slow wave sleep or delta sleep. After a brief return to stage N2, the individual then enters stage R (REM sleep). The first episode of REM sleep occurs after about 60–90 min and thereafter alternates with NREM sleep approximately every 90 min or so (Fig. 1.1). NREM sleep predominates in the

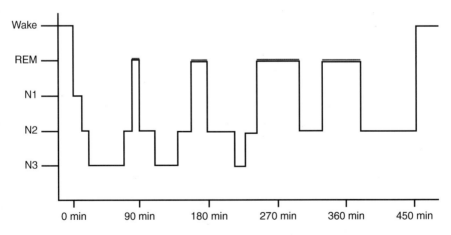

Fig. 1.1 Normal hypnogram: x axis = time in minutes from sleep onset. Y axis = sleep stages: Wake = wakefulness; Rem = Rapid Eye Movement Sleep; N1 = Non-REM Stage 1; N2 = Non REM Stage 2 and N3 = Non-REM Stage 3 (Slow wave sleep/Delta Sleep)

first third of the night. The amount of NREM sleep (delta power) decreases with the progression of the sleep period. REM sleep increases in frequency and length later during the sleep period. The first REM period of the night may be less than 10 min in duration, while the last may exceed 60 min. REM density (eye movements/time) is also greater in the second half of the night. Abnormal events (parasomnias) arising out of NREM sleep, such as sleep walking (somnambulism), are therefore more likely to occur in the first half of the night and events arising out of REM sleep, such as REM behaviour disorder, are more likely to occur in the second half of the night. In adults, the average sleep duration is about 8 h and 20 min; some individuals will need much less than this while others will need more to function optimally during the day.

Sleep in infants is quite different from sleep in the adult. Term infants enter sleep through REM sleep (active sleep). At that time, REM sleep comprises 50% of the total sleep time. Sleep cycles are 45–60 min in duration. Various EEG features emerge as the brain matures: sleep spindles appear at 2–3 months, K complexes appear at 4–6 months and slow wave activity appears at 4–5 months. By the time the infant is 6 months old, stage N1, N2 and N3 can be identified. Sleep across the lifespan is described in more detail below.

1.2.1   Stage Wake

The electrographic features of wakefulness were first described by Hans Berger in 1929. The electro-encephalogram (EEG) of stage wake with eyes open demonstrates low amplitude beta and alpha frequencies. Alpha rhythm activity (8–13 Hz) is usually demonstrated in the posterior regions of the head with eyes closed during relaxed wakefulness. A posterior dominant rhythm of less than 8 Hz is deemed pathological. It is important to be aware that the alpha rhythm of wakefulness is 1–2 Hz faster than the alpha rhythm which occurs during REM sleep. In addition to the EEG features of wakefulness, the electro-oculogram (EOG) may demonstrate rapid eye movements (REMs), blinks and reading eye movements. Slow eye movements (SEMs) may also be present. Chin electromyogram (EMG) activity could be normal or high. During wakefulness, respiratory activity is usually regular; but as with other physiological variables, it is also affected by external stimuli (Figs. 1.2 and 1.3).

1.2.2   Sleep Onset

The perception of sleepiness is all too familiar but the precise definition of sleep onset is still not so clear cut. Sleep onset is heralded by certain behavioural, EEG, EOG and electro-myographic (EMG) changes (Davis et al. 1938). As described above, stage wake is characterized by open eyes and low amplitude EEG activity (beta and alpha frequencies). REMs may be present. The EMG demonstrates muscle artefact and the chin EMG is usually relatively increased. As sleep onset

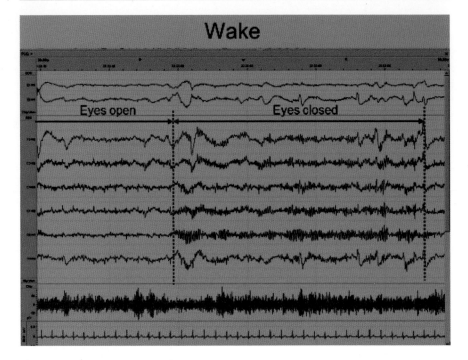

Fig. 1.2 Wakefulness

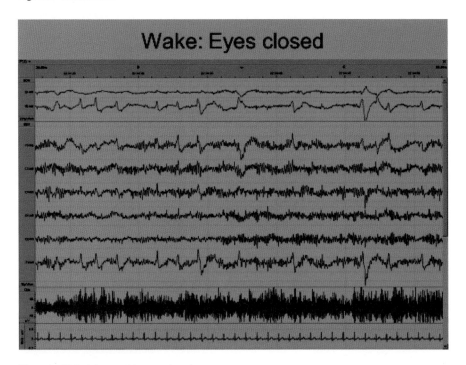

Fig. 1.3 Wakefulness with eyes closed

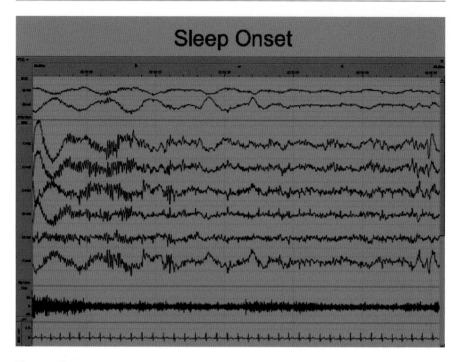

Fig. 1.4 Sleep onset

approaches, the EEG pattern of wakefulness is replaced by a low voltage mixed frequency pattern (Fig. 1.4). The EOG may show asynchronous eye movements and may also show SEMs. Generally, there is also a diminution in muscle tone on EMG. Behavioural features of sleep onset include eye closure and reduced attentiveness and responsiveness to external sensory input and stimuli; this could be visual, auditory, olfactory and indeed quite a number of other stimuli. Another curious but common phenomenon observed in healthy individuals at sleep onset is hypnic jerks (hypnic myoclonus) which are characterized by sudden muscle contractions. The hypnic jerks are not well understood but are non-pathological—although they tend to occur more frequently with stress, sleep deprivation and irregular sleep patterns.

1.2.3   Stage N1

Stage N1, the transitional stage, is characterized by a low-amplitude mixed-frequency (LAMF) EEG activity without sleep spindles and K-complexes (see below). The dominant EEG activity is in the 4–7 Hz range. Blinking stops and saccadic eye movements are absent. Vertex waves may be present but are not required to fulfil the criteria of stage N1. Chin EMG is of variable amplitude but is usually lower than in wake. Sudden muscle contractions (hypnic jerks) may occur and may

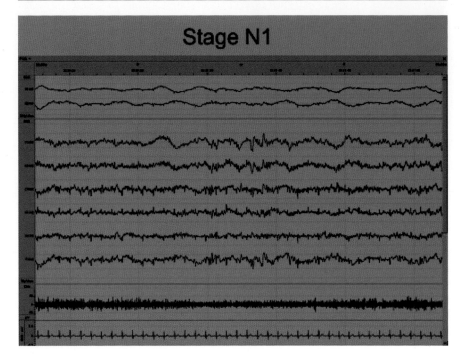

Fig. 1.5 Stage N1

jolt the individual awake. Individuals are easily woken up from stage N1 sleep as the arousal threshold is low. Stage N1 accounts for about 5% of total sleep time, but is increased in patients with a disturbed night's sleep. Such sleep is generally non-refreshing (Fig. 1.5).

1.2.4 Stage N2

Stage N2, the intermediate sleep stage, is characterized by the presence of K complexes which are not associated with arousals. These are brief (0.5 s) high voltage spikes on the EEG. Another hallmark of stage N2 is sleep spindles which are brief (0.5–1.5 s) bursts of high frequency (12–16 Hz) low amplitude waves which initially increase then decrease in amplitude. SEMs will have ended and usually no eye movements are seen on EOG. EMG demonstrates variable muscle tone which is usually lower than that of wakefulness. Stage N2 accounts for 50% of total sleep time (Fig. 1.6).

1.2.5 Stage N3

Stage N3—deep sleep—is characterized by the presence of slow wave (delta) activity of 0.5–2 Hz which is equal to or greater than 20% of an epoch. SEMs and REMs

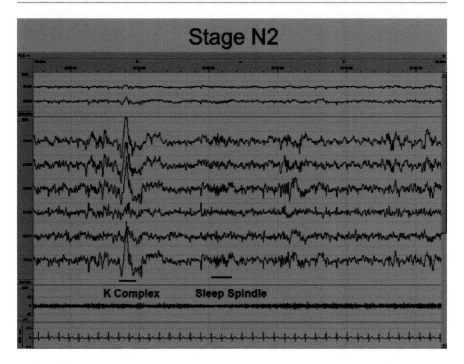

Fig. 1.6 Stage N2

are absent. The chin EMG is usually less than during wake. The arousal threshold is highest in stage N3; a larger stimulus is required to produce an arousal, hence the term deep sleep. This is the most restorative sleep stage. Most stage N3 sleep is during the first half of the night. Delta power decreases with each NREM cycle. Stage N3 accounts for 12.5–20% of total sleep time (Fig. 1.7).

1.2.6 Stage R

Stage R—REM sleep—is characterized by the presence of rapid eye movements (REMs), muscle atonia and EEG desynchronisation. The EEG background activity changes to a low voltage, mixed frequency activity not too dissimilar to that of wakefulness, but with alpha rhythm 1–2 Hz slower than the alpha rhythm of wakefulness. Saw tooth waves are frequently seen in stage R. The heart rate picks up and respiration becomes erratic. Blood brain flow increases as does brain metabolism. Penile tumescence occurs in males and vaginal engorgement in females. Muscle tone is lost (atonia) except for diaphragmatic activity that maintains respiration, the muscles controlling eye movements and the muscles of the middle ear. REM sleep has a baseline tonic component and intermittent phasic events (Table 1.1). This is the sleep stage associated with the most vivid and prolonged dreams. The purpose of REM atonia is presumably to stop the individual from acting out their dreams. Stage R

Stage N3

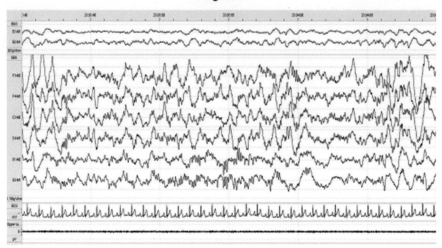

Fig. 1.7 Stage N3: Our sleep techs have offered the slide below as a better example of StageN3

Table 1.1 Physiological features of tonic and phasic REM sleep

Tonic features	Phasic features
1. Electro-encephalogram (EEG) desynchronization	1. Ponto-geniculo-occipital (PGO) waves
2. Saw tooth wave on EEG	2. Contraction of middle ear muscles
3. Muscle atonia	3. Irregular respiration and heart rate
4. Absence of thermoregulation	4. Rapid eye movements (REMs)
5. Penile tumescence in males and vaginal engorgement in females	
6. Pupil constriction	

typically follows epochs of N2. Stage R arising from stage N1 has recently been identified as a possible feature of narcolepsy (Drakatos et al. 2013). Muscle atonia is demonstrated by a low chin EMG tone. The arousal threshold in stage R is variable, but it is generally easier to wake someone from stage R than from stage N3. Episodes of REM sleep are longer in the second part of the night and REM density is also higher in the later episodes of REM sleep. Furthermore, arousals from stage R are usually complete and are not usually followed by post arousal confusion or disorientation. Stage R accounts for about 20–25% of sleep time (Figs. 1.8 and 1.9).

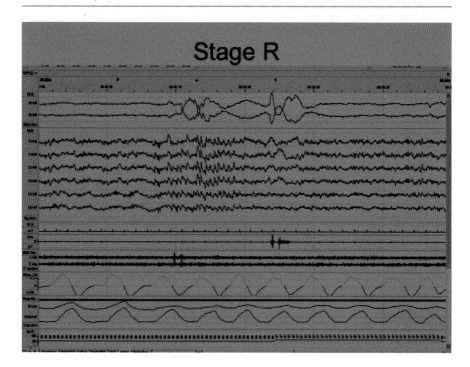

Fig. 1.8 Stage R: rapid eye movement sleep

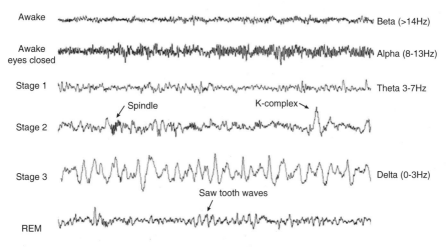

Fig. 1.9 Summary of the typical EEG features of the sleep stages

Most theories suggest a role for NREM sleep in energy conservation and in nervous system recuperation (Genzel et al. 2014; Chokroverty 1999; Scharf et al. 2008). The decreased metabolic rate in NREM sleep might help in the replenishment of glycogen stores. A role for NREM sleep in memory consolidation has also been suggested; the oscillating depolarizations and hyper-polarizations are presumed to consolidate sleep and remove redundant or excess synapses (Maquet 2001).

The functions of REM sleep and dreaming have been a subject of much debate since Sigmund Freud's publication of 'The Interpretation of Dreams'. It has been suggested that REM sleep, by its periodic brain activation, could have a role in localized recuperative processes and in emotional regulation (Hobson 2009; Horne 2000, 2013; Siegel 2011). However, deprivation of REM sleep, as occurs in patients on certain antidepressants, does not seem to have any significant adverse consequences (Espana and Scammell 2004). REM sleep might, so to speak, help expose the subject to situations and emotional experiences not commonly encountered; in other words, dreams might act as a rehearsal exercise. Others have suggested that REM sleep and dreams could be important in the processing and transfer of memories between the hippocampus and neocortex. On the other hand, Crick and Mitchison suggest that REM sleep serves as a way of degrading unhelpful neuronal activity during random cortical activation (Crick and Mitchison 1983). REM sleep might aid in the selection of brain networks that recover during NREM sleep and are ready for optimal functioning during the wake period. There has been some suggestion that REM sleep also plays a role in memory consolidation, but evidence supporting this is not strong. The periodic brain activation of REM sleep, which does not awaken the subject, allows sleep continuity.

1.3   The Two-Process Model of Sleep Regulation

In 1982 Alexander Borbély, a Swiss sleep researcher, proposed a two-process model of sleep regulation involving the homeostatic process (Process S) and the circadian process (Process C) (Achermann et al. 1993; Borbely 1982) (Fig. 1.10).

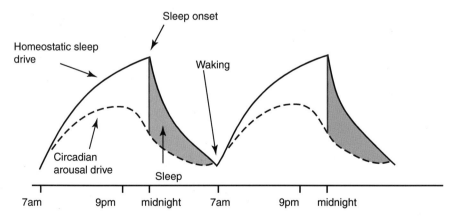

Fig. 1.10 Two-process model of sleep

1.3.1   The Homeostatic Process (Process S)

The propensity to sleep builds during the waking period and is dissipated during sleep, and so the longer an individual is awake, the higher is their propensity to sleep; conversely, the longer an individual is asleep, the lower their sleepiness (delta pressure on EEG is the surrogate of the sleep propensity) (Carskadon and Dement 1979). Adenosine has been identified as one of the possible somnogens responsible for the sleep propensity. The basal forebrain levels of adenosine progressively increase during wake periods. Adenosine is a breakdown product of adenosine triphosphate (ATP) which is the brain's metabolic substrate during wakefulness (adenosine inhibits the excitatory neurotransmitters acetylcholine and glutamate). In the basal forebrain, adenosine binds to A1 receptors thereby inhibiting the wakefulness signals which project to the cortex. In the ventrolateral preoptic area (VLPO), adenosine binds to A2 receptors to induce Fos expression and increase sleep. Caffeine, a non-specific adenosine receptor antagonist, is the most commonly used stimulant. There are most certainly other as-yet unidentified neurochemical pathways involved in homeostatic sleep regulation. The neuroanatomical and chemical basis of sleep will be described in greater detail later in the chapter.

The two-process model of sleep as proposed by Borbély considers the interaction of process S with the circadian drive (process C). As sleep pressure builds during the day, the circadian signal (see below) increases to help maintain alertness.

1.3.2   Circadian Rhythm (Process C)

Alongside the homeostatic process is an altogether different rhythmic variation in sleep propensity that is controlled by a circadian oscillator (Dijk and Czeisler 1995; Fisher et al. 2013). This circadian oscillator, or pacemaker, is in the suprachaismatic nucleus (SCN) which is located in the anterior hypothalamus. The SCN sets the body clock at 24.2 h by rhythmic expression of clock genes. The SCN is entrained to conform to the daily 24 h cycle by light using specialized retinal cells containing melanopsin. From these melanopsin-containing photosensitive retinal ganglion cells, the light stimulus reaches the SCN via the retinohypothalamic tract. The SCN then signals the pineal gland to inhibit melatonin production. It is important to note that blue light has the most potent effect. Light is the most important external stimulus or *zeitgeber* ('time giver') which helps maintain the 24 h sleep-wake cycle. Other external stimuli include social activities, exercise and eating habits.

Wake-promoting signals from the SCN increase during the day; this counters the increasing homeostatic sleep drive. The SCN has projections to the sleep-wake centres (the VLPO and lateral hypothalamus). During the night, the reduced light signal helps promote sleep. In addition to the control of the sleep-wake propensity, the SCN also controls the rhythm of core body temperature as well as the secretion of hormones such as melatonin and cortisol.

Melatonin is secreted in the darkness by the pineal gland when the inhibiting signals from the SCN have been removed. Melatonin promotes sleep by binding onto the SCN and inhibiting the alerting signal (the SCN and the pineal gland are mutually inhibitory.). In summary, light inhibits melatonin secretion and the absence of light (removal of this inhibition) allows secretion of melatonin.

Two important markers of the circadian phase are the dim light melatonin onset (DLMO) and the minimum of the core body temperature (CBTmin). As the ambient light falls, the melatonin begins to rise. The DLMO occurs about 2–3 h before the usual time of sleep onset. Salivary or plasma levels of melatonin are used in the measurement of DLMO. The CBTmin occurs at the peak of melatonin secretion which is about 2 h before the usual awakening time; usually around 4–5 am.

The interaction of the circadian rhythms and the homeostatic processes affect alertness. Human alertness is lowest around 4–6 am, after which it starts to increase. It decreases slightly around 2–4 pm and then rises again, peaking around 9 pm. During the first part of the day, the homeostatic drive is low due to prior sleep. During the second part of the day, the homeostatic drive is high and increasing due to prior wake, but the circadian alerting signal is also high. Once the circadian drive starts to drop in the late evening, the homeostatic drive to sleep becomes greater than the homeostatic drive to stay awake and the person falls asleep.

1.4   Sleep Across the Lifespan

It is not unusual to hear an older person yearning 'to sleep like a baby'. Sleep quality and quantity do indeed change across the lifespan. Chronological as well as physiological/biological age has a bearing on the quality and quantity of sleep. Pathological neuro-degenerative processes can affect the integrity of the neurons and nuclei important in the regulation of sleep and wakefulness. On the other hand, psychiatric as well medical co-morbidities also affect sleep, as do various drugs. Polysomnographic studies have demonstrated changes in various sleep parameters across the life span. Different studies have sometimes yielded conflicting results. Notable gender differences in sleep architecture have been reported by some researchers (Latta et al. 2005). It must also be appreciated that in-laboratory studies might yield results different from ambulatory home studies. Generally, total sleep time, sleep efficiency and slow wave sleep tend to decrease with age. The amount of wake after sleep onset (WASO) tends to increase with age.

1.4.1   The Infant

Sleep in the infant is quite different from sleep in the adult individual. A healthy term infant normally spends about two-thirds of the time asleep i.e. 16–18 h. REM sleep constitutes about 50% of the total sleep time and NREM sleep 50%. Active sleep in an infant corresponds to REM sleep and quiet sleep corresponds to NREM. The term infant normally enters sleep via stage R (active sleep) whereas sleep onset REM in adults might have pathological connotations and has been associated with conditions such as narcolepsy. The sleep cycle periodicity in an infant is

45–50 min, which is much shorter than the adult cycle of about 90–100 min. Infant sleep is interrupted by the need to wake up for feeds every 3 h or so. The percentage of REM sleep starts to gradually decrease at about 3 months of age. Appearance of sleep spindles at the age of 2–3 months and appearance of K complexes at the age of 4–6 months are some of the notable EEG milestones of the growing infant. By the age of 6 months, stage N1, N2 and N3 can be identified polysomnographically. The amount of NREM sleep increases as the amount of REM sleep declines. The latency to REM sleep also gradually increases during the first year. As the infant adapts to the light-dark cycle and its associated social cues, the amount of day sleep decreases and sleep begins to consolidate into longer night time sleep, much to the delight of the parents.

1.4.2 The Child

By the time the child is 4–5 years of age, daytime napping is no longer common. Total sleep time (TST) progressively decreases as the child matures (Table 1.2) Sleep latency is usually 5–10 min and sleep efficiency is quite high at 95%. Stage N1 is short. Stage N2 progressively increases as stage N3 decreases. REM sleep decreases progressively as the child grows. When the child is about 2 years old, REM sleep constitutes about 30% of total sleep time; this decreases further to about 20–25% of total sleep time by the time the child is about 5 years of age. Between the ages 5 and 10, the sleep architecture gradually takes the shape of an adult with

Table 1.2 Total sleep duration by age in normal children

Age	Sleep duration (hr ± SD)
6 months	14.2 ± 1.9
1 year	13.9 =/− 1.2
2 years	13.2 ± 1.2
3 years	12.5 ± 1.1
4 years	11.8 ± 1.0
5 years	11.4 ± 0.9
6 years	11.0 ± 0.8
7 years	10.8 ± 0.7
8 years	10.4 ± 0.7
9 years	10.1 ± 0.6
10 years	9.8 ± 0.6
11 years	9.6 ± 0.6
12 years	9.3 ± 0.6
13 years	9.0 ± 0.7
14 years	8.7 ± 0.7
15 years	8.4 ± 0.7
16 years	8.1 ± 0.7

SD = standard deviation. From Iglowstein I, Jenni OG, Largo RH: Sleep duration from infancy to adolescence: reference values generational trends. Paediatrics 2003; 111: 302–307 more stage N3 in the first half of the night and more REM sleep in the second half of the night. The percentage of REM sleep will remain relatively stable until adulthood. Social circumstances, parental discipline, cultural habits (such as bed sharing) and the need to wake up early for school all have a bearing on sleep in children. In their meta-analysis, Ohayon and colleagues concluded that in children 5 years and older and in adolescents, the apparent decrease in TST with age might be related to environmental factors rather than to biologic changes (Ohayon et al. 2004). For instance, TST was not associated with age when studied on non-school days.

1.4.3 The Adolescent

Biological and hormonal changes of puberty have an impact on the sleep of the adolescent. School schedules are usually out of sync with the natural tendency towards a phase delayed sleep pattern of the adolescent (Carskadon and Dement 1987; Carskadon et al. 1998). The intrinsic biological clock in adolescents dictates sleep onset times of around 11 pm to midnight, but they still have to get up before 7 am to prepare to go to school or college. This leads to chronic sleep deprivation with its associated daytime sleepiness. Sleep latency remains much the same and sleep efficiency also remains quite good and unchanged from childhood to adolescence. There is a significant decline in stage N3 with the onset of puberty. Stage N2 sleep may increase as Stage N3 declines. REM constitutes about 25% of total sleep time. Total sleep time averages between 7 and 8 h, but can be much reduced because of social and academic commitments. The sleep architecture gradually develops into the pattern seen in adults.

1.4.4 The Adult

As the adult ages, sleep efficiency becomes reduced and the number of arousals increase. Sleep latency, stage N1 and WASO all increase. Some studies have reported significant gender differences in adults. There is a greater association between declining sleep efficiency and ageing among women, though Redline and colleagues reported an increase in Stage N1 sleep with age in men but not in women (Redline et al. 2004). They also found stage N2 to increase with age in men but not in women. Stage N3 continues to decline as Stage N2 increases. In the meta-analysis by Ohayon and co-workers, the decrease of stage N3 with age was also noted; the effect size was greater in men than women (Ohayon et al. 2004). Redline and colleagues noted a decrease in stage N3 sleep in men only (Redline et al. 2004). Stage N3 is much more prominent in the first half of the night whereas stage R and stage N2 are more prevalent in the second half of the night. REM latency decreases with age. There is a decrease in Stage R as a percentage of TST in both men and women (Floyd et al. 1995, 2007). The decrease in stage R is more prominent after the age of 50. TST remains at about 7–8 h on average, but does tend to decrease with ageing. A greater association between declining TST and ageing is seen among women.

1.4.5 The Older Person

Sleep in older people is affected not only by the chronological age but also by the neuro-pathological processes and medical co-morbidities prevalent in that age group (Anderson et al. 2014; Carskadon et al. 1982). Use of medications, including sleeping pills, is also quite high in this age group. Sleep problems such as insomnia, intrusive early morning waking, restless leg syndrome and sleep disordered breathing are much more prevalent in the older person. In a meta-analysis of sleep parameters across the life span, Ohayon et al. concluded that sleep latency increases with age (Ohayon et al. 2004). The change with age is more apparent when young adults are compared to elderly individuals. The overall increase in sleep latency between ages 20 and 80 years was, however, not too impressive (less than 10 min).

1.4.6 Conclusion

In summary, all parameters of sleep change with ageing. Total sleep and sleep efficiency decrease with age. Sleep latency increases with age; this change is much more apparent in the older person. Wake after sleep onset (WASO) also increases quite significantly in adulthood and going into old age. Percentage of stage N1 increases with age across adulthood and more significantly going into old age. Stage N2 significantly increases with age in men with a corresponding decrease in stage N3. There is a modest decrease in the percentage of REM sleep and REM latency in adults.

1.5   Neuroanatomical and Neurochemical Basis for Sleep

Complex neurochemical circuitry is involved in the generation of wakefulness and sleep. Knowledge of this complex but exciting field is rapidly expanding and, with time, there will be a better understanding of the neurochemical basis of sleep. It is essential for a practising psychiatrist or sleep physician to have a basic knowledge of the neurobiology of sleep in order to understand the pathogenesis of sleep disorders and the mechanisms of action of various drugs.

Multiple excitatory and inhibitory neurotransmitters and neuromodulators are involved in sleep-wake regulation. Brain centres important in the promotion of wakefulness include the pons, midbrain and posterior hypothalamus. Wake-promoting neurotransmitters include acetylcholine, norepinephrine, dopamine, serotonin, histamine and orexin/hypocretin. The preoptic area in the anterior hypothalamus and the adjacent forebrain are important in the generation of NREM sleep. Gamma-aminobutyric acid (GABA) and galanin are the neurotransmitters which inhibit the arousal systems. On the other hand, pontine and adjacent midbrain structures are important in the generation of REM sleep with acetylcholine, glutamate and glycine being some of the important neurotransmitters in this process.

1.5.1 Historical Perspectives of the Neurobiology of Sleep

Our current understanding of neurobiology has evolved tremendously over the past century. The first insights into the neurobiology of sleep arose from the encephalitis lethargica epidemic of 1915–1920. Von Economo observed that patients with damage to the posterior hypothalamus had severe hypersomnolence, while those with damage to the anterior hypothalamus had insomnia (Von Economo 1930). He then hypothesized that the anterior hypothalamus contained sleep-promoting neurons whereas the posterior hypothalamus contained wake-promoting neurons. The first description of the ascending reticular activating system was by Mogoun and Moruzzi who demonstrated that stimulation of the reticular formation led to electrographic changes similar to those of arousal (Moruzzi and Magoun 1949). Kleitman and Aserinsky went on to describe REM sleep in the mid-1950s (Aserinsky and Kleitman 1953). Jouvet and others established that the REM sleep state is driven by circuitry in the pons (Jouvet 1962). A lot of work has gone on in the past few decades into elucidating the regions and circuitry important in the regulation of wakefulness, NREM sleep and REM sleep.

1.5.2 Hypothalamic Areas

The key hypothalamic areas in sleep neurobiology are the lateral hypothalamus, the ventrolateral preoptic (VLPO) nucleus and the tuberomammillary (TMN) nucleus.

1.5.2.1 The Lateral Hypothalamus

The neurons in the lateral and posterior hypothalamus secrete the wake-promoting peptides hypocretin 1 (also known as orexin A) and hypocretin 2 (orexin B). These excitatory hypocretin neurons project widely to areas that include the wake-promoting dorsal raphe nucleus (DRN), the locus coeruleus (LC) and the TMN. These three monoaminergic areas in turn send back inhibitory projections to the hypocretin areas. The DRN has receptors for both hypocretin 1 and hypocretin 2, whereas the LC nucleus exclusively expresses hypocretin 1 and the TMN exclusively expresses hypocretin 2. Hypocretin also has an excitatory influence on the basal forebrain cholinergic neurons leading to enhanced cortical arousal. Hypocretin stabilizes wake-sleep transitions. Deficiency of hypocretin results in loss of sleep-wake control with resultant unstable transitions between wake, NREM and REM sleep. Hypocretin neurons discharge during active waking but are relatively inactive during quiet waking. They are silent during NREM sleep and tonic REM but have some activity during phasic REM.

Clinical and Pharmacological Correlates

Loss of the hypocretin-secreting neurons leads to narcolepsy (Siegal et al. 2001). In patients with narcolepsy with cataplexy, cerebrospinal fluid hypocretin is either very low or undetectable. Research into pharmacotherapy using hypocretin receptor agonists and antagonists to treat narcolepsy/hypersomnolence and insomnia respectively has gathered pace in the last two decades. Almorexant, a hypocretin antagonist, has been shown to promote sleep and exacerbate cataplexy in a murine model of narcolepsy.

1.5.2.2 The Ventrolateral Preoptic Nucleus (VLPO)

The VLPO nucleus neurons are active during both NREM and REM sleep, but are silent during wakefulness. These neurons contain the neurotransmitters GABA and galanin and are activated by sleep-inducing factors such as adenosine and prostaglandin D2. A group of VLPO neurons, called the VLPO cluster, has an inhibitory projection to the TMN. Another group of neurons, called the extended VLPO neurons, has inhibitory projections to the DRN and the LC. The DRN, LC and TMN, in turn, have inhibitory projections on the VLPO. There is thus reciprocal inhibition. The median preoptic nucleus neurons are also sleep active and discharge during both NREM and REM sleep. They also discharge during prolonged wakefulness, thereby contributing to sleep pressure.

Clinical and Pharmacological Correlates

Lesions in the VLPO area result in sleep impairment. Benzodiazepines exert their anxiolytic effect by binding to a specific site on the GABA-receptor, thus potentiating the effect of the inhibitory neurotransmitter GABA.

1.5.2.3 The Tuberomammillary Nucleus (TMN)

The TMN is found in the posterior hypothalamus and contains excitatory histaminergic neurons. The neuronal projections are quite wide and include projections to the cerebral cortex, amygdala, substantia nigra, DRN, LC and nucleus of the solitary tract. The TMN receives stimulatory input from the hypocretin neuronal projections from the lateral hypothalamus. The TMN is the sole source of brain histamine. The histaminergic neurons are wake-active, less active during NREM sleep and silent in REM sleep. Although silent in REM sleep, interestingly, the firing rate is high during attacks of cataplexy (REM intrusion into wakefulness). Cerebrospinal fluid levels of histamine are low in patients with narcolepsy.

Clinical and Pharmacological Correlates

Drugs that reduce histaminergic signalling, such as the H_1 receptor antagonists like diphenhydramine and low dose doxepin, increase NREM and REM sleep. Cerebrospinal fluid histamine levels are low in narcoleptics with and without cataplexy and in patients with idiopathic hypersomnolence. H_3 receptors are auto-inhibitory; H_3 receptor agonists therefore cause sleepiness by decreasing histamine release whereas H_3 receptors antagonists will do the opposite and promote wakefulness. Pitolasant is a selective histamine H_3 receptor inverse agonist and shows promise as an additional wake-promoting agent in the management of narcolepsy.

1.5.3 Brainstem Regions

The main sleep-relevant brain dopaminergic areas are the substantia nigra and the ventral tegmental area. Their firing rates do not seem to be that sleep-stage dependant, but the dopaminergic neurons in the ventral periaqueductal grey are wake-active.

1.5.3.1 Clinical and Pharmacological Correlates

In Parkinson's disease, where there is nigrostriatal degeneration leading to the loss of dopaminergic neurons, sleepiness is a common problem. Amphetamines increase wakefulness by increasing dopamine signalling. Dopamine antagonists such as Chlorpromazine and Haloperidol induce sleepiness whereas dopamine agonists, such as Ropinirole and Pramepexole also induce sleepiness by reducing dopamine signalling through activation of auto-inhibitory D_2/D_3 receptors.

1.5.4 Reticular Formation

The ascending reticular activating system plays a major role in the maintenance of wakefulness. It has two main pathways: the dorsal reticular activating system and the ventral reticular activating system. Although the reticular activating system is a useful anatomical way of localizing the arousal system, recent research has shown that there are a number of neural groupings that act in concert to promote arousal.

The dorsal reticular activating system is made up of lateral dorsal tegmentum (LDT) and pedunculopontine tegmentum (PPT) cholinergic neurons. Some of these neurons discharge during wake and REM (Wake/REM-on) whereas others discharge during REM only (REM-on). They are inactive during NREM sleep. Neurons from these two areas have axonal projections to the subcortical centres including the thalamus, hypothalamus and the midbrain, which in turn project to the cortex leading to the characteristic EEG features of wakefulness and REM.

The ventral reticular activating system ascends through the lateral hypothalamus and the forebrain. It terminates in the substantia innominata, medial septum, magnocellular preoptic nucleus and diagonal band of Broca. These neuronal regions in turn project to the cortex leading to cortical arousal. The ventral reticular activating system receives neuronal projections from the DRN and the LC.

1.5.5 Dorsal Raphe Nucleus (DRN)

Neurons in the DRN produce serotonin. These neurons project to the preoptic area, the basal forebrain hypothalamus and thalamus. They promote wakefulness and suppress REM sleep. The firing rates of these serotonergic neurons are highest during wakefulness, lower in NREM sleep and lowest in REM sleep. The actions of serotonin are complex as there are at least 15 different types of serotonin receptors with varied effects.

1.5.5.1 Clinical and Pharmacological Correlates

Some serotonin receptor agonists increase wakefulness and, in clinical practice, selective serotonin reuptake inhibitors such as fluoxetine and citalopram similarly increase wakefulness and reduce REM sleep. Drugs such as Agomelatine which block serotonin ($5\text{-}HT_2$) receptors may induce NREM sleep and might therefore be helpful in managing insomnia.

1.5.6 Locus Coeruleus (LC)

The LC is the main brain source of noradrenaline, although noradrenaline is produced by many other nuclei. These noradrenergic neurons project widely in the brain with mostly stimulatory effects. The firing rates are highest during wake, lower in NREM sleep and absent in REM sleep. The LC activity is inhibited by noradrenaline acting on the alpha 2 receptors.

1.5.6.1 Clinical and Pharmacological Correlates

Excessive noradrenergic tone can cause agitation, anxiety and insomnia. The alpha 1 antagonist Prazosin can reduce the noradrenergic tone and has found some use in the management of post-traumatic stress disorder (PSTD) nightmares. Alpha 2 antagonists like clonidine induce sleepiness by inactivating the LC neuronal discharge.

1.5.7 Basal Forebrain

The basal forebrain has both cholinergic and GABAergic neurons. Basal forebrain cholinergic neurons project to the cortex to promote arousal. The GABAergic neurons disinhibit cortical neurons and thus augment arousal.

1.5.8 Control of NREM Sleep

During wakefulness, there are high neuronal firing rates from the wake-promoting cholinergic (basal forebrain) and monoaminergic nuclei (TMN, the DRN and the LC) and hypocretin neurons (lateral hypothalamus). During NREM sleep, the VLPO neurons are active and release GABA which inhibits the neuronal discharge from these arousal systems. The GABAergic neurons of the VLPO are themselves inhibited by the cholinergic and monoaminergic systems. This mutual inhibition operating in a 'flip-flop' manner facilitates a stable transition between wake and NREM sleep (Espana and Scammell 2004; Brown et al. 2012; Saper et al. 2001; Schwartz and Roth 2008; Sigel 2009; Super et al. 2001).

1.5.9 Control of REM Sleep

As previously discussed, the hallmarks of REM sleep are EEG desynchronization, ocular saccades, muscular atonia and dreaming (Table 1.1). The noradrenergic (LC), serotonergic (DRN), and histaminergic (TMN) neurons are active during wake, less active during NREM sleep and much less active or completely inactive during REM sleep. For some time, the understanding has been that cholinergic and monoaminergic systems interact to produce REM sleep. It is now known that the neurotransmitters of the REM-on neurons include acetylcholine, glutamate, GABA

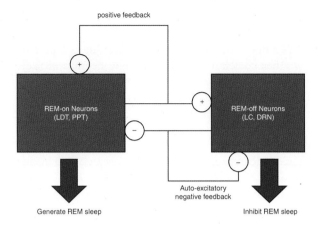

Fig. 1.11 Reciprocal interaction REM model

and glycine. On the other hand, neurotransmitters of the REM-off cells include noradrenaline, adrenaline, serotonin, histamine and GABA.

Although REM sleep was identified some decades ago, the neuro-circuitry behind its control is still very much a subject of on-going debate. Different models for the control of REM have been proposed. There is no doubt that there will be further advances in the understanding of REM sleep control. The anatomical sites important in the generation of REM sleep are the pons and the caudal midbrain. McCarley and colleagues proposed a REM sleep model based on reciprocal interaction between REM-on neurons in the LDT/PPT area and REM-off neurons in the LC and DRN] (McCarley 2007). This model has undergone some modifications. John Lu and co-workers back in 2006 proposed a putative flip-flop switch for control of REM (Fuller et al. 2007; Lu et al. 2006). Another version of the flip-flop circuit was proposed by Sapin et al. (2009) only to be later modified by Grace et al. (2014). Still more theories about REM sleep control are being proposed (Luppi et al. 2013; Vetrivelan et al. 2009). The keen reader might want to look up all these fascinating models (Fig. 1.11).

1.5.10 Muscle Atonia

REM-on neurons in the LDT/PPT area have an excitatory projection to neurons in the medial medulla. These neurons in turn project to the ventral horn motor neurons and release inhibitory GABA and glycine which lead to hyperpolarization and atonia. In addition to this glycinergic and GABAergic inhibition, there is also reciprocal dysfacilitation as a result of reduced excitatory monoaminergic activity (noradrenaline and serotonin) during REM sleep. There are, of course, other versions of the REM atonia mechanisms which have been proposed.

1.5.10.1 Clinical and Pharmacological Correlates

Narcolepsy is one clinical entity in which the control of REM sleep is impaired. There can be a lag of the disengagement from atonia when an individual wakes up from REM sleep leading to sleep paralysis. There can also be intrusion of REM paralysis into wakefulness leading to cataplexy.

In REM sleep behaviour disorder, the absence of REM atonia may lead to dream enactment behaviour.

Conclusion

Although our understanding of sleep has expanded greatly in the past seven decades, sleep is still very much a complex phenomenon which is still not yet fully understood. Digital polysomnography has greatly improved sleep staging and monitoring. A lot of research has gone into understanding the mechanisms and role of NREM and REM sleep. Although it has been suggested that sleep is essential for learning and memory consolidation, the underlying role of sleep in learning and memory has yet to be precisely characterized. Sleep neurobiology, although extremely fascinating, is still only partly understood. A better understanding of sleep neurobiology will help in the development of pharmacological agents and management strategies of various sleep and psychiatric disorders. Factors which affect sleep across the life span still need to be fully understood.

References

Achermann P, Dijk DJ, Brunner DP, Borbely AA. A model of human sleep homeostasis based on EEG slow wave activity: quantitative comparison of data and simulations. Brain Res Bull. 1993;31(1–2):97–113.

Anderson KN, Catt M, Collerton J, Davies K, von Zglinicki T, Kirkwood TB, et al. Assessment of sleep and circadian rhythm disorders in the very old: the Newcastle 85+ cohort study. Age Ageing. 2014;43(1):57–63. https://doi.org/10.1093/ageing/aft153.

Aserinsky E, Kleitman N. Regularly occurring periods of eye motility, and concomitant phenomena, during sleep. Science. 1953;118:273–4.

Banks S, Dinger DF. Behavioral and physiological consequences of sleep restriction. J Clin Sleep Med. 2007;3(5):519–28.

Borbely AA. A two process model of sleep regulation. Hum Neurobiol. 1982;1(3):195–204.

Brown RE, Basheer R, McKenna JT, Strecker RE, McCarley RW. Control of sleep and wakefulness. Physiol Rev. 2012;92:1087–187.

Carskadon MA, Dement WC. Effects of total sleep loss on sleep tendency. Percept Mot Skills. 1979;48:495–506.

Carskadon MA, Dement WC. Sleepiness in the normal adolescent. In: Guilleminault C, editor. Sleep and its disorders in children. New York: Raven Press; 1987. p. 53–66.

Carskadon MA, Dement WC. Normal human sleep: an overview. In: Kryger MH, Roth T, Dement WC, editors. Principles and practice of sleep medicine. Philadelphia: W.B. Saunders Company; 1994. p. 16–25.

Carskadon MA, Brown ED, Dement WC. Sleep fragmentation in the elderly: relationship to daytime sleep tendency. Neurobiol Aging. 1982;3:321–7.

Carskadon MA, Wolfson AR, Acebo C, et al. Adolescent sleep patterns, circadian timing, and sleepiness at a transition to early school days. Sleep. 1998;21:871–81.

Chokroverty S. Physiologic changes in sleep. In: Sleep disorders medicine. Boston: Butterworth-Heinemann; 1999. p. 95–126.

Cirelli C, Tononi G. Is sleep essential? PLoS Biol. 2008;6(8):e216.

Crick F, Mitchison G. The function of dream sleep. Nature. 1983;304(5922):111–4.

Davis H, Davis PA, Loomis AL, et al. Human brain potentials during the onset of sleep. J Neurophysiol. 1938;1:24–38.

Dement W, Kleitman N. Cyclic variations in EEG during sleep and their relation to eye movements, body motility, and dreaming. Electroencephalogr Clin Neurophysiol. 1957;9:673–90.

Dijk DJ, Czeisler CA. Contribution of the circadian pacemaker and the sleep homeostat to sleep propensity, sleep structure, electroencephalographic slow waves, and sleep spindle activity in humans. J Neurosci. 1995;15(5 Pt 1):3526–38.

Drakatos P, Kosky CA, et al. First rapid eye movement sleep periods in sleep-stage sequencing of hypersomnias. Sleep Med. 2013;14(9):897–901.

Durmer JS, Dinges DF. Neurocognitive consequences of sleep deprivation. Semin Neurol. 2005;25:117–29.

Espana RA, Scammell TE. Sleep neurobiology for the clinician. Sleep. 2004;27:811–20.

Fisher SP, Foster RG, Peirson SN. The circadian control of sleep. Handb Exp Pharmacol. 2013;217:157–83.

Floyd JA, Janisse JJ, Jenuwine ES, et al. Changes in REM-sleep percentage over the adult lifespan. Sleep. 2007;30:829–36.

Foley DJ, Monjan AA, Borwn SL, et al. Sleep complaints among elderly persons: an epidemiologic study of three communities. Sleep. 1995;18:425–32.

Fuller PM, Saper CB, Lu J. The pontine REM switch: past and present. J Physiol. 2007;584:735–41.

Gangwisch JE, Heymsfield SB, Boden-Albala B, Buijs RM, Kreier F, Pickering TG, Rundle AG, Zammit GK, Malaspina D. Short sleep duration as a risk factor for hypertension. Analyses of the first national health and nutrition examination survey. Hypertension. 2006;47:1–7.

Genzel L, Kroes MC, Dresler M, Battaglia FP. Light sleep versus slow wave sleep in memory consolidation: a question of global versus local processes? Trends Neurosci. 2014;37:10–9.

Grace KP, Vanstone LE, Horner RL. Endogenous cholinergic input to the pontine REM sleep generator is not required for REM sleep to occur. J Neurosci. 2014;34:14198–209. https://doi.org/10.1523/JNEUROSCI.0274-14.2014.

Hobson JA. REM sleep and dreaming: towards a theory of protoconsciousness. Nat Rev Neurosci. 2009;10(11):803–13.

Horne JA. REM sleep—by default? Neurosci Biobehav Rev. 2000;24(8):777–97.

Horne J. Why REM sleep? Clues beyond the laboratory in a more challenging world. Biol Psychol. 2013;92(2):152–68.

Iber C, Ancoli-Israel S, Chesson AL, Quan SF. The AASM manual for the scoring of sleep and associated events: rules, terminology and technical specifications. Westchester, IL: American Academy of Sleep Medicine; 2007.

Jouvet M. Research on the neural structures and responsible mechanisms in different phases of physiological sleep. Arch Ital Biol. 1962;100:125–206.

Knutson KL, Spiegel K, Penev P, VanCauter E. The metabolic consequence of sleep deprivation. Sleep Med Rev. 2007;11(3):163–78.

Latta F, Leproult R, Tasali E, et al. Sex differences in delta and alpha EEG activities in healthy older adults. Sleep. 2005;28:1525–34.

Loomis AL, Harvey EN, Hobart G. Distribution of disturbance-patterns in the human EEG with special reference to sleep. J Neurophysiol. 1938;1:413–30.

Lu J, Sherman D, Devor M, Saper CB. A putative flip-flop switch for control of REM sleep. Nature. 2006;441:589–94. https://doi.org/10.1038/nature04767.

Luppi PH, Peyron C, Fort P. Role of MCH neurons in paradoxical (REM) sleep control. Sleep. 2013;36:1775–6. https://doi.org/10.5665/sleep.3192.

Maquet P. The role of sleep in learning and memory. Science. 2001;294:1048–52.

McCarley RW. Neurobiology of REM and NREM sleep. Sleep Med. 2007;8:302–30.

Moruzzi G, Magoun H. Brain stem reticular formation and activation of the EEG. Electroencephalogr Clin Neurophysiol. 1949;1:445–73.

Ohayon MM, Carskadon MA, Guilleminault C, et al. Meta-analysis of quantitative sleep parameters from childhood to old age in healthy individuals: developing normative sleep values across the human lifespan. Sleep. 2004;27:1255–73.

Oliver SJ, Costa RJ, Laing SJ, et al. One night of sleep deprivation decreases treadmill endurance performance. Eur J Appl Physiol. 2009;107:155–61.

Rechtschaffen A, Kales A. A manual of standardized terminology, techniques and scoring system for sleep stages of human subjects. In: Rechtschaffen A, Kales A, editors. Brain information service, brain research institute, University of California, los Angeles. California: University of California; 1968. p. 1–57.

Redline S, Kirchner HL, Quan SF, et al. The effects of age, sex, ethnicity, and sleep-disordered breathing on sleep architecture. Arch Intern Med. 2004;164:406–18.

Saper CB, Chou TC, Scammell TE. The sleep switch:hypothalamic control of sleep and wakefulness. Trends Neurosci. 2001;24:726–31.

Sapin E, Lapray D, Berod A, Goutagny R, Leger L, Ravassard P, et al. Localization of the brainstem GABAergic neurons controlling paradoxical (REM) sleep. PLoS One. 2009;4:e4272. https://doi.org/10.1371/journal.pone.0004272.

Scharf MT, Naidoo N, Zimmerman JE, Pack AI. The energy hypothesis of sleep revisited. Prog Neurobiol. 2008;86(3):264–80.

Schwartz JR, Roth T. Neurophysiology of sleep and wakefulness: basic science and clinical implications. Curr Neuropharmacol. 2008;6:367–78.

Sejnowski TJ, Destexhe A. Why do we sleep? Brain Res. 2000;886(1–2):208–23.

Siegal JM, Moore R, Thannickal T, et al. A brief history of hypocretin/orexin and narcolepsy. Neuropsychopharmacology. 2001;25:S14–20.

Siegel JM. Clues to the functions of mammalian sleep. Nature. 2005;437(7063):1264–71.

Siegel JM. REM sleep: a biological and psychological paradox. Sleep Med Rev. 2011;15(3):139–42.

Sigel JM. The neurobiology of sleep. Semin Neurol. 2009;29:277–96.

Thomas M, Sing H, Belenky G. Neural basis of alertness and cognitive performance impairments during sleepiness. II. Effects of 48–72 hours of sleep deprivation on waking human regional brain activity. Thalamus Relat Syst. 2003;2:199–229.

Thorne D, Thomas M, Russo M, et al. Performance on a driving-simulator divided attention task during one week of restricted nightly sleep. Sleep. 1999;22(Suppl 1):301.

Vetrivelan R, Fuller PM, Tong QA, Lu J. Medullary circuitry regulating rapid eye movement sleep and atonia. J Neurosci. 2009;29:9361–9.

Von Economo CP. Sleep as a problem of localisation. J Nerv Ment Dis. 1930;71:249–59.

Welsh A, Thomas M, Thorne D, et al. Effect of 64 hours of sleep deprivation on accidents and sleep events during a driving simulator. Sleep. 1998;21(Suppl 3):234.

Range and Classification of Sleep Disorders

2

Helen S. Driver and Muhannad Hawari

The recognition and growth of sleep medicine as a clinical specialty is manifested by the inclusion of sleep disorders in disease classification systems from the 1970s. The task of developing a classification system for sleep disorders has been undertaken by three organizations, namely, the World Health Organization (WHO), the American Psychiatric Association (APA) and associations and societies involved in sleep medicine as a clinical discipline, most recently the American Academy of Sleep Medicine (AASM). Three different classification systems have evolved: first, with sleep disorders being added to a general coding system, the International Classification of Diseases (ICD)(World Health Organization 1977, 1994, 2011); second, designed for use by mental health professionals, the Diagnostic and Statistical Manual of Mental Disorders (DSM)(American Psychiatric Association 1994, 2013); and third, developed by and for specialists in sleep medicine, the International Classification of Sleep Disorders (ICSD)(Association of Sleep Disorders Centers 1979, 1990, 1997; American Academy of Sleep Medicine 2005, 2014). A summary of the development of these three nosologies from the 1970s to the present is summarized in Table 2.1. In examining their development, it is important to recognize how the classification systems should, and do, evolve in response to other classification systems, as well as advances in scientific knowledge and clinical experience.

H. S. Driver, Ph.D. (✉) · M. Hawari, M.D.
Queen's University and Kingston General Hospital, Kingston, ON, Canada

King Faisal Specialist Hospital and Research Center, Riyadh, Saudi Arabia
e-mail: Helen.Driver@kingstonhsc.ca; MHawari@kfshrc.edu.sa

© Springer-Verlag GmbH Germany, part of Springer Nature 2018
H. Selsick (ed.), *Sleep Disorders in Psychiatric Patients*,
https://doi.org/10.1007/978-3-642-54836-9_2

Table 2.1 Development of three different sleep disorder classification systems over 40 years from the 1970s–2010s

	World Health Organization (WHO)	American Psychiatric Association (APA)	Sleep Associations/Societies
	International Classification of Disease (ICD) codes	*Diagnostic and Statistical Manual of Mental Disorders (DSM)*	*International Classification of Sleep Disorders (ICSD) Diagnostic and Coding Manual*
1970s and 1980s	1980 and 1994: ICD-9 and *ICD-9-CM* Sleep disorders characterized as endogenous, i.e. organic, or exogenous, i.e. nonorganic **Organic 780.**5x Insomnia 780.52 Hypersomnolence 780.54 **Nonorganic 307.**4x Sleepwalking 307.46 Shift work 307.45 Other disease categories: Narcolepsy 347.0x RLS 333 Breathing disorders 327.2x Cheyne-Stokes breathing 786.04	1987: *DSM-III-R* Dyssomnias (intrinsic/**organic**) Primary vs. Secondary Parasomnias	1979: *Diagnostic Classification of Sleep and Arousal Disorders* Association of Sleep Disorders Centres (ASDC) and Association for the Psychophysiological Study of sleep, published in the journal SLEEP 1. DIMS (Disorders of Initiating and Maintaining Sleep) 2. DOES (Disorders of Excessive Daytime Sleepiness) 3. Sleep-wake schedule disorder 4. Parasomnia
1990s and 2000s	1994 to present: *ICD-10* Chapter VI (G) **diseases of the nervous system Sleep disorders G47** Insomnia G47.00 Hypersomnolence G47.10 Shift work G47.26 Narcolepsy G47.4xx Breathing disorders G47.3x RLS G25.81 Chapter V (F) **mental and behavioural disorders F51** Sleepwalking F51.3 Cheyne-Stokes breathing R06.3	1994: *DSM-IV* Four major categories according to presumed aetiology, identify whether primary or secondary 1. Primary sleep disorders (a) Dyssomnias (b) Parasomnias 2. Sleep disorder related to another mental disorder 3. Sleep disorder related to general medical condition 4. Substance induced *2000: DSM-IV-TR* "text revision". Included ICD numeric code for each category of disorder	*1990: ICSD and 1997 ICSD-R* American Academy of Sleep Medicine (AASM) 1. Dyssomnias (a) Intrinsic sleep disorders (b) Extrinsic sleep disorders (c) Circadian rhythm sleep disorders 2. Parasomnias (a) Arousal disorders (b) Sleep-wake transition disorders (c) Parasomnias usually associated with REM sleep (d) Other parasomnias 3. Sleep disorders associated with (a) mental, (b) neurological or (c) other medical disorders 4. Proposed sleep disorders 2005: *ICSD-2* Specify if concurrent with non-sleep disorder but not primary or secondary 1. Insomnia 2. Sleep-related breathing disorders 3. Hypersomnias of central origin 4. Circadian rhythm sleep disorders 5. Parasomnias 6. Sleep-related movement disorders 7. Isolated symptoms that are apparently normal variants and unresolved issues 8. Other sleep disorders

Table 2.1 (continued)

2010s	2017: ICD-11 (pending)	2013: DSM-5	2014: ICSD-3
		1. Insomnia disorder	1. Insomnia (3 disorders)
		2. Hypersomnolence disorder	2. Sleep-related breathing disorders (19 disorders) 5 subcategories
		3. Narcolepsy	(a) Obstructive (2) adult and paediatrics
		4. Breathing-related sleep disorder	(b) Central syndromes (8)
		5. Circadian rhythm sleep-wake disorders	(c) Hypoventilation (6)
		6. Parasomnias	(d) Hypoxemia(1)
		7. RLS	(e) Isolated symptoms and normal variants (2)
		8. Substance–/ medication-induced sleep disorder Others and unspecified	3. Central disorders of hypersomnia (8 disorders)
			4. Circadian rhythm sleep disorders (7 disorders)
			5. Parasomnias (14 disorders) three subcategories
			(a) NREM (4)
			(b) Rem (3)
			(c) Others (6)
			(d) Isolated (1) sleep talking
			6. Sleep-related movement disorders (10 disorders)
			(a) Isolated symptoms that are apparently normal variants and unresolved issues (3 disorders)
			Other sleep disorders

2.1   Why Develop a Classification System?

There are four main reasons for clinical classification systems in that they provide (1) a standardized coding system used worldwide by healthcare systems and third-party payers, (2) standardized definitions and diagnostic criteria to differentiate between a set of related disorders and (3) descriptions of the disorders and their course, with (4) a view to treatment. Standard definitions are based on unambiguous pathology and defined aetiology that rely on scientific research and evidence to describe symptom presentation and relevant physiological measures. Initially research driven, the classification evolves with clinical practice and experience. Thus the clinical utility of the classification system is derived from research, expert opinion and consensus.

2.2   The Evolution of Sleep Disorder Classifications

During the 1970s sleep disorders began to appear in disease classification systems (Edinger and Morin 2012) (Table 2.1). The first inclusion of sleep disorders was in 1977 in the International Classification of Diseases (ICD) published by the WHO.

2.2.1   The International Classification of Diseases (ICD)

The WHO oversees the International Classification of Diseases (ICD) revisions and the allocation of numeric and alphanumeric codes to designate disease diagnoses and health problems for electronic storage, retrieval and analysis of data (World Health Organization 1977, 1994, 2011). ICD codes are given to every diagnosis, description of symptoms and cause of death attributable to human beings. This is the international standard for defining and reporting diseases and health conditions. The most current version of the ICD in use is the 10th revision, the ICD-10[3]. The ICD-10 was developed from 1983 and completed in 1992 and is used by more than 100 countries around the world. The 2010 edition of ICD-10 includes updates that came into effect between 1998 and 2010 and is also referred to as the 4th edition of ICD-10. Work on the 11th revision of the classification is underway and due for release in 2018. National versions of the ICD, for example, in the USA called Clinical Modifications ICD-10-CM, frequently include much more detail and some-times have separate sections for procedures. Given the extensive use of the ICD codes in healthcare and for statistical analysis in the era of electronic health records, it is vital that these codes be included in the classification of sleep disorders.

In early versions of the ICD, some sleep disorders such as narcolepsy, restless legs syndrome (RLS) and sleep-related breathing disorders had already been listed under clinical sections, and they have remained under these original categories in more recent revisions. The ICD-9-CM[2] included sleep disorders under two major subheadings, namely, "Specific Disorders of Sleep of Nonorganic Origin" (ICD code #307.4) and "Sleep Disturbances" (ICD code# 780.5). The nonorganic disorders included those con-sequent to phase-shifting of the sleep-wake cycle, for example, shift work (307.45-1) or jet lag (307.45-0), as well as types based on the chronicity of the complaint as transient or persistent, for example, inadequate sleep hygiene (307.41-1) and persistent disorder of initiating or maintaining sleep (307.42). Also included in the nonorganic subtype were some parasomnias such as nightmares (307.47-0) and sleep talking (307.47-3), whereas other parasomnias such as sleep paralysis (780.56-2) and REM sleep behaviour disorder (780.59-0) were categorized under the (organic) category of sleep disturbances.

2.2.1.1 Sleep Disturbance/Disorder Categorization Based on Aetiology

A major consideration in the ICD-9 diagnostic categorization of sleep disorders was the distinction of whether the aetiology was "organic" (i.e. "true" or endogenous sleep disturbances) or "nonorganic" (i.e. due largely to external factors), which in practice is often a challenge to distinguish with sleep disorders (Edinger and Morin 2012). Recognizing that sleep problems may evolve from a combination of endog-enous and exogenous factors, the initial classification system of the Association of Sleep Disorders Centres in 1979 for sleep specialists made no attempt to utilize the scheme of organic versus nonorganic (Association of Sleep Disorders Centers 1979). The subsequent classification system for sleep specialists (ICSD) (American Sleep Disorders Association 1990, 1997) opted to use the subdivisions of "intrinsic" (coming from within the body) or "extrinsic" (produced primarily by factors outside the body), but this was eliminated in the second and third edition of ICSD. The early editions of the APA's classification also included a diagnostic distinction of sleep disorders based on aetiology, but in this case as "primary" or "secondary" (American Psychiatric Association 1994), while in the current DSM-5, this distinction no longer applies (American Psychiatric Association 2013).

2.2.2   The Diagnostic and Statistical Manual of Mental Disorders (DSM)

The 1970s also brought in a refinement of diagnostic criteria for mental disorders as incorporated in the 8th revision of the ICD. Building on this work, starting with the 3rd revision of the Diagnostic and Statistical Manual of Mental Disorders (DSM) published in 1980 by the APA, there was an effort to align their nomenclature to be more consistent with that of the ICD. Published in 1987, the DSM-III-R was the first time sleep disorders appeared in the DSM (Edinger and Morin 2012). However, with regard to sleep disorders, these two classification systems, ICD and DSM, presented two different nosological frameworks (see Table 2.1).

In the DSM-IV published in 1994, sleep disorders were organized into four major sections according to presumed aetiology (American Psychiatric Association 1994).

1. Primary sleep disorders are those in which none of the aetiologies listed below (i.e. another mental disorder, a general medical condition or a substance) is responsible.
2. Sleep disorder related to another mental disorder.
3. Sleep disorder related to a general medical condition.
4. Sleep disorder induced by a substance.

These latter three groups form separate sleep disorder categories. Under the category of "sleep disorder related to another mental disorder", the two subtypes were based on the essential feature of either insomnia (307.42) or hypersomnia (307.44). When a disturbance to sleep was severe enough to warrant independent clinical attention and was due to a general medical condition, it would be classified under "sleep disorder related to a general medical condition" (780.xx) with four subtypes of insomnia, hypersomnia, parasomnia or mixed. These four subtypes were also used under the category of "sleep disorder induced by a substance" along with the applicable substance type, for example, alcohol, amphetamine or sedative hypnotic.

The "primary sleep disorders" were subdivided into dyssomnias (characterized by abnormalities in the amount, quality or timing of sleep) and parasomnias (characterized by abnormal behavioural or physiological events occurring in association with sleep, specific sleep stages or sleep-wake transitions). Dyssomnias included primary insomnia (307.42), primary hypersomnia (307.44), narcolepsy (347) and breathing-related sleep disorder (780.59) leading to excessive sleepiness or insomnia. Dyssomnias also included circadian rhythm disorder (307.45) which included delayed sleep phase (780.55-0), jet lag (307.45-0), shift work (307.45-1) or unspecified type. Finally, dyssomnia not otherwise specified (307.47) included those due to environmental factors, or attributable to sleep deprivation, RLS or periodic limb movements (PLMS) also known as nocturnal myoclonus. The subcategory of parasomnias included nightmare disorder (307.47) formerly known as dream anxiety disorder, sleep terror disorder (307.46), sleepwalking disorder (307.46) and parasomnia not otherwise specified (307.47), for example, REM sleep behaviour disorder (RBD) and sleep paralysis.

It is important to recognize that the DSM was prepared for use by mental health and general clinicians, not experts in sleep medicine, and therefore represented an effort to simplify sleep-wake disorder classification by aggregating diagnoses under broad labels. In contrast to this clustering approach, the classification system for sleep specialists includes a large number of highly specific sleep disorder diagnoses.

2.2.3 Diagnostic Classification of Sleep and Arousal Disorders

Adding to the mix, in 1979 a third nosological framework entirely different than those of the ICD and DSM was presented by professional sleep societies—the Association of Sleep Disorders Centres (ASDC) and the Association for the Psychophysiological Study of Sleep—and published in the journal Sleep (Association of Sleep Disorders Centers 1979). Unique to this nosology, prepared by researchers and clinicians specializing in sleep, was the inclusion of the term "arousal" in a manual entitled the *Diagnostic Classification of Sleep and Arousal Disorders*. This classification system was based on four categories grouped into disorders of initiating and maintaining sleep (DIMS), disorders of excessive daytime sleepiness (DOES), sleep-wake schedule disorders and parasomnias.

2.2.4 The International Classification of Sleep Disorders (ICSD)

Introduced in 1990 and revised in 1997, the International Classification of Sleep Disorders (ICSD) manual was produced by the American Academy of Sleep Medicine (AASM) in collaboration with the European Sleep Research Society (ESRS), the Japanese Society of Sleep Research and the Latin American Sleep Society (American Sleep Disorders Association 1990, 1997). The ICSD was developed as a revision and update of the 1979 Diagnostic Classification of Sleep and Arousal Disorders. In general, it was agreed that the first two categories, namely, the disorders of initiating and maintaining sleep (DIMS) and the disorders of excessive somnolence (DOES), were very helpful in considering the differential diagnosis of patients presenting with one or both of those major sleep symptoms. However, complaints of insomnia or excessive sleepiness could also be the result of disorders listed within the other two sections—disorders of the sleep-wake schedule (DSWS) and the parasomnias. Furthermore, some diagnostic entries were listed in more than one section. This updated classification system was based on a pathophysiological and symptom-based organization to facilitate a multidisciplinary approach. Comprised of four categories, the ICSD listed 88 sleep disorders. As with the DSM-IV, in the ICSD the primary sleep disorders were classified under two groups—dyssomnias and parasomnias. The remaining two categories were sleep disorders associated with mental, neurological or other medical disorders and proposed sleep disorders.

Published in 2005, the 2nd edition of the ICSD (ICSD-2) (American Academy of Sleep Medicine 2005) reflected the science and opinions of the sleep specialist community and was prepared for use by specialists in sleep medicine. The ICSD-2 included 81 highly specific sleep disorders and 8 major categories as summarized in Table 2.1. The eight categories were insomnia, sleep-related breathing disorders, hypersomnias of central origin, circadian rhythm sleep disorders, the parasomnias, sleep-related movement disorders, isolated symptoms that are apparently normal variants and unresolved issues and other sleep disorders. Interestingly, the second edition was a return to a classification system based on phenomenology resembling the 1979 system.

2.3   Classification Systems Currently in Use

As noted above, the development of new releases of classification systems takes years; for example, it was a 12-year process to develop the 5th edition of the Diagnostic and Statistical Manual of Mental Disorders (DSM-5) (American Psychiatric Association 2013). This project began in 1999 and included hundreds of medical, scientific and clinical professionals, followed by field trials, and then public and professional input, before the publication of the DSM-5 in 2013. With this revision, the APA and the WHO collaborated to harmonize their classification systems as much as possible. Harmonization with the ICD codes is also a goal of the AASM; particularly from the year 2001, panellists from the AASM have been working with the WHO to secure more extensive ICD codes for sleep disorders. The ICD-9 and ICD-10 codes were incorporated into the ICSD-3 published by the AASM in 2014.

2.3.1   International Classification of Diseases (ICD-10)

The ICD-10 alphanumeric codes (World Health Organization 1994, 2011) are different from their ICD-9 numeric counterparts. These alphanumeric codes are broken down into chapters and subchapters. They are comprised of a letter identifying groups of diseases, followed by two digits, a decimal point and then one digit (e.g. G47.3 for sleep apnoeas). For example, all codes preceded by "F" indicate mental and behavioural disorders (Chapter V). Under this coding, for example, "nonorganic" sleep disorders such as insomnia and the parasomnia of sleepwalking begin with the code F51 (see Table 2.2), whereas the coding for nocturnal enuresis only is F98.0.00 as it falls under "other behavioural and emotional disorders with onset usually occurring in childhood and adolescence".

Codes preceded by a "G" indicate diseases of the nervous system (Chapter VI). Most of the sleep disorders in ICD-10 are coded under G47 "episodic and paroxysmal disorders". These categories are closely aligned with the 1979 *Diagnostic Classification of Sleep and Arousal Disorders* categories of DIMS, DOES and circadian rhythm disorders (sleep-wake schedule disorders).

Table 2.2 The ICD-10 Chapter V (F) nonorganic sleep disorders

Classification of mental and behavioural disorders including the classification of nonorganic sleep disorders (F51) (World Health Organization)
F51.0 Nonorganic insomnia
F51.1 Nonorganic hypersomnia
F51.2 Nonorganic disorder of the sleep-wake schedule
F51.3 Sleepwalking [somnambulism]
F51.4 Sleep terrors [night terrors]
F51.5 Nightmares
F51.8 Other nonorganic sleep disorders
F51.9 Nonorganic sleep disorder, unspecified

2.3.1.1 Sleep Disorders G47

- G47.0 Disorders of initiating and maintaining sleep (insomnias)
- G47.1 Disorders of excessive somnolence (hypersomnias)
- G47.2 Disruptions in circadian rhythm (including jet lag)
- G47.3 Sleep apnoea
- G47.4 Narcolepsy and cataplexy
- G47.5 Parasomnias
- G47.6 Sleep-related movement disorders

2.3.2 Diagnostic and Statistical Manual of Mental Disorders, 5th Edition (DSM-5) 2013

As with DSM-IV, the approach taken to the classification of sleep-wake disorders in DSM-5 can be understood within the context of grouping similar disorders, so-called lumping or clustering, versus the more expansive list based on specialist criteria or "splitting" (American Psychiatric Association 2013). In the DSM-5, sleep-wake disorders are classified under ten disorders, or disorder groups, as summarized in Table 2.3.

2.3.3 International Classification of Sleep Disorders, 3rd Edition (ICSD-3) 2014

The third edition of the ICSD follows the same general structure as the second edition so that the major clinical divisions remain unchanged (American Academy of Sleep Medicine 2014). In this edition, 64 highly specific sleep disorders are described under six categories. A further six sleep-related disorders are listed in an appendix category of "sleep-related medical and neurological disorders"; these include fatal familial insomnia, sleep-related epilepsy, headache, laryngospasm, gastro-oesophageal reflux and myocardial ischaemia.

Table 2.4 shows the ICSD-3 classification of sleep disorders by categories and subtypes including the numeric ICD-9-CM and alphanumeric ICD-10-CM codes. The most notable change is the collapse of all previous chronic insomnia diagnoses

Table 2.3 The DSM-5 Classification of Sleep-Wake Disorders

Insomnia disorder 780.52 G47.00	Difficulty initiating sleep, maintaining sleep or early morning awakening. Causes significant distress. Occurs at least 3 nights per week despite adequate opportunity to sleep. Present for at least 3 months; acute and short term if present for less than 3 months Specify if: With non-sleep disorder mental comorbidity, with other comorbidity or other sleep disorder Specify if: Episodic (>1 < 3 months), persistent (3 months +) or recurrent (2+ episodes in 1 year)
Hypersomnolence disorder 780.54 G47.10	Specify if: With non-sleep disorder mental comorbidity (including substance abuse), with medical condition or with other sleep disorder Specify if: Acute, subacute or persistent Specify current severity: Mild, moderate, severe
Narcolepsy 347.00 G47.419 347.01 G47.411 347.00 G47.419 347.00 G47.419 347.10 G47.429	Specify current severity: Mild, moderate, severe Narcolepsy without cataplexy but with hypocretin deficiency Narcolepsy with cataplexy but without hypocretin deficiency Autosomal dominant cerebella ataxia, deafness and narcolepsy Autosomal dominant narcolepsy, obesity and type 2 diabetes Narcolepsy secondary to another medical condition
Breathing-related sleep disorders	

327.21 G47.33
 	
327.21 G47.31
786.04 R06.3
780.57 G47.37
 	
327.24 G47.34
327.25 G47.35
327.26 G47.36
	Obstructive sleep apnoea-hypopnea (current severity: Mild, moderate, severe)
	Central sleep apnoea:
	    Idiopathic central sleep apnoea
	    Cheyne-Stokes breathing
	    Complex sleep apnoea comorbid with opioid use
	Sleep-related hypoventilation:
	    Idiopathic hypoventilation
	    Congenital central alveolar hypoventilation
	    Comorbid sleep-related hypoventilation

Circadian rhythm sleep-wake disorders specify if: Episodic, persistent or recurrent	
307.45 G47.21 307.45 G47.22 307.45 G47.23 307.45 G47.24 307.45 G47.26 307.45 G47.20	Delayed sleep phase type Advanced sleep phase type Irregular sleep-wake type Non-24 h sleep-wake type Shift work type Unspecified type

Parasomnias
307.46 F51.3
 	
307.46 F51.4
307.47 F51.5
 	
327.42 G47.52
	Non-rapid eye movement arousal disorders
	    Sleepwalking type. Specify if: With sleep-related eating, sexsomnia
	    Sleep terror type
	Nightmare disorder. Specify if: With associated non-sleep disorder, with other medical condition or with other sleep disorder
	Rapid eye movement sleep behaviour disorder

333.94 G25.81	Restless Legs Syndrome (RLS)
Substance−/medication-induced sleep disorder	Alcohol, caffeine, cannabis, opioid, sedatives/hypnotics/anxiolytics, amphetamines, cocaine, tobacco or other (unknown) substances

(continued)

Table 2.3 (continued)

780.52 G47.09	Other specified insomnia disorder, e.g. brief insomnia disorder, nonrestorative sleep
780.52 G47.00	Unspecified insomnia disorder
780.54 G47.19	Other specified hypersomnolence disorder
780.54 G47.10	Unspecified hypersomnolence disorder
780.59 G47.8	Other specified sleep-wake disorder
780.59 G47.9	Unspecified sleep-wake disorder

Diagnostic and Statistical Manual of Mental Disorders 5th edition (DSM-5) Classification of Sleep Disorders 2013

Table 2.4 The ICSD-3: Classification of sleep disorders by categories and sub-types including the numeric ICD-9-CM and alphanumeric ICD-10-CM codes in brackets (ICD-9-CM; ICD-10-CM)

Insomnia	1. Chronic insomnia disorder (307.42; F51.01)
	2. Short-term insomnia disorder (307.41; F51.02)
	3. Other insomnia disorder (307.49; F51.09)
	4. Isolated symptoms and normal variants:
	Excessive time in bed
	Short sleeper
Sleep-related breathing disorders	1. **Obstructive sleep apnoea disorders:**
	(a) obstructive sleep apnoea, adults (327.23; G47.33)
	(b) obstructive sleep apnoea, paediatrics (327.23; G47.33)
	2. **Central sleep apnoea syndromes:**
	(a) central sleep apnoea with Cheyne-Stokes breathing (786.04; R06.3)
	(b) central sleep apnoea due to a medical disorder without Cheyne-Stokes breathing (327.27; G47.37)
	(c) central sleep apnoea due to high-altitude periodic breathing (327.22; G47.32)
	(d) central sleep apnoea due to medication or substance (327.29; G47.39)
	(e) primary central sleep apnoea (327.21; G47.31)
	(f) primary central sleep apnoea of infancy (770.81; P28.3)
	(g) primary central sleep apnoea of prematurity (770.82; P28.4)
	(h) treatment emergent central sleep apnoea (327.29; G47.39)
	3. **Sleep-related hypoventilation:**
	(a) obesity hypoventilation syndrome (278.03; E66.2)
	(b) congenital central alveolar hypoventilation syndrome (327.25; G47.35)
	(c) late-onset central hypoventilation with hypothalamic dysfunction (327.26; G47.36)
	(d) idiopathic central alveolar hypoventilation (327.24; G47.34)
	(e) sleep-related hypoventilation due to a medication or substance (327.26; G47.36)
	(f) sleep-related hypoventilation due to a medical disorder (327.26; G47.36)
	4. **Sleep-related hypoxemia disorder:**
	Sleep-related hypoxemia (327.26; G47.36)
	5. **Isolated symptoms and normal variants:**
	(a) snoring (786.09; R06.83)
	(b) Catathrenia

Table 2.4 (continued)

Central disorders of hypersomnia	1. Narcolepsy type 1 with cataplexy (347.01; G47.411) 2. Narcolepsy type 2 without cataplexy (347.00; G47.419) 3. Idiopathic hypersomnia (327.11; G47.11) 4. Kleine-Levin syndrome (327.13; G47.13) 5. Hypersomnia due to a medical disorder (327.14; G47.14) 6. Hypersomnia due to medication or substance 7. Hypersomnia associated with psychiatric disorder (327.15; F51.13) 8. Insufficient sleep syndrome (307.44; F51.12) 9. Isolated symptoms and normal variants: Long sleeper
Circadian rhythm sleep-wake disorders	1. Delayed sleep-wake phase disorder (327.31; G47.21) 2. Advanced sleep-wake phase disorder (327.32; G47.22) 3. Irregular sleep-wake rhythm disorder (327.33; G47.23) 4. Non-24-hour sleep-wake rhythm disorder (327.34; G47.24) 5. Shift work disorder (327.36; G47.26) 6. Jet lag disorder (327.35; G47.25) 7. Circadian sleep-wake disorder not otherwise specified (327.30; G47.20)
Parasomnias	**1. NREM-related parasomnias**: Disorders of arousals (from NREM sleep) (a) Confusional arousals (327.41; G47.51) (b) sleepwalking (307.23; F51.3) (c) sleep terrors (307.23; F51.4) (d) sleep-related eating disorders (327.40; G47.59) **2. REM-related parasomnias:** (a) REM sleep behavioural disorder (327.42; G47.52) (b) recurrent isolated sleep paralysis (327.43; G47.51) (c) nightmare disorder (307.47; F51.5) **3. Other parasomnias:** (a) exploding head syndrome (327.49; G47.59) (b) sleep-related hallucinations (368.16; H53.16) (c) sleep enuresis (788.36; N39.44) (d) Parasomnias due to a medical disorder (327.44; G47.54) (e) Parasomnias due to a medication or substance (f) Parasomnias, unspecified (327.40; G47.50) **4. Isolated symptoms and normal variants:** Sleep talking
Sleep-related movement disorders	1. Restless legs syndrome (333.94; G25.81) 2. Periodic leg movement disorder (327.51; G47.61) 3. Sleep-related leg cramps (327.52; G47.62) 4. Sleep-related bruxism (327.53; G47.63) 5. Sleep-related rhythmic movement disorder (327.59; G47.69) 6. Benign myoclonus of infancy (327.59; G47.69) 7. Propriospinal myoclonus at sleep onset (327.59; G47.69) 8. Sleep-related movement disorders due to a medical disorder (327.59; G47.69) 9. Sleep-related movement disorder due to medication or substance 10. Sleep-related movement disorder, unspecified (327.59; G47.69) 11. Isolated symptoms and normal variants: (a) excessive fragmentary myoclonus (b) hypnagogic foot tremor and alternating leg muscle activation (c) sleep starts

Other sleep disorder

Adapted from the American Academy of Sleep Medicine. The International Classification of Sleep Disorders: Diagnostic and Coding Manual (3rd ed) into a single chronic insomnia disorder category. Within the central disorders of hypersomnolence, the nomenclature for narcolepsy has been changed to narcolepsy type 1 (with cataplexy) and type 2 (without cataplexy). The expansion of disorders listed within the sleep-related breathing disorders category reflects the increased awareness and research, as well as technological and therapeutic advances, in this area of sleep medicine.

2.4   Technical Publications and Specifications for Recording and Scoring Sleep and Sleep Disorders

Along with clinical diagnostic criteria, standardized and internationally accepted criteria for recording and measuring sleep are required. The first technical manual for recording sleep or polysomnography (PSG) which incorporated EEG, EOG and EMG was published in 1968. This manual for recording and scoring sleep, edited by Rechtschaffen and Kales, was only updated in 2007 by the AASM. In addition to sleep recording specifications, the AASM manual included technical specifications and rules for recording and scoring associated physiological events such as respiration, limb movements and electrocardiogram. Prior to the combination of these associated monitoring rules into a single manual, separate technical publications were used for detailing specific parameters such as EEG arousals, periodic leg movements or respiratory disorders as outlined in Table 2.5. The technical manual for sleep disorder laboratories that is currently in use was published by the AASM in 2012 (Berry et al. 2012), with version 2.3 released online on April 1, 2016 and version 2.4 released in April 2017.

For sleep medicine practice in Europe, the European Sleep Research Society (ESRS) has published three guideline documents and a textbook on sleep medicine. In 2006, guidelines were published for the accreditation of sleep medicine centres in Europe, which defined the characteristics of multidisciplinary sleep medicine centres and requirements regarding staff, operational procedures and logistics (Steering Committee for the European Sleep research Society 2006). These guidelines were followed in 2009 with guidelines for the certification of professionals in sleep medicine (Pevernagie et al. 2009) and in 2012 with standard procedures for adults in accredited sleep medicine centres in Europe (Fischer et al. 2012). In 2014, the ESRS published a comprehensive textbook on sleep medicine (Bassetti et al. 2014).

Table 2.5 Technical publications for the recording and scoring of sleep and sleep disorders

Year	Technical publication
1968	Rechtschaffen A, Kales A. A manual of standardized terminology, techniques and scoring system for sleep stages of human subjects. Bethesda, MD: National Institutes of Health (NIH Publ. No. 204)
1992	American Sleep Disorders Association (ASDA). EEG arousals: Scoring rules and examples. A preliminary report from the sleep disorders atlas task force of the American sleep disorders association. *Sleep* 1992; 15: 174–184.
1993	The atlas task force. Recording and scoring leg movements. *Sleep* 1993; 16: 748–759
1999	American Academy of Sleep Medicine (AASM) task force. Sleep-related breathing disorders in adults: Recommendations for syndrome definition and measurement techniques in clinical research. *Sleep* 1999; 22: 667–689.
2006	Steering Committee for the European Sleep Research Society (ESRS). European guidelines for the accreditation of sleep medicine centres. *Journal of Sleep Research* 2006; 15 (2): 231–238 http://www.esrs.eu/publication-standards.html
2007	The AASM manual for the scoring of sleep and associated events: Rules, terminology and technical specifications, 1st ed. Westchester, Illinois
2012	Standard procedures for adults in accredited sleep medicine centres in Europe *Journal of Sleep Research* 2012; 21 (4): 357–368 http://onlinelibrary.wiley.com/doi/10.1111/j.1365-2869.2011.00987.x/full
2012	The AASM manual for the scoring of sleep and associated events: Rules, terminology and technical specifications, version 2. Darien, Illinois
2016	The AASM manual for the scoring of sleep and associated events. Version 2.3 http://www.aasmnet.org/scoringmanual/default.aspx
2017	The AASM manual for the scoring of sleep and associated events: Rules, terminology and technical specifications. Version 2.4 https://aasm.org/clinical-resources/scoring-manual/

2.5   Summary

The three different nosologies developed by the WHO, psychiatric (APA) and sleep specialists (AASM) for the classification of sleep disorders have evolved over the last 45 years. In the most recent revision of the ICD, most of the sleep-wake disorders fall under diseases of the nervous system, and their unique alphanumeric codes are preceded by the letter G, under G47 "episodic and paroxysmal disorders". The classification system for sleep specialists is comprised of a greater number of highly specific disorders compared with the system developed for psychiatry. The DSM's grouping of similar disorders, or "lumping" approach, versus "splitting" into highly specific disorders was an effort to simplify the classification of sleep-wake disorders for non-sleep specialists by aggregating diagnoses under broad labels. There has been a convergence of the categories used in the current systems, namely, ICD-10, ICSD-3 and DSM-5, based on pathophysiology. The six common groups are insomnia, hypersomnia, circadian rhythm disorders, sleep-related breathing disorders (apnoea), the parasomnias and sleep-related movement disorders. An exception to the lumping approach is narcolepsy, which has its own category in the ICD and DSM but in the ICSD is included with the hypersomnias. As is reflected in the expansion of sleep-related breathing disorders listed in the most recent system for sleep specialists, the ICSD-3, classification systems evolve with advances in the understanding, recognition and treatment of disorders.

References

American Academy of Sleep Medicine. International classification of sleep disorders (ICSD-2): diagnostic and coding manual. 2nd ed. Westchester: American Academy of Sleep Medicine; 2005.

American Academy of Sleep Medicine. International classification of sleep disorders (ICSD-3): diagnostic and coding manual. 3rd ed. 2014. www.aasm.org.

American Psychiatric Association. Diagnostic and statistical manual of mental disorders 4th edition (DSM-IV). Washington, DC: American Psychiatric Association; 1994.

American Psychiatric Association. Diagnostic and statistical manual of mental disorders 5th edition (DSM-5). Washington, DC: American Psychiatric Association; 2013.

American Sleep Disorders Association. International classification of sleep disorders (ICSD): diagnostic and coding manual. Rochester: Diagnostic and Classification Steering Committee; 1990.

American Sleep Disorders Association. International classification of sleep disorders, revised (ICSD-R): diagnostic and coding manual. Rochester: American Sleep Disorders Association; 1997.

Association of Sleep Disorders Centers. Diagnostic classification of sleep and arousal disorders. Prepared by the Sleep Disorders Classification Committee, Roffwarg HP. Sleep. 1979;2:1–137.

Bassetti C, Dogas Z, Peigneux P. Sleep medicine textbook. Regensburg: European Sleep research Society (ESRS); 2014. http://www.esrs.eu/esrs/sleep-medicine-textbook.html

Berry RB, et al. for the American Academy of Sleep Medicine. The AASM manual for the scoring of sleep and associated events: rules, terminology and technical specifications, version 2. Darien, IL: AASM; 2012. www.aasmnet.org.

Edinger JD, Morin CM. Sleep disorders classification and diagnosis. In: Morin CM, Espie CA, editors. The Oxford handbook of sleep and sleep disorders. Oxford: Oxford University Press; 2012.

Fischer J, et al. Standard procedures for adults in accredited sleep medicine centres in Europe. J Sleep Res. 2012;21(4):357–68. http://onlinelibrary.wiley.com/doi/10.1111/j.1365-2869.2011.00987.x/full

Pevernagie D, et al. European guidelines for the certification of professionals in sleep medicine: report of the task force of the European Sleep Research Society. J Sleep Res. 2009;18(1):136–41. http://onlinelibrary.wiley.com/doi/10.1111/j.1365-2869.2008.00721.x/abstract

Steering Committee for the European Sleep research Society. European guidelines for the accreditation of Sleep Medicine Centres. J Sleep Res. 2006;15(2):231–8. http://www.esrs.eu/publication-standards.html

World Health Organization. International classification of diseases, ninth revision (ICD-9), vol. 1. Geneva: World Health Organization; 1977.

World Health Organization. ICD-9-CM international classification of diseases, clinical modification, 4th edition, ninth revision. Salt Lake City: Medicode; 1994.

World Health Organization. ICD-10 international classification of diseases and health related problems, 4th edition, ten revision, vol. 2. Geneva, Switzerland: World Health Organization; 2011. http://www.who.int/classifications/icd/ICD10Volume2_en_2010.pdf?ua=1 Accessed 18 Feb 2014

Taking a Sleep History

3

Hugh Selsick

3.1 Introduction

Taking a sleep history can at first seem a daunting task. After all, much of what we are asking about is occurring when the patient is asleep. As a result, it can be tempting to bypass the history and rely on objective sleep studies such as the polysomnogram (PSG). However, there is no substitute for a good history, and the majority of sleep disorders can be diagnosed on history alone, with objective studies often being used simply for confirmation or to look for complicating and exacerbating factors.

There are generally two types of sleep history: a screening history and an indepth history. Often the purpose of the history is simply to screen for sleep disorders, and this is something that should ideally be done in every psychiatric patient. The screening history is necessarily brief and should take no more than a few minutes. However, if a potential sleep disorder is identified, or when patients present to a clinician with a complaint of a sleep disorder, a much more detailed history is warranted. In this chapter, I will first address the detailed sleep history and then demonstrate an efficient way of quickly screening for sleep disorders that can be incorporated into a psychiatric history.

3.2 Main Complaint

It may sound obvious, but it is essential to allow the patient to explain what it is that distresses them and why they are seeking help. This not only informs your history taking but allows you to direct your treatment plan to address the patient's concerns. Often patients will be referred to a specialist with a request from the referrer to

H. Selsick
Insomnia Clinic, Royal London Hospital for Integrated Medicine, London, UK
e-mail: hugh@selsick.net

© Springer-Verlag GmbH Germany, part of Springer Nature 2018   41
H. Selsick (ed.), *Sleep Disorders in Psychiatric Patients*,
https://doi.org/10.1007/978-3-642-54836-9_3

address a particular problem, but that may not be the problem that particularly worries the patient. In particular, it is helpful to determine whether it is the patient, the bed partner, the employer or a physician who has raised the concern.

Patients presenting with sleep disorders may present with a very clear description of their problem, but this is not always the case. They may describe their problem in layman's terms which are at odds with the terminology we use. For example, they will often confuse nightmares and night terrors, and therefore it is essential to ask the patient to describe their symptoms in more detail.

In terms of how you take a history, the presenting complaint will likely fall into one of three categories:

- Difficulty initiating and/or maintaining sleep or sleeping at the wrong time. The common differential diagnoses are insomnia, restless legs and circadian rhythm disorders.
- Excessive daytime sleepiness and/or snoring with or without observed apnoeas. Diagnoses to consider include obstructive sleep apnoea (OSA), periodic limb movements (PLMs), narcolepsy and idiopathic hypersomnia (IH).
- Unusual behaviours or unpleasant experiences at night. These include the parasomnias, nocturnal epilepsy and nocturnal panic attacks.

3.3   Timeline of Symptoms

Explore when the symptoms were first noticed, how they developed over time and whether they vary from night to night. It is particularly important to establish whether the onset of symptoms had any relationship with starting or stopping medication or whether medications exacerbate or improve the symptoms. In the context of psychiatric patients, determine whether the sleep disorder preceded the psychiatric disorder or vice versa and whether the patient feels that one contributes to the other. Numerous disorders, particularly insomnia and some of the parasomnias, may be particularly sensitive to anxiety and mood changes and understanding that relationship allows one to focus on managing those precipitants.

Some sleep disorders may vary in intensity or frequency across the year. The reasons for this are likely to be multifactorial. The amount of light exposure is certainly relevant in more northerly latitudes, but other factors to consider are cycles of work stress, increased alcohol consumption in holiday periods or decreased sleep opportunity at certain times of the year.

3.4   Typical Night

Ask the patient to describe in some detail a typical night's sleep. Beware that, when asked this, patients will often describe their most recent night's sleep regardless of whether or not it is typical or they will describe the worst-case scenario. If the sleep pattern is very variable, record what good and bad nights look like. Similarly, if they take hypnotics, ask them to describe a night with the hypnotic and a night without it. However, as most hypnotics can cause rebound insomnia, the first few nights after stopping the hypnotic may not be representative of their baseline sleep. Therefore, one may need to obtain information about a night during the rebound period and a night during a more sustained period of hypnotic abstinence.

There are a number of specific questions to ask if the patient does not volunteer the information in their description of the night:

- What time do they go to bed, and what do they do when they go to bed, i.e. do they read, watch TV, watch a video on their laptop, etc.?
- How long does it take to fall asleep? This will give you an estimate of their sleep onset latency (SOL). A SOL greater than 20 min in children and young adults, or 30 min in middle aged or elderly adults, is indicative of insomnia (American Academy of Sleep Medicine AASM 2014).
- How many times do they wake during the night, and what wakes them? How long does it take for them to get back to sleep each time? This gives an estimate of the time awake during the night. Ask what time the awakenings occur and what they do during these awakenings, e.g. do they get up, eat, read or lie in bed trying to sleep?
- What time do they wake up? Is this to an alarm or spontaneously? Are they waking earlier than they would like and, if so, how much earlier? This information can be combined with the time awake during the night (see above) to estimate the wakefulness after sleep onset (WASO). WASO greater than 20 min in children and young adults, or 30 min in middle aged or elderly adults, is indicative of insomnia (AASM 2014).
- What time do they rise? Note that this is the time they actually climb out of bed, not the time they wake up. Knowing the rising time and the bedtime will allow you to calculate the time in bed (TIB). Generally, this calculation ignores any time spent out of the bed during awakenings in the middle of the night.
- Ask the patient how long they feel they sleep in total. Often patients will answer this by giving you the time of their longest individual sleep period during the night, so it is important to check that the patient is giving you the total of all their sleep periods. This is their total sleep time (TST) and there is no normal value for this. It can be interesting to compare their estimated TST with the TST calculated from their TIB, SOL and WASO, i.e. TST = TIB – SOL – WASO; if their estimated TST and calculated TST are very different, explore why that is. The ratio of the TST to TIB expressed as a percentage is called sleep efficiency (SE) and can be a very useful measure, particularly in insomnia treatment (see the Chap. 9 on cognitive behavioural therapy for insomnia for more details).
- If the main complaint involves specific events such as parasomnias, panic attacks, etc., then find out how long after sleep onset they occur. This will be expanded upon later.

Table 3.1 Summary of sleep parameters and calculations

Lay terms	Technical terms	Calculations
Time taken to fall asleep	Sleep onset latency (SOL)	SOL = time from lights out to falling asleep
Wakefulness during the night	Wakefulness after sleep onset (WASO)	WASO = sum of time awake during awakenings + time awake in the morning before the alarm
Time from going to bed to rising	Time in bed (TIB)	TIB = rising time – bedtime
Time asleep	Total sleep time (TST)	Either estimated by patient or calculated as TST = TIB – SOL – WASO
Proportion of time in bed spent asleep	Sleep efficiency (SE)	SE (%) = TST/TIB x 100

3.5   Typical Day

3.5.1   Effect on Daytime Functioning

In most sleep disorders, it is not the night-time symptoms that cause the most distress but rather the impact of the disorder on daytime mood, alertness and cognitive function. Therefore it is important to establish how the disorder affects your patient during the day.

3.5.2   Sleepiness and Fatigue

One of the essential skills needed to take a good sleep history is the ability to differentiate between fatigue and sleepiness. Fatigue has many causes—one of which is poor sleep—whereas sleepiness is more likely a sign of a sleep disorder. Patients who report feeling tired may be talking about fatigue, sleepiness or both. Fatigue is a state of reduced subjective energy, motivation, concentration, etc., while sleepiness is difficulty staying awake and a strong desire to sleep. It is essential to ask patients which of these they mean by 'tiredness'. In this context, the Epworth Sleepiness Scale (ESS) (Appendix A) is often helpful (see below for more detail on the ESS). This scale asks the patient the likelihood of falling asleep in eight scenarios, and this forces the patient to think about their degree of sleepiness separately from their fatigue.

The majority of patients with OSA and clinically significant PLMs will score highly on the ESS; practically all narcolepsy and hypersomnia patients will have high ESS scores. The situation with insomnia is more complex. Some insomnia patients will have high ESS scores, but many will have normal, or indeed very low scores. Insomnia patients with hypervigilance will not only be unable to sleep well at night but will be unable to feel sleepy during the day despite having significant fatigue.

In addition to performing an ESS with the patient, one should ask if they nap during the day, how often and for how long. Some sleepy patients have a low ESS because they take planned naps and will therefore only score high on the question that asks about napping but will score low on the other questions.

One should also ask about when the patient feels most fatigued or sleepy and when they feel most alert. The importance of this will be expanded upon in the section on circadian rhythm disorders.

3.5.3   Occupation and Driving

At this point it is worth determining the impact of the sleepiness/fatigue on driving and occupational functioning. Here again, the ESS can be useful as it asks a specific question about the likelihood of falling asleep when in a stationary car. However, one should also ask directly about sleepiness when driving, especially long distances. In many countries, sleepiness due to a sleep disorder needs to be reported to the relevant licencing authority, and patients must be made aware of this. However, once patients become aware of this legal requirement, they may be reluctant to disclose sleepiness when driving for fear of losing their licence. It is useful therefore to reassure them that most sleep disorder patients are permitted to drive once their condition is treated.

The relationship between sleep disorders and occupation is bidirectional. Understanding how the sleep difficulty impacts on work attendance, performance and safety is central to determining how urgent treatment is and which risks need to be managed. For example, untreated OSA can effectively end the career of a trucker or taxi driver, while a shift work sleep disorder might affect the safety of a doctor working on a rotating shift pattern. Conversely, work stress, shift work and irregular working hours can all have a negative impact on sleep, while it is not uncommon for parasomnia patients to report a reduction in symptom frequency when not working and an increase in frequency when working long hours. Ironically, the sedentary lifestyle of occupational drivers predisposes them to obesity which may cause the OSA which then threatens that occupation.

3.6   Assessing Insomnia, Restless Legs and Circadian Rhythm Disorders

Patients with these disorders will typically present with a complaint of difficulty initiating sleep, maintaining sleep or of sleeping at the wrong time. When a patient complains of difficulty initiating or maintaining sleep, it is tempting to assume that the problem is insomnia and leave it at that. However, while insomnia is the commonest cause of sleep initiation or maintenance problems, circadian rhythm disorders or restless legs are not infrequently the underlying problem; indeed, almost any sleep disorder can present with insomnia symptoms. Therefore, a complaint of insomnia should be a trigger to take a comprehensive sleep history. A more detailed description of the insomnia assessment is to be found in Chap. 7.

3.6.1 Insomnia

Much of the relevant history in insomnia will already have been articulated in the description of a typical night. However, one should look for exacerbating and perpetuating factors for their insomnia. Clearly caffeine, nicotine and alcohol consumption are relevant here. Ask the patient to describe what strategies they have tried to tackle the insomnia and what impact medications have had on their sleep. Pain, asthma, gastro-oesophageal reflux and other physical complaints can impair sleep. It is informative to find out if they sleep better or worse when not in their own bed. Some patients have no difficulty falling asleep on the couch but struggle to sleep in their bed, and this may indicate that they have a conditioned response to the bed which wakes them.

Ask the patient why they feel they can't sleep. Is there an external, environmental factor such as noisy neighbours, a snoring bed partner or bright light that is preventing their sleep? If so, the problem may in fact be sleep deprivation due to an environmental factor rather than an inherent sleep disorder. Many patients will describe having an overactive mind at night, particularly once they get into bed. This is common in psychophysiological insomnia and can be a sign of a dysfunctional conditioned association of the bed with wakefulness.

3.6.2 Restless Legs Syndrome (RLS)

Given the degree of distress caused by restless legs, it is striking how few patients will spontaneously volunteer this symptom. Most RLS patients present with a complaint of insomnia. It is therefore critical that you specifically enquire about it. Restless leg patients will usually have difficulty describing the discomfort, but they are usually able to describe where in the body they feel it. This difficulty in describing the discomfort is also a useful way of differentiating it from cramps, which are usually described as such. In RLS, the discomfort can occur anywhere in the body but is most often localized to the lower limbs. A single question has been shown to have 100% sensitivity and 96.8% specificity for RLS in a neurology outpatient population (Ferri et al. 2007): 'When you try to relax in the evening or sleep at night, do you ever have unpleasant, restless feelings in your legs that can be relieved by walking or movement?'

In psychiatric patients on medication, particularly antipsychotics, it can sometimes be a challenge to differentiate between restless legs and akathisia as both can present with discomfort in the limbs and an irresistible urge to move the legs. Some akathisia patients will describe a mental unease which may be less common in RLS. Perhaps the best differentiator is the timing of the symptoms. Restless legs characteristically occur at night with a reduction, or complete absence, of symptoms during the day (as RLS gets worse, the onset of symptoms may occur earlier in the day, but there will still usually be a clear diurnal pattern). Akathisia severity is more likely to vary with the timing of the medication, being worse after taking a dose of that medication. Of course, there is no reason that a patient cannot have both akathisia and restless legs!

3.6.3 Circadian Rhythm Disorders

Circadian rhythm disorders are best diagnosed with the aid of a sleep diary (Appendix C) which can show the trend in sleep-wake times across several weeks. In the absence of a sleep diary, one should enquire about the patient's habitual bed and rising times and what times they fall asleep and wake up. In the most common circadian rhythm disorder—delayed sleep-wake phase disorder (DSWPD)—the patient will typically report being unable to initiate sleep until well after midnight and, if left to their own devices, would sleep late into the morning or afternoon.

Ask what would happen if they tried to change their bedtimes and rising times, for example, by going to bed earlier. Typically, in circadian rhythm disorders, it would have little or no impact on their sleep times. It is also critical to enquire about daytime symptoms and how they vary across the day. Patients with a DSWPD will feel worst in the mornings and progressively more alert as the day progresses; they feel most alert and energetic late at night when everyone else is going to sleep. Many patients will have tried hypnotics, and, even if they succeed in falling asleep earlier, the daytime symptoms will still follow the pattern described above. Of course, in advanced sleep-wake phase disorder (ASWPD), the patient will be most alert early in the morning and most sleepy at night, and their sleep times will be advanced. In a non-24-h sleep-wake rhythm disorder, the sleep time will rotate around the clock, usually getting progressively later each day.

It is often very difficult to elicit a clear history of a circadian rhythm disorder in someone who has waking times imposed on them by outside commitments such as school or work. It is helpful to ask the patient to describe what happens when they are on an extended holiday and these commitments are removed. When external constraints are removed, most patients with a circadian rhythm disorder will revert to their innate sleep pattern and report an improvement in daytime symptoms. The Morningness-Eveningness Questionnaire (Horne and Ostberg 1976) (Appendix B), which asks the patient about their typical pattern of alertness in the day and preferred sleep pattern, can also be helpful to confirm the diagnosis.

3.7 Assessing Parasomnias and Other Night-Time Events

It is tempting to think that the diagnosis of parasomnias requires specialist investigations such as PSG with video monitoring, and it is true that these studies can be helpful. However, a good history will yield the correct diagnosis in most cases, and the studies are usually done purely to confirm the diagnosis or screen for any exacerbating factors such as OSA or PLMs. Furthermore, as these events can be sporadic, parasomnias are often not observed during a one-night PSG.

Parasomnias fall into two broad categories: REM sleep parasomnias and non-REM sleep parasomnias which usually arise from slow-wave (N3) sleep. Understanding the basic phenomenology and distribution of the different sleep stages across the night is vital in making a diagnosis. Slow-wave sleep is a very deep stage of sleep, with a high arousal threshold and very little dreaming or complex mentation. It occurs primarily in the first half of the night and is increased in sleep deprivation. REM sleep is a lighter stage of sleep with a lower arousal threshold and is associated with detailed, vivid dreaming. It occurs primarily in the second half of the night. Therefore, in assessing unusual behaviours at night, one should determine the time of night they occur, how much the patient recalls about them, whether they recall vivid dreams or only vague fragments, whether they get out of bed and how organized the behaviour is (Table 3.2).

3.7.1 Sleepwalking

In sleepwalking, the diagnosis is generally very clear on history. The person typically gets out of bed and walks around the room or the home. They are able to turn door handles, open drawers, arrange objects, etc. fairly skilfully. However, although the individual actions are coordinated, the sum of the actions is often not. For example, the sleepwalker may open a drawer in the dresser, carefully rearrange the clothes and then urinate in the drawer or may eat a solid block of butter on a plate with a knife and fork. They may return to bed or continue sleeping in another location without waking up. If woken during an episode, they may describe feelings of confusion or panic, sometimes accompanied by hypnopompic hallucinations. As these episodes occur early in the sleep period, they may be witnessed by other members of the household, and therefore a collateral history is often available. If there is no one to give a collateral history, the patient will usually still be able to report symptoms and clues which are suggestive of sleepwalking, including waking up in a different place, finding household objects rearranged or unexplained bruises on the legs (from bumping into coffee tables, etc.).

Table 3.2 Comparison of non-REM and REM parasomnias

	Non-REM (slow-wave) sleep parasomnias	REM sleep parasomnias
Timing	First half of night	Second half of night
Arousal threshold	High	Low
Dreaming	Vague, fragmentary or none	Frequent, detailed, vivid
Recall of events on waking	Little or none	More frequent
Behaviour	Coordinated, may get out of bed, manipulate objects, etc. Eyes open	Uncoordinated, generally stay in bed. thrash around and hit out but rarely manipulate objects. Eyes closed
Onset	Often start in childhood, though nature of parasomnia may evolve through the years, e.g. it may start as sleep walking and progress to night terrors or sleep sex	Nightmares may start in childhood but can occur at any time; REM behaviour disorder starts in middle or old age

3.7.2   REM Sleep Behaviour Disorder

In contrast, REM sleep behaviour disorder (RBD) occurs in the second half of the night, is often violent in nature, appears less coordinated and is associated with vivid dreams and nightmares. It is very rare for the patient to leave the bed during an episode of RBD. In very extreme cases, they may jump out of the bed but will then wake immediately. Because they rarely leave the bed, it will often go undetected for many years if there is no bed partner to witness the events. However, a common presentation is when the patient throws a punch in their sleep and, in the process, throw themselves out of bed. They either wake up on the floor or hit their head on the bedside table on the way down! RBD can also lead to significant injury or even death of the bed partner. The author has encountered two patients who have been misdiagnosed with a personality disorder as they injured bed partners during their sleep and the psychiatrists, unaware of the RBD, presumed they were cases of domestic abuse.

A single screening question for REM sleep behaviour disorder has been shown to have a sensitivity of 93.8% and a specificity of 87.2% in a sleep clinic population: 'Have you ever been told, or suspected yourself, that you seem to "act out your dreams" while asleep (e.g. punching, flailing your arms in the air, making running movements, etc.)?' (Postuma et al. 2012).

3.7.3   Nocturnal Epilepsy

If a patient has nocturnal epilepsy, this is likely to be detected when you are enquiring about sleepwalking and RBD. There is a great deal of variability in the presentation of nocturnal epilepsy, but there are a number of factors that would raise the suspicion of seizure activity. The presence of daytime seizures and classic signs of seizure activity such as tongue biting or incontinence should make one consider the possibility that unusual night-time events are epileptic in nature. Try to get an impression of how frequent the events are and whether they occur more than once a night. Slow-wave sleep parasomnias are often sporadic, while epilepsy tends to be more consistent, and multiple episodes per night make epilepsy the more likely diagnosis. Unlike parasomnias, the offset of seizures is often abrupt and may be followed by an awakening. Stereotyped movements are more likely with epilepsy, while organized activity and leaving the bedroom are less likely. However, some epileptic patients do experience nocturnal wandering as part of their condition, and so leaving the room does not preclude a diagnosis of epilepsy.

3.7.4   Confusional Arousals

Confusional arousals may occur independently or following an episode of sleep walking or a night terror. The patient reports being confused and disorientated. This usually resolves within a few minutes, either with the person waking up fully or going back to sleep. Partners may report that the patient says odd things and looks confused.

3.7.5   Sleep Terrors

Sleep terrors are sometimes reported by the patient's family rather than the patient. The patient may have little or no recollection of the events, but their dramatic nature can be distressing for bed partners and may adversely affect their sleep. A good collateral history is therefore very important. The bed partner will typically report that the patient sits up suddenly in the bed, their eyes are usually open wide and they will scream or cry. It can take several seconds or minutes for the patient to calm down, and they are generally very resistant to reassurance and consolation. In more dramatic episodes, they may jump out of the bed in a panic before coming to. Sleep terrors tend to occur in the first hour or two of the sleep period.

Where the sleep terrors are frequent, the patient is likely to be aware of some episodes. The disruption to their sleep may lead to daytime fatigue and sleepiness, and the unpleasant experience of the sleep terrors may lead to anxiety about sleep with secondary insomnia. They may report hypnopompic hallucinations during the episodes (see below).

3.7.6   Nightmares

Nightmares are frightening or deeply upsetting vivid dreams that often leave patients with a sense of loss, sadness or fear extending into the day. Patients who suffer from frequent nightmares may develop considerable anxiety about going to sleep leading to insomnia, sleep avoidance or choosing to sleep during the day. Of all the sleep disorders, nightmares are the strongest predictor of suicide (Bernert and Nadorff 2015), and so it is surprising how rarely they are asked about in routine psychiatric interviews. Taking a history of nightmares is complicated by the very different expectations that patients have about what normal dreaming entails. Some patients will be distressed by dream content that most people simply accept as part of normal dreaming. For example, it is common for people that we have not seen or thought about in years to appear in our dreams, yet some people find this very disturbing. However, one would not normally consider this a nightmare. Similarly, a very high proportion of normal dreams have a negative emotional tone, but this alone would not qualify them as nightmares.

Therefore, in order to determine if the patient is experiencing nightmares as opposed to negative or strange dreams, one needs to take a very detailed history. One can ask the patient if they feel the dreams are actual nightmares as opposed to anxious, unpleasant dreams, and some patients may be able to differentiate between the two. However, it is generally more useful to ask the patient to describe a typical dream; it is then much easier to get an impression of the content and emotional intensity of the dreams and determine whether they should be classified as nightmares.

Once again, as nightmares are REM phenomena, they are more likely to occur in the second half of the night.

3.7.7 Panic Attacks

Finally, one must also consider the possibility of panic attacks which arise from sleep. These are similar in presentation to daytime panic attacks but can be difficult to differentiate from parasomnias, especially sleep terrors. As with sleep terrors, they are not preceded by dream mentation and generally arise from non-REM sleep (Krystal et al. 2015). Unlike non-REM parasomnias, where the patient's recall for the event may be incomplete or absent, and where they may go back to sleep at the end of the episode, panic attacks are typically clearly recalled and can lead to a prolonged awakening. However, the diagnosis of nocturnal panic does not preclude a sleep disorder; the panic may well be precipitated by an obstructive apnoea, for example.

3.7.8 Hypnagogic and Hypnopompic Hallucinations

These are brief hallucinations that occur either at sleep onset (hypnagogic) or waking (hypnopompic). They can be in any sensory modality, but common hallucinations are a sense of there being an intruder or malign presence in the room, hearing the doorbell or their name being called, seeing spiders or snakes or seeing the walls and ceiling collapsing in on them. They are very often unpleasant in nature (Iranzo et al. 2009).

Patients will often describe these experiences as dreams or nightmares, and one needs to elicit more details to differentiate them from dreams. In hallucinations, the person experiences the hallucination superimposed on the real world. They will usually be aware that they are in their bed and in their room and will see, hear or feel the hallucination within the room. So they may feel as if someone is behind their bed, see a figure in the corner of the room or see snakes coming out of their cupboard. The hallucinations are generally short-lived, fragmentary experiences and dissipate as soon as the person is fully awake. In contrast, dreams occur in a 'dream space'. The person dreams that they are in the kitchen, at school, out on the street, etc. The dreams are usually longer and more detailed and involve a sequence of events.

It is also important to differentiate these hallucinations from those found in psychotic disorders. This author has encountered numerous patients who have been put on antipsychotic medications as it was supposed that their hallucinations were a sign of schizophrenia. A careful history will reveal that the hypnagogic/hypnopompic hallucinations occur exclusively at the junctures of sleep and wakefulness, whereas those found in psychotic disorders can occur at any time of the day. Sleep-related hallucinations tend to dissipate rapidly when the lights are turned on, which would be unusual in psychosis. Once they are fully awake, most patients with sleep-related hallucinations rapidly become aware that the hallucinations are not real. Another clue that these are sleep-related hallucinations rather than psychosis is if they are accompanied by sleep paralysis (see below).

The situation is more complex, however, in patients with learning disabilities or dementia who may not always be able to articulate when they experience the hallucinations. This is especially true if they have severe excessive daytime sleepiness, such as in narcolepsy. As these patients drift in and out of sleep many times a day, they may experience hypnagogic/hypnopompic hallucinations throughout the day.

3.7.9   Sleep Paralysis

Sleep paralysis is the experience of being paralysed on waking or, less commonly, on falling asleep. Sleep paralysis is the intrusion of the normal REM atonia and paralysis into wakefulness. The most important task in taking a history of sleep paralysis is to differentiate sleep paralysis from sleep inertia, which is the difficulty waking up fully and is often accompanied by difficulty moving due to fatigue and sleepiness.

In sleep paralysis, the paralysis generally affects the entire body, and the person cannot speak, though they may be able to generate simple vocalizations such as grunts or squeaks. If the patient feels they have difficulty breathing, or have a sense of something pressing on their chest, then sleep paralysis is more likely. Similarly, hypnagogic/hypnopompic hallucinations during the episode mitigate in favour of sleep paralysis. Understandably, most patients describe sleep paralysis as a frightening experience, though some patients who suffer from frequent episodes may get used to them and find them less distressing. Sleep paralysis can occur at sleep onset, though many patients only experience it on waking, and in many patients it occurs more frequently in the supine position. It usually resolves suddenly, often in response to a light touch by the bed partner (Vaughn and D'Cruz 2017). Some patients will report experiencing paralysis during dreams rather than wakefulness; commonly the dream is distressing, and they need to flee or fight but cannot move. It is likely that this is the awareness of normal REM sleep paralysis being incorporated into the dream and is not in itself pathological.

Sleep inertia occurs on waking. It is not accompanied by difficulty breathing, and hallucinations are rare. The patient subjectively experiences intense fatigue and weakness rather than fear. With effort, they are able to move and speak. It is not related to body position and tends to resolve very gradually, over the space of several minutes or even hours (Table 3.3).

When asking about sleep paralysis, some patients will report having temporary paralysis or loss of sensation in a limb, usually an arm. This is not sleep paralysis and is likely due to extended pressure on the limb from lying on it.

If you have diagnosed sleep paralysis, then establish the frequency of episodes. Sporadic episodes are not uncommon and are generally benign, but frequent episodes can be a sign of isolated sleep paralysis, and frequent episodes in the context of sleepiness may be a sign of narcolepsy.

Table 3.3 Comparison of sleep paralysis and sleep inertia

	Sleep paralysis	Sleep inertia
Timing	Usually on waking but can be at sleep onset	On waking
Movement	Can only move eyes and diaphragm	Able to move, at least a little, but with significant effort
Speech	No; may be able to grunt or squeak	Able to speak though may be difficult
Duration	Seconds to minutes	Minutes to hours
Resolution	Sudden, complete resolution	Very gradual; often has lingering sleepiness after rising
Subjective sensations	Difficulty breathing, frightening, hallucinations	Exhausted, drained, heavy, sleepy

3.8 Assessing Excessive Daytime Sleepiness

This is a common presenting complaint and has a wide differential diagnosis.

3.8.1 Insufficient Sleep Syndrome

Before making a diagnosis of another sleep disorder, one needs to be sure that the patient is not sleepy due to inadequate sleep opportunity. The description of a typical night and the sleep diary may demonstrate that the patient frequently has inadequate time in bed. If a patient sleeps significantly longer on weekends than during the week, this is likely a sign they are getting insufficient sleep during the week. As these patients accumulate a sleep debt which cannot be paid off with one or two longer nights' sleep, one wouldn't necessarily expect them to feel less sleepy when they try to catch up sleep on weekends. Therefore, ask the patient whether they feel less sleepy when they have had an extended period of longer sleep, such as on holiday.

3.8.2 Obstructive Sleep Apnoea (OSA)

Ask the patient if they snore. A collateral history is particularly helpful here, but not absolutely necessary. Most patients, even those who live alone, will know if they have significant snoring. They may wake themselves up snoring or describe embarrassing snoring when falling asleep on buses, in hotel rooms, etc. Other clues include regularly waking with a sore throat or their voice becoming more gravelly. If there is a bed partner, ask if they have ever reported a cessation of the patient's breathing during the night. Apnoeas can be quite alarming, and the bed partner will usually try to rouse the patient the first few times it happens. If there is no bed partner, ask if the patient ever wakes up choking or gasping for breath. Sleep apnoea may cause significant night sweats and marked nocturia (though other causes such as diuretics need to be taken into account). Another sign to ask about is the presence of frequent morning headaches. Finally, apnoea patients commonly—but not universally—experience excessive daytime sleepiness. The assessment of sleepiness is described in more detail below.

It should be noted that many OSA patients may be completely unaware of any of these features. They may feel they sleep solidly through the night and deny any difficulties with breathing or sleep continuity. The only clues may be daytime fatigue or sleepiness and the physical examination. OSA is more common in men, the older age group and those who are overweight, have retrognathia, an enlarged tongue, a thick neck or enlarged tonsils. Despite this, it is important to remember that OSA can occur in young, slim individuals with no facial abnormalities. Weight gain is a common problem with numerous psychiatric medications, and increasing frequency or severity of the sleep disorder with increasing weight may be an indicator that OSA is the underlying problem, or at least an exacerbating factor.

3.8.3 Periodic Limb Movement Syndrome (PLMS)

Periodic limb movement syndrome (PLMS) (repetitive, stereotyped limb movements in sleep) is probably the most difficult sleep disorder to detect on history and is very much a diagnosis of exclusion. PLMS should be suspected if the patient has disrupted sleep and/or excessive daytime sleepiness, but there is a low probability of OSA, or in patients who have OSA which is being effectively treated but who continue to experience disrupted sleep or daytime sleepiness. It should also be suspected if the patient has predisposing factors such as low iron, kidney failure and neuropathy or is on antidepressants, antipsychotics or lithium (AASM 2014). The patient is usually unaware of the leg movements, and they can be so subtle that the bed partner may be unaware of them as well. In severe cases, the partner will complain of repetitive leg movements, or the patient may experience leg twitches at night prior to sleep onset. These need to be differentiated from sleep starts (hypnic jerks) which are more rapid, usually involve the entire body and occur singly rather than repetitively. Many patients with PLMS will have a positive personal or family history of restless legs (AASM 2014). In the absence of these signs and symptoms, one can ask if there are signs of restless sleep, such as blankets tangled round the legs or the bottom of the fitted sheet pulled out. PLMS patients whose pets sleep on their bed may notice that the pets have abandoned the bed in the morning. However, history alone does not have the sensitivity or specificity to make a diagnosis of PLMS, and ultimately a polysomnogram will be required (AASM 2014).

3.8.4 Central Hypersomnolence

If there are no clear indications of an underlying sleep disorder, such as OSA or PLMS, then one should consider the possibility of a central disorder of hypersomnolence.

If the sleep quantity seems adequate, then the two most likely diagnoses to investigate are narcolepsy and idiopathic hypersomnia (IH). Although these will require actigraphy, a PSG and a multiple sleep latency test to confirm the diagnosis, there are a number of clues in the history that make one suspect narcolepsy or IH and help differentiate between the two.

In both narcolepsy and IH, patients report significant sleepiness, often described as irresistible. Most of these patients will nap during the day, either taking planned naps or falling asleep unintentionally. In narcolepsy, these naps are often refreshing, and the person wakes feeling quite alert; sleepiness then gradually increases in intensity leading up to the next sleep episode. Many narcoleptic patients will report vivid dreaming even in brief naps and may experience sleep paralysis and hypnagogic/hypnopompic hallucinations. In IH, naps tend to be longer than in narcolepsy—often longer than an hour—and are usually unrefreshing; IH patients often report that they feel worse after naps rather than better (AASM 2014).

The night-time sleep of many narcoleptics is very fragmented, and they have a higher rate of parasomnias such as RBD. In IH the sleep is typically long, subjectively deep and consolidated, yet unrefreshing. 36%–66% of IH patients experience severe sleep inertia on waking and will require multiple alarms and prompts, and often several hours, before they are able to get out of bed. In contrast, long sleepers (people who simply need more sleep than the mean for their age) will wake feeling refreshed and alert if they have had adequate sleep (AASM 2014).

Age of onset of the symptoms is also informative. Whilst OSA and PLMS become more frequent with increasing age, narcolepsy typically starts between ages 10 and 25. Similarly, the peak age of onset for IH is 16.6–21.2 years (AASM 2014).

Although sleep paralysis and hypnagogic/hypnopompic hallucinations can occur in IH, if they occur frequently, they are much more likely to be a sign of narcolepsy. Sleep paralysis at sleep onset is less common than on waking and may be indicative of narcolepsy.

Cataplexy is rarely observed in the clinic, and so a good history is needed to determine if it is present. Its presentation varies across individuals and between episodes; it can also evolve across time. It is a brief loss of muscle tone and control without loss of consciousness. In mild episodes, it can manifest as the head dropping forward or nodding, the jaw sagging and slurred speech. In more severe episodes, the patient may drop to the ground. It is usually precipitated by emotion, particularly by laughter, and patients may learn to avert attacks by avoiding emotional stimuli and reining in their emotions. The muscle weakness is generally bilateral though there may be greater weakness on one side than the other. It starts suddenly but usually builds in intensity over a few seconds, which sometimes allows the patient to minimize the risk of injury (AASM 2014).

When asked about cataplexy, many patients will report episodes of head nodding or their head dropping forward, but they are often describing sleep episodes rather than cataplexy. One must establish very clearly whether these events are happening when dozing or in full consciousness. In addition, many non-cataplectic people will experience muscle weakness when laughing for a prolonged period, when angry or when scared. It is therefore more indicative of cataplexy if these physical symptoms are precipitated by milder emotions and/or positive emotions or are clearly visible to observers. As cataplexy symptoms can be controlled by REM-suppressing antidepressants, this symptom may be masked in patients on these drugs. If the patient is on, or has ever been on, an antidepressant one should enquire about whether cataplexy was present before starting on the antidepressant and whether the antidepressant improved the cataplexy. If patients experience a significant and rapid improvement in symptoms on starting an antidepressant, or a rebound of symptoms on stopping it, this makes a diagnosis of cataplexy more likely.

In any patient with suspected central hypersomnolence, one needs to screen for psychiatric disorders. Hypersomnia associated with a psychiatric disorder accounts for 5–7% of hypersomnolence (AASM 2014). In cases where the hypersomnolence is precipitated by depression, the hypersomnolence may persist once the mood has stabilized (AASM 2014). Therefore, one should ask about mood and other psychiatric disorders at the time the sleepiness started, even if there is no psychiatric comorbidity at present.

Mood symptoms may be common in narcolepsy, and patients report that these symptoms lead to significant daytime dysfunction. Anxiety disorders, particularly panic attacks and social phobia, are also more common in narcolepsy, but the anxiety symptoms are not always volunteered by the patients; therefore one needs to specifically ask about them (Fortuyn et al. 2010).

3.9   Sleep Diaries

There are few tools more useful in assessing sleep disorders than a sleep diary. Obviously, the utility of the diary will depend on the patient keeping a reasonably accurate record of their behaviours and their subjective experience of sleep. A basic sleep diary (Appendix A) will record time to bed and rising time, time in bed, sleep onset latency, number of awakenings, wakefulness after sleep onset and total sleep time. It can be helpful to instruct the patient to fill in TIB, SOL, WASO and TST in minutes rather than hours as it is then easier to calculate an average for the week. The TIB and SOL can be used to calculate the sleep efficiency as described above. One can also ask patients to record parasomnias such as night terrors or nightmares, whether they took a sleeping pill, daytime caffeine and alcohol, exercise, etc.

If one suspects a circadian rhythm disorder, it may be more helpful to utilize a visual diary with the day divided into blocks of 30 min. The patient colours in blocks a different colour depending on whether they were predominantly asleep or awake during that time (see Fig. 3.1). If they are asleep for only part of that time, they colour the block according to whether they spent more time asleep or awake in that epoch. For example, if they wake from sleep at 7:10, the 7:00 to 7:30 epoch is coloured as awake; if they wake at 7:20, the epoch is coloured as asleep. This allows one to see patterns and changes more clearly. One can of course use smaller blocks of time, but the inherent inaccuracy of all sleep diaries means this is rarely useful.

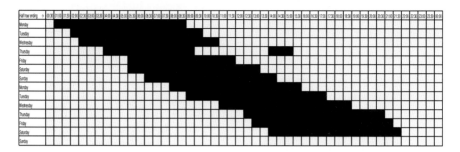

Fig. 3.1 Visual sleep diary showing a non-24-h sleep-wake rhythm. The light blocks indicate wakefulness, and the dark blocks indicate sleep

3.9.1   Using Scales

There are numerous scales that have been developed for sleep medicine over the years. However, very few of them are used in clinical practice, and they tend to be used more in research or audit settings. When used in a clinical context, the choice of scale will depend on the specific clinical setting. For example, the type of questionnaire used to screen for OSA in primary care will likely be one with a high sensitivity but poor specificity in order to screen for patients that require further investigations. Once those patients have been channelled to a sleep clinic, it may be more useful to administer questionnaires with a high specificity to clarify the diagnosis.

One problem that affects most scales is that they have not been validated in the psychiatric population. This is problematic as there is often significant overlap between psychiatric symptoms and the symptoms of sleep disorders. For example, fatigue, irritability and difficulty concentrating could be symptoms of depression, schizophrenia, OSA, insomnia, PLMS or circadian rhythm disorders. One therefore needs to interpret any scales used with the psychiatric co-morbidities in mind.

3.9.2   Epworth Sleepiness Scale (ESS)

(See Appendix A).

The one scale that is almost ubiquitous is the Epworth Sleepiness Scale (ESS) which measures the degree of sleepiness experienced during waking hours (Johns 1991). This scale asks the patients how likely they are to fall asleep in eight different situations in recent times. If they haven't been in a particular situation recently, then they are asked to imagine how likely they would be to fall asleep if they had been in that situation. This is not always easy for patients, particularly with regard to the last question which asks about falling asleep while stationary in a car. In countries where there are large numbers of people who have never learned to drive, many patients find this a very difficult question to answer. Despite this, the ESS has been validated in numerous countries and languages and can be a very helpful measure.

The cut-off between normal and abnormal sleepiness on the ESS is an area of debate, but 10 or 11 out of 24 is generally considered to mark the transition from normal to abnormal sleepiness (Johns and Hocking 1997). It can be really useful to get partners/parents, etc. to also fill in an Epworth for the patient and, if there is a significant difference, to explore why. This is also important when there may be a reason for the patient to give an artificially high score (e.g. if drug seeking or looking to be signed off from work) or an artificially low score (e.g. if their driving licence is at risk). One should also view the Epworth in the context of the patient's history. It is not uncommon for patients to have a low Epworth score but describe significant sleepiness in their history. Some patients who are sleepy learn to manage their sleepiness, for example, by taking a nap every afternoon. They will therefore score 3/3 for the question on whether they would sleep if they lie down in the afternoon, but score low on other questions. It is therefore important when looking at the Epworth score to not only look at the total but also at each individual question. Clearly there is a big difference between someone who has a high chance of falling asleep when lying down and someone who would fall asleep while talking to someone. Insomnia patients tend to have a low Epworth score, but this is not always the case. Interestingly, insomnia patients will often report falling asleep easily while watching TV, sitting quietly after lunch, etc. but score 0/3 on the question about lying down in the afternoon. This demonstrates that there is strong psychological element to the insomnia as they are capable of falling asleep easily except when actually trying to fall asleep.

Another very useful aspect of the ESS is that it helps the patient (and the clinician) to differentiate between sleepiness and fatigue/tiredness. Most sleep disorder patients experience fatigue, but not all are sleepy. For example, many insomnia patients have crippling fatigue but are not sleepy. By getting the patient to focus on whether they would actually fall asleep as opposed to feeling tired, one can gain an insight into their sleep propensity.

It is common practice in sleep clinics to do an Epworth on every visit. This allows one to monitor the response to treatment, and, if a person's Epworth does not drop into the normal range with treatment, one should consider whether there is an additional cause for their sleepiness that may have been missed. Once again, be aware that patients may give an artificial score once they understand what the implications of their diagnosis are in terms of treatment, work and driving. A sudden drop in the Epworth score before treatment is initiated should raise the suspicion that this may be a factor.

3.10 Assessing Sleep in a Psychiatric Inpatient Setting

When a patient is admitted to hospital, it presents an opportunity to more fully assess their sleep over a period of time, but one needs to look out for certain pitfalls. The acutely unwell patient may have a very different sleep pattern from when they are in remission and living at home, and this is further confounded by the fact that medications are often being titrated and changed. The psychiatric ward can be a very unnatural, and sometimes frightening, environment for patients. The fact that there are so many staff and other patients in a confined space means they are often quite noisy.

Nevertheless, it is still potentially fruitful to assess patients' sleep. If nothing else, asking about a patient's sleep can be a good way of building rapport. In patients with psychotic disorders or mania, there may be a great deal of disagreement between the clinician and the patient about the nature and importance of their symptoms. But the patient and the clinician are likely to agree on the importance of good sleep, and patients are often extremely grateful when someone takes an interest in their sleep. Secondly, an inpatient stay does create an opportunity to detect sleep disorders that might otherwise be missed. Many patients with chronic and severe mental illness live alone, and there is often no one to provide a collateral sleep history. When they are staying on a ward, there is a rare opportunity to observe their sleep. Having a systematic and effective way of doing this makes these observations more useful.

Sleep reports are commonly collected by ward staff on night duty. However, these are usually reports of behaviour rather than observations about sleep. A common example is that patients may be reported to have had 'a settled night'. This is more of a statement of how long they were in bed and how frequently they were seen out of bed rather than an observation about their sleep. When staff check on patients in the night, they will usually record them as being asleep if they are in bed with the lights off, though they may well be awake in the bed. It should be borne in mind that the act of making these observations may in itself disrupt the patients' sleep.

There is therefore a lot to be gained from training ward staff to be exact in their use of terminology, e.g. differentiating between 'the patient was asleep' and 'the patient was in bed' as well as training them to report more detailed sleep information. For example, night staff should report if patients were heard snoring so that their doctor can be alerted to the possibility of OSA. Similarly, sleepiness in the day often goes unnoticed as the patient is quiet and not demanding attention, so day staff should be encouraged to report periods of sleep during the day.

Finally, although staff may be keeping a log of the patient's sleep, there is no reason that the patient cannot keep a sleep diary for themselves when on the ward. This can be compared to the staff log and may provide useful clinical information. It also encourages the patient to be actively involved in the management of their sleep and allows them to monitor their own progress as the therapeutic interventions take effect.

3.11 Taking a Brief Sleep History

There are numerous scenarios where taking a full and detailed sleep history is unnecessary or impractical. For example, in primary care or during a psychiatric assessment, one may only have a few minutes to enquire about sleep. What follows is a simple format for taking a brief sleep history for screening purposes, or to decide whether and where to refer someone with a sleep complaint. Each box addresses an aspect of the history and suggests some useful questions to elicit that history.

3.11.1 Brief Sleep History Template

Epworth sleepiness score: _____

Main Complaint
- How do you sleep?
- How long has this been a problem?
- What do you think is causing the problem?

Typical Night
- What time do you go to bed?
- What time do you fall asleep?
- How many times do you wake during the night?
- How long are you awake for during these awakenings?
- What time do you wake up? (this is the final awakening after which the patient does not return to sleep)
- What time do you need to get up?
- What time do you get up?
- How much sleep do you think you get in total on a typical night?

Daytime Symptoms
- How do you feel during the day?
- Do you feel tired or sleepy?
- Do you nap intentionally or unintentionally during the day?
- What time of day do you feel most alert and most sleepy?

Previous Treatments
What remedies have you already tried (behavioural and medical); what effects did they have?

Sleep Apnoea
- Do you snore?
- Has anyone said you stop breathing in your sleep?
- Do you ever wake up choking?
- Do you sweat a lot in your sleep?
- How many times do you have to pass water at night?
- Do you often wake with a headache?

Restless Legs
- When you try to relax in the evening or sleep at night, do you ever have unpleasant, restless feelings in your legs that can be relieved by walking or movement?
- Do you get these feelings in the day as well? If so are they worse during the day or the night?

Periodic Limb Movements
- Have you ever been told you kick or fidget your legs in your sleep?
- Do your legs twitch repeatedly late at night when you are sleepy?
- When you wake up, are there signs that you have been very restless during the night?

Nightmares and Night Terrors
- Do you regularly suffer from nightmares?
- Do you recall the nightmares vividly on waking?
- Are these awful, frightening dreams or anxious unpleasant dreams?
- What time of the night do they occur?

Unusual Behaviours in the Night
- Have you ever been told, or suspected yourself, that you seem to 'act out your dreams' while asleep (e.g. punching, flailing your arms in the air, making running movements, etc.)?
- Do you sleep walk?
- How often does the behaviour occur?
- Is the behaviour the same each time or does it vary?
- What time of the night does it occur?

Hypnagogic/Hypnopompic Hallucinations
- When you are drifting into or out of sleep, do you ever see or hear or feel things that aren't there, e.g. a sensation that there is someone in the room, seeing shadowy figures or faces or hearing your name called?
- If so, how often?

Sleep Paralysis
- When you fall asleep or wake up, do you ever find you are completely paralysed?
- Do you feel that you cannot breathe during these episodes?
- Are you able to talk during these episodes?
- Do they resolve suddenly or gradually?

Cataplexy
- When you are **awake**, if something makes you laugh, makes you angry or surprises you, do you suddenly feel very weak, so you can't hold your head up or your legs turn to jelly?
- Do you feel weak but alert, or do you feel sleepy?

References

American Academy of Sleep Medicine. International classification of sleep disorders. 3rd ed. Darien: American Academy of Sleep Medicine; 2014.

Bernert RA, Nadorff MR. Sleep disturbances and suicide risk. Sleep Med Clin. 2015;10(1):35–9. https://doi.org/10.1016/j.jsmc.2014.11.004.

Ferri R, et al. A single question for the rapid screening of restless legs syndrome in the neurological clinical practice. Eur J Neurol. 2007;14(9):1016–21. https://doi.org/10.1111/j.1468-1331.2007.01862.x.

Fortuyn HAD, et al. Anxiety and mood disorders in narcolepsy: a case–control study. Gen Hosp Psychiatry. 2010;32(1):49–56. https://doi.org/10.1016/j.genhosppsych.2009.08.007.

Horne JA, Ostberg O. A self-assessment questionnaire to determine morningness-eveningness in human circadian rhythms. Int J Chronobiol. 1976;4(2):97–110. https://doi.org/10.1177/0748730405285278.

Iranzo A, Santamaria J, Tolosa E. The clinical and pathophysiological relevance of REM sleep behavior disorder in neurodegenerative diseases. Sleep Med Rev. 2009;13(6):385–401. https://doi.org/10.1016/j.smrv.2008.11.003.

Johns MW. A new method for measuring daytime sleepiness: the Epworth sleepiness scale. Sleep. 1991;14(6):540–5. https://doi.org/10.1016/j.sleep.2007.08.004.

Johns M, Hocking B. Daytime sleepiness and sleep habits of Australian workers. Sleep. 1997;20(10):844–9.

Krystal A, Stein M, Szabo S. Chapter 136: anxiety disorders and posttraumatic stress disorder. In: Principles and practice of sleep medicine. Philadelphia: Elsevier; 2015. p. 1341–51.

Postuma RB, et al. A single-question screen for rapid eye movement sleep behavior disorder: a multicenter validation study. Mov Disord. 2012;27(7):913–6. https://doi.org/10.1002/mds.25037.

Vaughn BV, D'Cruz OF. Chapter 58—Cardinal manifestations of sleep disorders. In: Principles and Practice of Sleep Medicine. Philadelphia, PA: Elsevier; 2017. p. 576–586.e3. https://doi.org/10.1016/B978-0-323-24288-2.00058-1.

Sleep Investigations

4

Christopher Kosky

4.1 Introduction

Investigations have a key role in the diagnosis of sleep disorders because the patient remembers little whilst asleep. In most medical conditions, the patient's history and examination is paramount in the process of reaching a diagnosis. During sleep, amnesia makes the patient's history incomplete or unreliable. Memory during sleep can also be distorted. The hypnagogic hallucinations associated with narcolepsy or the confusional arousals in non-rapid eye movement (NREM) sleep parasomnias leave the patient unsure of what is real and what was dreamed. Often the clinician relies on a collateral history from the patient's bed partner if one is available, but the bed partner may have moved out of the room because their own sleep is disturbed by the patient's snoring, restlessness, limb movements or parasomnia. Moreover, when examining the patient, there are few clinical signs of an underlying sleep disorder. For these reasons, investigations are an essential part of the diagnostic criteria of many sleep conditions.

Investigations in sleep medicine have become standardized with published practice parameters (Berry et al. 2014; Morgenthaler et al. 2017). Countries at the forefront of sleep medicine require sleep laboratories, medical staff and sleep scientists or technicians to be accredited to national or international standards. Accreditation ensures uniform quality of data, allows comparison of centres by peer review and assists in research.

C. Kosky, MBBS, FRACP, FRCP.
Department of Pulmonary Physiology and Sleep Medicine, Sir Charles Gairdner Hospital, Nedlands, WA, Australia

University of Western Australia, Crawley, WA, Australia

West Australian Sleep Disorders Research Institute, Queen Elizabeth 2 Medical Centre, Nedlands, WA, Australia
e-mail: Chris.Kosky@health.wa.gov.au

© Springer-Verlag GmbH Germany, part of Springer Nature 2018
H. Selsick (ed.), *Sleep Disorders in Psychiatric Patients*,
https://doi.org/10.1007/978-3-642-54836-9_4

This century, the world faces a great burden of sleep disorders. Obesity is driving an epidemic of obstructive sleep apnoea in both developed and emerging economies. Inadequate sleep is common due to pressures to work and the lures of electronic entertainment. Insomnia remains the commonest sleep disorder. To meet this demand, cost-effective high-quality investigations for sleep disorders are required. However there is also a need for investigations that go beyond a superficial understanding of a patient's structure of sleep and tell us about the function and quality of an individual's sleep and the interplay of environment, neurobiology, chemistry and genetics.

In patients with psychiatric disease, the incidence of sleep disorders is thought to be very high; yet investigating these patients can be difficult. Obstructive sleep apnoea, circadian rhythm disorders, insomnia and hypersomnia are probably under-recognized amongst patients with psychiatric disease. Performing detailed in-laboratory polysomnography may not be possible in agitated, delusional or involuntary patients. In addition, the interpretation of tests such as the multiple sleep latency test for hypersomnia can be confounded by psychiatric disease and medication. Smaller portable sleep studies and actigraphy may offer novel ways of identifying sleep disorders, allowing for assessment in the patient's home or hospital ward.

Here I have given a description of each of the common sleep investigations from a clinician's perspective. More detailed and technical information is available from the references.

4.2   In-Laboratory Polysomnography

Polysomnography (PSG) performed in a sleep laboratory with an attendant sleep technologist remains the 'gold standard' in the investigation of sleep disorders. It allows for a detailed assessment of a patient's physiology during sleep. It is useful in the assessment of sleep-disordered breathing, titration of non-invasive ventilation and identification of periodic limb movement disorder (PLMD). The addition of synchronized high-definition video allows assessment of parasomnias and movement disorders. An extended montage electroencephalogram (EEG) allows for assessment of sleep-related epilepsy. PSG requires an inpatient stay in a sleep laboratory and skilled technicians for set-up, scoring and interpretation of the polysomnography.

4.2.1   Technique

A laboratory polysomnograph measures multiple channels of physiological parameters focused on sleep stage, body position, respiration and muscle tone. The information is recorded digitally by computer software. An infrared camera and a microphone allow the technician to see and communicate with the patient. A sleep technician makes notes during the recording and manually scores the data, dividing the study into 30-s epochs.

Sleep stage is determined by global neural activity (measured by EEG), eye movements (measured by electroculogram) and muscle tone (measured by submental electromyogram [EMG]). Sleep onset is characterized by slow eye rolling movements and a slowing of EEG activity with alpha waves (8–13 Hz). Stage 2 NREM sleep is defined as the presence of sleep spindles (oscillations of 12–14 Hz) or K complexes (high amplitude, biphasic waves of at least 0.5 s in duration). Stage 3 NREM sleep is characterized by slow (delta) waves which are high amplitude broad waves. REM sleep is characterized by sharp phasic eye movements on electroculogram and a reduction in muscle tone on submental EMG. In REM sleep, the EEG may have a sawtooth pattern or a low-voltage, mixed-frequency pattern which may be difficult to differentiate from stage 1 NREM sleep.

The polysomnograph provides a detailed assessment of respiration during sleep. Nasal prongs connected to a pressure transducer can detect subtle airflow limitation. Hypopnoeas are scored using the nasal prongs trace. Nasal prongs fail to detect airflow if the patient breathes through their mouth during sleep. To overcome this, an oronasal thermal airflow sensor is used to confirm a complete cessation in airflow (an apnoea). A microphone, piezoelectric sensor or nasal pressure transducer are used to detect snoring. The oxygen saturation of haemoglobin is measured by continuous pulse oximetry. Respiratory effort is detected by bands placed around the chest and abdomen. The bands contain respiratory inductive plethysmography or piezo electrodes, which detect movement of the chest and abdomen during respiration. Transcutaneous carbon dioxide can be added to detect sleep hypoventilation. Alternatives include measuring arterial carbon dioxide or end tidal carbon dioxide. Hypoventilation during sleep can occur in neuromuscular disorders or severe obesity (obesity hypoventilation syndrome). A rise of more than 10 mmHg of transcutaneous carbon dioxide from baseline at the beginning of the study usually indicates nocturnal hypoventilation.

Periodic limb movements in sleep are detected by a leg EMG positioned on the anterior tibialis muscle. Periodic limb movements (PLMs) are repetitive dorsiflexions of the big toe, with fanning of the small toes accompanied by flexion of ankle, knees and thighs that occur at regular intervals of 5–90 s. A limb movement is defined as an increase in leg EMG amplitude by at least 8 μV from baseline with a duration of between 0.5 and 10 s (Berry et al. 2014). Periodic limb movements can be associated with symptoms such as sleep maintenance insomnia or excessive daytime sleepiness.

Other physiological parameters are measured on PSG. Electrocardiogram allows determination of pulse rate and arrhythmias. Body position is measured using a position sensor and is also recorded by the technician in attendance.

Additional modalities can be added to the polysomnography to help detect specific conditions. Synchronized high-definition video is useful in detecting parasomnias and movement disorders and to characterize seizures. Current software allows high-definition video to be included and synchronized with the polysomnography data. As mentioned above, an extended montage of EEG can be added to help detect epileptic activity during sleep.

When performing a polysomnography, the patient's usual sleep behaviours are encouraged. Patients are asked to come to the sleep laboratory in the early evening and to sleep at their usual time. They should avoid caffeine and take their usual medication. There is no consensus on alcohol. On the one hand, it is argued that the sleep study should be performed with the patient's usual intake of alcohol, as alcohol makes sleep apnoea worse and changes sleep architecture. This needs to be balanced with patient and staff safety. Shift workers should have the PSG performed during their usual sleep time.

The PSG should be performed in a sound-proofed room. Set-up of the leads usually takes about an hour and is followed by a series of calibration tests. The sleep study is attended by one or more sleep technicians who sit in a control room. The role of the overnight sleep scientist is to observe the patients on video, ensure signals from each of the physiological channels are of good quality, introduce non-invasive therapies if required and attend to patients during the night. The study usually finishes at about 6 am. The PSG is manually scored by a sleep scientist. Software packages can assist in scoring of the sleep study. Scoring usually requires identification of the sleep stage and respiratory and limb movements during each 30-s epoch. This may take between 1 and 3 h. The overnight sleep study may be followed immediately by a multiple sleep latency test (MSLT) or maintenance of wakefulness test (MWT) performed during the day.

4.2.2 Patterns of Disease

Obstructive sleep apnoea is characterized on polysomnography by episodes of airflow reduction with continued effort as the upper airway occludes. An apnoeic event is usually followed by a reduction in oxygen saturations of haemoglobin and/or a cortical arousal on EEG.

The American Association of Sleep Medicine (AASM) defines an apnoea as a greater than 90% reduction in airflow from baseline on an oronasal temperature transducer with a duration equal to or greater than 10 s (Berry et al. 2014). Airflow signal on a positive airway pressure device or an alternative sensor can also be used. An obstructive apnoea is characterized by absent airflow with continued or increased respiratory effort throughout the duration of the apnoea (Fig. 4.1). A central apnoea is defined as an absence of airflow with absent chest wall movement throughout the period of the apnoea. A mixed apnoea is characterized by absent inspiratory effort in the initial part of the apnoea and resumption of inspiratory effort in the second part of the apnoea.

A hypopnoea is defined as a 30% reduction in airflow lasting 10 s or longer, associated with a 3% or greater oxygen desaturation or an arousal. Hypopnoeas can be further classified into obstructive or central. In obstructive events there is snoring and increased flattening of airflow; there may also be paradoxical or seesawing movement of the chest compared to the abdomen. In central hypopnoeas there is an absence of snoring and absence of paradoxical respiratory effort.

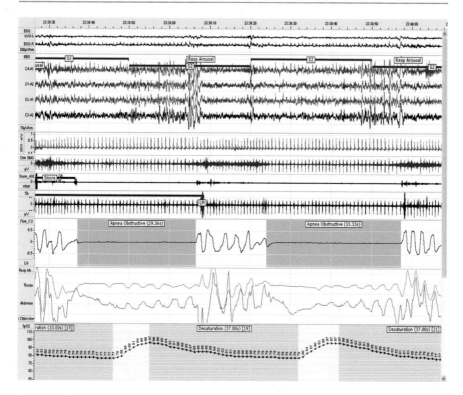

Fig. 4.1 Showing two obstructive apnoeas on polysomnography. There is an absence of airflow associated with an oxygen desaturation and cortical arousal. Note also paradoxical movement of the chest wall and abdomen, with the chest moving inwards whilst the abdomen moves outwards

Obstructive sleep apnoea is a polysomnographic diagnosis based on the apnoea-hypopnoea index (AHI): the average number of apnoeas and hypopnoeas per hour of sleep. Mild obstructive sleep apnoea (OSA) is defined as an AHI of 5–15 events per hour, moderate OSA as 15–30 events per hour and severe OSA as greater than 30 events per hour.

Central sleep apnoea is diagnosed when the majority of apnoeas are central. Central sleep apnoea is commonly due to opiates, but other causes include heart failure and brainstem disease affecting the respiratory centres. Cheyne-Stokes breathing is a special form of central sleep apnoea with waxing and waning periods of apnoea and hyperventilation with a cycle length of approximately 1 min. Cheyne-Stokes respiration is associated with heart failure and stroke. Biot's breathing is a pattern of rapid breaths of roughly equal depth separated by central apnoeas and is seen in brainstem lesions.

Nocturnal hypoventilation has a different respiratory trace to sleep apnoea on polysomnography. It is characterized by prolonged periods of oxygen desaturation and a rise in transcutaneous carbon dioxide lasting several minutes to hours. Nocturnal hypoventilation can occur in severe obesity, parenchymal lung disease and neuromuscular disease. When nocturnal hypoventilation first begins, it is isolated to REM sleep. This is because, during REM sleep, there is paralysis (hypotonia) of all skeletal muscles except for the diaphragm and muscles of the eye. Chest wall muscles that assist ventilation are inactive. This leaves ventilation during REM sleep reliant upon a diaphragm that is weakened by neuromuscular disease, loaded by obesity or whose mechanics are altered by lung disease. As these diseases progress, ventilatory failure occurs in NREM sleep and then later into wakefulness resulting in daytime respiratory failure.

Periodic limb movements in sleep are characterized by bursts of increased leg EMG activity occurring periodically. Some leg movements may also be detected on video. Often the limb movements are associated with cortical or autonomic arousal.

PSG can be helpful for identification of parasomnias. REM sleep behaviour disorder is characterized by dream enactment, often with injury to self or bed partners. It is characterized by loss of the REM muscle atonia, often with movement (Fig. 4.2). The PSG of patients with NREM parasomnias is often normal. Confusional arousals may occur in which the patient wakes from slow-wave sleep and appears confused before falling asleep. Sleep deprivation prior to the sleep study has been shown to increase the probability of the patient sleep walking during the sleep study (Zandra et al. 2008).

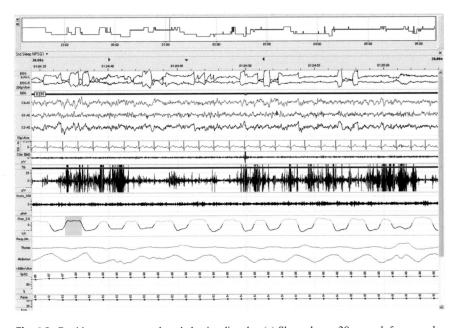

Fig. 4.2 Rapid eye movement sleep behavior disorder. (a) Shows loss a 30 s epoch from a polysomnography showing loss of the muscle atonia during rapid eye movement (REM) sleep. Normally the tibialis EMG (labeled Tib) is flat during REM sleep, in this case there is activity. Synchronized high-resolution video (not shown) was showed the patient punching during REM sleep

Polysomnography with extended montage can be helpful in the identification of seizures that occur during sleep. Interictal spike activity may be seen, although these can occur in normal subjects as well. Prior to seizures, spike activity may occur showing recruitment, but the EEG during motor seizures may be obscured by movement artefact. In frontal lobe seizures, the EEG is frequently normal because of the depth of the frontal lobes. Video demonstrating repeated stereotyped posturing or movement may be more helpful in diagnosing sleep-related epilepsy than the EEG.

4.2.3 Advantages

PSG has a number of advantages such as discrimination of the type of sleep-disordered breathing, detection of periodic limb movements and characterization of sleep-related movement disorders. It also provides a picture of the patient's sleep architecture, wake after sleep onset, depth of sleep, slow-wave and REM sleep pressure and sleep fragmentation that no other sleep investigation can yet replicate.

The other great advantage of PSG is that it allows the introduction and fine-tuning of non-invasive ventilation in real time whilst the patient is asleep. Non-invasive ventilation is the collective term for therapies such as continuous positive airway pressure (CPAP) or bi-level positive airway pressure (BiPAP). The aim of a titration polysomnography is to abolish sleep-disordered breathing and return a normal pattern of tidal breathing. The pressure of continuous positive airway pressure is gradually increased, whilst the patient is asleep to overcome airflow limitation and stop obstructive apnoeic events. In a similar fashion, BiPAP pressures are increased to abolish both apnoeic events and hypoventilation. Oxygen can be added if the patient remains hypoxic despite non-invasive ventilation.

Many centres have found it cost-effective to perform a split night PSG for suspected obstructive sleep apnoea. A split night sleep study avoids the need for two sleep studies, one for diagnosis and one for titration of CPAP. In a split night study, the first few hours of the study are diagnostic. The second part of the study allows CPAP to be introduced and titrated to control sleep apnoea. Usually CPAP will only be introduced if the patient has moderate or severe obstructive sleep apnoea. It's important that REM and supine sleep are seen on the diagnostic part of the study, as this is when sleep apnoea is most severe. Failure to include REM or supine sleep on the diagnostic portion of the sleep study can lead to an underestimate of OSA severity.

A respiratory PSG is a form of limited polysomnography performed at some centres. A respiratory PSG is a laboratory PSG without EEG, EMG and EOG. Sleep can therefore not be identified. The advantage of a respiratory PSG is a reduced set-up time, reduced scoring time and less equipment with possibly fewer disturbances to the patient's sleep. There is a sleep technician available if there is a lead failure and patient problems or if non-invasive ventilation is to be introduced. Limited polysomnography will be discussed further in the home-based polysomnography section.

4.2.4 Disadvantages

Cost and the time required are the main disadvantages to the laboratory PSG. Costs are predominantly those associated with an overnight stay in a single room and the labour costs associated with set-up, running, manual scoring and reporting of a sleep study. A laboratory PSG requires highly skilled staff and should be performed in accredited centres.

The patient's sleep architecture in the sleep laboratory may not be the same as at home. The hospital setting may feel foreign and artificial for patients and is not always conducive to sleep. The wires and monitoring equipment often force the patient to sleep in the supine position. Meals, alcohol and medication normally taken at home may vary in the environment of the sleep laboratory. Sleep routines and zeitgebers (time cues) may be different in the sleep laboratory compared to the patient's home. Noise, light and interruptions in the laboratory may disturb the patient's sleep. Another relevant factor is the absence of bed partners. Many of these factors have led to a growing interest in home-based sleep studies, which is discussed later.

4.2.5 Reliability

A manually scored in-laboratory PSG is currently considered the gold standard in sleep investigation. However it is not without problems. There can be night-to-night variability in the severity of obstructive sleep apnoea, resulting in an underestimate of sleep apnoea (Meyer et al. 1993). The unfamiliar sleep environment may lead to a 'first night effect' characterized by sleep initiation and sleep maintenance insomnia. One study found that patients having an in-laboratory PSG had a higher micro-arousal frequency, increased percentage of wake and reduced slow-wave and REM sleep compared to a PSG at home (Kingshott and Douglas 2000). However this did not significantly affect objective measures of daytime sleepiness. In addition, leads can be affected by artefact (e.g. sweat or electrical artefact) or may migrate from original position.

4.3 Multiple Sleep Latency Test

The multiple sleep latency test (MSLT) is an objective test for excessive sleepiness. Excessive sleepiness is defined as sleepiness that occurs at times during the day when it would not usually be expected. The MSLT is the principal diagnostic test for narcolepsy and idiopathic hypersomnia (IH).

4.3.1 Technique

The MSLT measures a patient's sleep latency during five daytime naps. Sleep latency is the time from lights out to the time the patient falls asleep. Sleep latency is a measure of the patient's drive to sleep and is usually decreased in sleep disorders that cause excessive sleepiness such as narcolepsy and sleep apnoea.

The MSLT follows a standard protocol developed by the American Academy of Sleep Medicine (Littner et al. 2005). Two weeks prior to the MSLT, the patient should stop any drugs that may affect sleep architecture. Antidepressants, antipsychotics, benzodiazepines and stimulants should be stopped if it is safe to do so. A sleep diary (Appendix C) or actigraphy is helpful 2 weeks prior to the sleep study to ensure sleepiness is not due to behaviourally induced inadequate sleep syndrome (BIISS). Urine drug testing should be performed at the beginning of the study to screen for undisclosed drugs that may affect the sleep study. A PSG is performed the night before the MSLT to exclude other causes of sleepiness such as sleep apnoea or periodic limb movement disorder. The PSG is used also to ensure the patient has had 6 h of sleep prior to the MSLT. Sleep for less than 6 h prior to the MSLT invalidates the results as daytime sleepiness may be due to inadequate sleep time prior to the study.

The patient undergoing MSLT is placed in a dark, quiet room. EEG, electroculogram and submental EMG are measured so that sleep and REM sleep onset can be objectively identified. The MSLT is started 1.5–3 h after the end of the PSG. It consists of five naps in which the lights are turned off and the patient is asked to go to sleep. Sleep is defined as three 30-s epochs of stage 1 sleep or any other stage of sleep. If sleep is detected, the test is continued for another 15 min to detect REM sleep. If the patient does not go to sleep, the test is terminated after 20 min. An average time to sleep onset, or mean sleep onset latency, is established for sleep of any stage and REM sleep.

4.3.2 Patterns of Disease

The MSLT is useful in supporting the diagnosis of narcolepsy or IH. Narcolepsy is characterized by mean sleep latency equal to or less than 8 min and two of five naps containing REM sleep. A sleep onset REM period (SOREMP) within 15 min on the preceding nocturnal polysomnograph may replace one of the SOREMPs on the MSLT (Fig. 4.3). Idiopathic hypersomnia is characterized by sleep latency equal to or less than 8 min and no more than one of five naps containing REM sleep. The patient must have had sufficient sleep the night before and a negative urine test for drugs that may cause sleepiness. Typical sleep latencies are 0–3 min for narcolepsy with cataplexy, 3–5 min for narcolepsy without cataplexy and 5–8 min for IH and probably reflect the severity of sleepiness. During the MSLT, REM sleep as the first sleep stage emerging from wake or from stage 1 sleep is unusual, and one should suspect narcolepsy with cataplexy, again perhaps reflecting the pressure or instability of REM sleep (Drakatos et al. 2013).

The MSLT may also be helpful in other situations where an objective measure of sleepiness is required, for example, in those patients who remain sleepy despite CPAP where a stimulant medication is being considered as an adjunct treatment.

Summary Graph

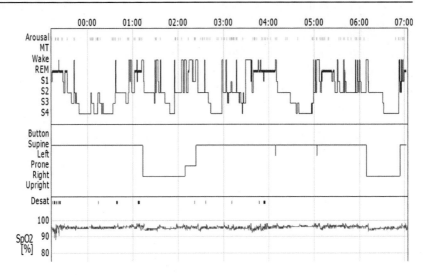

Fig. 4.3 Hypnogram from nocturnal polysomngram in a patient with narcolepsy with cataplexy. This shows a reduced sleep latency and a sleep onset REM period (SOREMP) occurring within the first 15 min of sleep onset. Sleep onset REM from wake or stage 1 NREM sleep has a high predictive value for narcolepsy

4.3.3 Reliability

MSLT is confounded by both false-positive and false-negative results. Pathological sleepiness (mean sleep latency less than 8 min) and sleep onset REM can occur in obstructive sleep apnoea, periodic limb movement disorder, depression and BIIS or by medication and drugs. In addition, sleep latency under 8 min with two sleep onset REM episodes can occur within the normal population, particularly those whose body clocks favour sleeping late at night. Typically in these patients, the reduced sleep latency and sleep onset REMs occur in the morning naps when they would normally be having REM sleep. A number of measures can be taken to reduce false positives for narcolepsy or IH. Depression can be screened for by careful history or a validated questionnaire; nocturnal PSG is used to exclude OSA and PLMD. Urine drug testing can be used to exclude medications or drugs that can cause sleepiness. A sleep diary and actigraphy can be used to ensure sleepiness is not a consequence of sleep deprivation.

False negatives also occur with the MSLT. About 25% of patients with narcolepsy do not fulfil the MSLT criteria for narcolepsy. Exercise or smoking between naps may affect the results, as can anxiety. Repeating the MSLT may be helpful, particularly in reducing the 'first night effect' of sleeping in the sleep lab. MSLT has a high false-negative rate in the diagnosis of patients with IH with long sleep time (Vernet and Arnulf 2009). Typically, the patient with IH with long sleep time regularly sleeps for greater than 10 h in a 24-h period and reports excessive daytime sleepiness. The diagnosis can be supported objectively by a 24-h PSG or 7 days of actigraphy where the patient can sleep freely (ad libitum).

4.3.4   Maintenance of Wakefulness Test

This study is used to examine whether a patient can remain awake after their usual sleep period. The patient is asked to sleep normally the night before the study. A PSG is often used to ensure at least 6 h of sleep. The following day, the patient undergoes a series of four tests at 2-h intervals where they are asked to stay awake in a quiet, dimly lit room for 40 min. Sleep is monitored by EEG and is defined as three epochs of stage 1 or one epoch of any other stage of sleep. Different protocols exist but the one given above is the standard (Kingshott and Douglas 2000).

The maintenance of wakefulness test may be helpful when an objective measure of the ability to stay awake is required. It is often used in patients with sleep disorders when assessing treatment efficacy, particularly when deciding fitness to drive. It may also be helpful when there is a disparity between what the patient reports ('I'm not sleepy doctor') and what is observed (asleep in the waiting room).

Difficulty arises in the interpretation of the test. Being able to stay awake for 40 min in all four naps is reassuring that the patient can maintain wakefulness. A mean sleep onset latency of 8 min or less is abnormal, and the patient is deemed to be unable to maintain wakefulness. The grey period is between 8 and 40 min, and there is little consensus on how to interpret these results.

Also difficult to interpret is the presence of microsleeps, where brief sleep comprising less than 50% of the epoch is observed. These episodes are scored as wakefulness according to the standard scoring rules. These patients may officially be reported as staying awake for all 40 min in all the trials but may still present a significant risk when driving.

4.4   Portable Sleep Studies

Portable sleep studies can be performed in the patient's home or in a hospital bed. Principally, they have been used to detect obstructive sleep apnoea. Home-based polysomnography is gaining popularity in many countries as it can be a cost-effective alternative to polysomnography with equivalent accuracy. Pulse oximetry and actigraphy are both forms of portable monitoring and are discussed separately.

4.4.1   Technique

Portable sleep studies vary in the number of channels of physiological information that can be collected: from two-channelled pulse oximetry to a detailed polysomnography including EEG in the patient's home. The AASM categorizes sleep-monitoring devices into four types (Collop et al. 2007; Ferber et al. 1994). Type 1 sleep studies are in-laboratory technician-attended overnight polysomnography studies. Type 2 is polysomnography, which records the same information as type 1 but can be performed unattended at the patient's home or in a hospital bed. Type 3 portable sleep studies record four channels of information, typically two respiratory variables (airflow and respiratory movement), one cardiac variable (heart rate or ECG) and pulse oximetry. Type 4 devices record one to three channels and include pulse oximetry. As technology becomes more sophisticated, these categories blur, with sometimes multiple variables recorded from a single monitor.

It is recommended that a sleep technician sets up or teaches the patient how to apply the monitoring leads. The device may be set up in the clinic, and the patient then goes home wearing the device. The following day the data is downloaded in the sleep laboratory. The raw data should be analysed by a qualified sleep practitioner. The sleep study may be manually scored and reported in the same manner as a polysomnograph.

4.4.2   Advantages

The main advantages of a portable sleep study are that it can be performed in the patient's home and has a lower cost. A portable sleep study can also be performed in a psychiatric hospital bed if the patient is unable to have an in-laboratory polysomnography. A portable sleep study avoids the need for staff to be present during the night. Sleeping in one's home may offer a more accurate reflection of the patient's sleep habits.

4.4.3   Disadvantages

The main disadvantage of portable devices (particularly types 3 and 4) is the possibility of misinterpretation of the data that may lead to an incorrect diagnosis. Most portable devices have been compared to in-laboratory PSG. As the number of channels is reduced, the sensitivity and specificity fall. Generally they are useful in patients with a moderate to high pretest probability of obstructive sleep apnoea. Type 3 and 4 devices may not detect respiratory effort-related arousals (RERAs) if they do not monitor cortical activity. Also, it may be difficult to distinguish between central and obstructive apnoeas if respiratory effort is not recorded.

The other disadvantage of portable devices is the potential for data or lead failure. Unlike a laboratory-based sleep study, leads that fail or have a poor signal cannot be corrected immediately. Non-invasive ventilation cannot be titrated in real time. Usually video is not possible but this may become possible in the future.

4.4.4   Reliability

Studies comparing home vs laboratory sleep studies have had conflicting results, with some showing domiciliary studies to be inferior, whilst others show equivalence. The United States, Australia and Canada have recognized domiciliary PSG for Medicare or equivalent rebate. Interestingly, studies looking at CPAP compliance in patients with OSA have found equivalent or superior results when the patient is studied and set up at home compared to within the laboratory (Rosen et al. 2012).

4.5 Nocturnal Pulse Oximetry

4.5.1 Use

Nocturnal pulse oximetry can be a useful case-finding tool to detect sleep-disordered breathing and is usually performed in the patient's home (Zamarrón et al. 2003). A pulse oximeter is typically the size of a wristwatch and provides continuous information on two channels—oxygen saturation and pulse—overnight. Its small size allows the device to be posted to patients.

4.5.2 Technique

The oximeter resembles a wristwatch with an oximetry probe attached to the finger. The oximeter records oxygen saturation (SaO_2) and pulse rate every 1–6 s. The recording is started by the patient pressing a button, and it can be turned off in the morning so that two or three nights' worth of data can be collected. Typically the oximeter collects about 6–18 h of data. Information from the device is downloaded and provides both numerical data and a trace of pulse rate and oxygen saturations. The oxygen desaturation index (ODI) and the pattern of the trace are both used in the identification of disease.

4.5.3 Patterns of Disease

A normal pulse oximetry trace is flat with oxygen saturations between 94% and 98% during the recording. There is a small reduction (1–3%) in oxygen saturation at the onset of sleep compared to wake. There is an increase in heart rate variability during REM sleep.

Obstructive sleep apnoea (OSA) is characterized by repetitive dips in oxygen saturation for part or all of the recording (Fig. 4.4). Oxygen desaturation occurs because of obstruction of the patient's upper airway, apnoea and hypoxia. Desaturation is usually accompanied by a rise in heart rate, but occasionally there can be an associated bradycardia. The fall in oxygen saturation is followed by a return of oxygen saturations back to baseline. If there is a persistent failure of oxygen saturations, to return to baseline, then hypoventilation should be suspected. Evidence of hypoventilation is often associated with daytime respiratory failure and may indicate a more severe form of obstructive sleep apnoea called obesity hypoventilation syndrome (Pickwickian syndrome).

Severity of obstructive sleep apnoea can be approximated using the ODI. The 3% oxygen desaturation index (3% ODI) has been shown to most closely resemble the

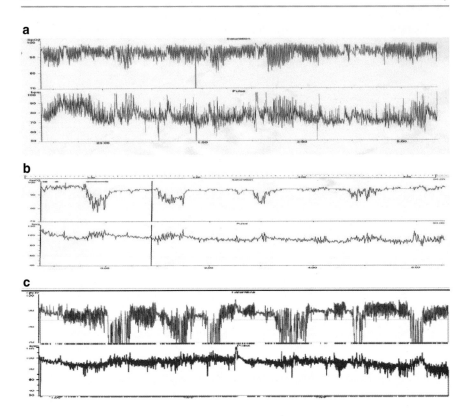

Fig. 4.4 Patterns of Nocturnal Pulse Oximetry. (Images courtesy of Dr. Nicholas Hart) The top trace shows oxygen saturations of haemoglobin (SaO_2), the bottom trace shows pulse rate. (**a**) shows a patient with obstructive sleep apnoea with repetitive oxygen dips that return to baseline accompanied by an increase in heart rate. (**b**) shows a patient with nocturnal hypoventilation from respiratory muscle weakness, with normal baseline oxygen saturations of haemoglobin but with prolonged periods of desaturation lasting approximately 30 min. These periods of desaturation probably correspond to REM sleep when hypoventilation is most severe. (**c**) Is a patient with obesity hypoventilation syndrome with both repetitive desaturations of obstructive sleep apnoea and evidence of nocturnal hypoventilation-where there is a failure of oxygen saturations to recover to baseline

apnoea hypopnea index in obese patients (Ling et al. 2012). A 3%ODI of 5–14/h accords with mild OSA, 15–29/h with moderate OSA and ≥30/h with severe OSA.

Clusters of desaturations that occur during only part of the recording suggest sleep apnoea that is related to body position, head position or sleep stage. Sleep apnoea is typically worse in the supine position and REM sleep and can be isolated to these times.

Other disease can have distinct oximetry trace patterns. The pulse oximetry in Cheyne-Stokes respiration shows even and regularly spaced desaturations with the resaturations often above the baseline. However, it can be difficult to distinguish central from obstructive apnoeas despite the different pattern (Sériès et al. 2005). Neuromuscular disease (motor neurone disease, diaphragm weakness, muscular dystrophy) is characterized by periods of prolonged desaturation for 30–90 min due to REM hypoventilation. This occurs because during REM sleep, the accessory muscles that support respiration are lost due to REM sleep muscle atonia. Chronic lung disease (chronic obstructive lung disease, asthma) is characterized by low baseline saturations, usually less than 90%.

Periodic limb movements in sleep also have a characteristic trace on pulse oximetry. There is large pulse rate variability with a normal oxygen saturation trace (Krishnaswamy et al. 2010). Heart rate variability is probably due to autonomic arousal.

4.5.4 Advantages

The great advantage of pulse oximetry is its ease of use, small size and low cost. Its ease of use means the patient can put it on at home, whilst other home-based sleep studies require a technician to set up the leads. Its small size means that pulse oximetry can be posted to patients. It can also be used outside the sleep lab such as in a general or psychiatric hospital bed. It is a cost-effective way of screening patients with symptoms of obstructive sleep apnoea by avoiding a more detailed and expensive sleep study. Pulse oximetry has been shown to reduce the number of inpatient PSGs for patients referred to a sleep centre with symptoms of OSA (Chiner et al. 1999).

4.5.5 Disadvantages

The main limitation of pulse oximetry is that it provides only two channels of data (SaO_2 of haemoglobin and pulse rate). Sleep and wake states cannot be differentiated nor does it provide information regarding sleep stage or position. A sleep diary completed during the oximetry study can help to identify the patient's sleep times. Pulse oximetry is not helpful in the assessment of parasomnias or narcolepsy unless comorbid sleep-disordered breathing is suspected. Oximetry can miss sleep-disordered breathing in patients with normal healthy lungs who arouse when their airway is partly obstructed but do not desaturate (upper airway obstructive syndrome).

4.5.6 Reliability

Nocturnal pulse oximetry lacks sensitivity and specificity in the detection of obstructive sleep apnoea when compared with (the gold standard) nocturnal PSG. The sensitivity and specificity of nocturnal oximetry varies in studies due to differences in methods, limiting the ability to pool results. Older studies used oximetry devices that had less frequent sampling times, which may have affected the sensitivity of the device to detect obstructive sleep apnoea. However, Ling et al. analysed 11,448 patients undergoing polysomnography. They established that 3% ODI performed best, and this index most closely approximated the apnoea hypopnea index (Ling et al. 2012). Pulse oximetry has a higher sensitivity to detect severe obstructive sleep apnoea compared with mild or moderate OSA. False-positive results for OSA may occur in patients with chronic lung disease, as they are more prone to oxygen desaturation. False-negative results may occur in patients who are of normal body mass index and have healthy lungs. Oximetry should be used with caution in these two groups.

We recommend two consecutive nights of data collection to improve assessment of the severity of obstructive sleep apnoea (Wallberg et al. 2010). Current devices have sufficient memory for 2–3 nights' recording. If pulse oximetry is not diagnostic and there is high clinical suspicion for OSA, then one should proceed to nocturnal PSG.

4.6   Actigraphy

Wrist actigraphy is a way of measuring sleep over days to weeks. Actigraphy records movement to allow sleep and wake schedules to be inferred.

The actigraphy watch is a small device, like a wristwatch, that the patient wears on their wrist during the day and night. They usually also complete a sleep diary recording sleep and wake times, naps, meals, alcohol and caffeinated drinks. Optimal recording time is not known, but one week of wrist actigraphy recording provides similar data to a 2-week recording, despite subtle differences between the weeks (Briscoe et al. 2014).

The current International Classification of Sleep Disorders recommends the use of actigraphy as a diagnostic tool where a single night of PSG is insufficient for the diagnosis, specifically to assess sleep patterns over time (American Academy of Sleep Medicine 2005). Actigraphy is particularly useful in the assessment of disorders of the human body clock (circadian rhythm disorders). Emerging evidence suggests that circadian rhythm disorders accompany many psychiatric disorders (Wulff et al. 2012; Jagannath et al. 2013).

4.6.1   Patterns of Disease

The AASM has produced an evidence-based review of the use and indications for actigraphy (Morgenthaler et al. 2017). Actigraphy is indicated to assist in the evaluation of advanced sleep phase syndrome (ASPS) where sleep onset is in the early evening delayed sleep phase syndrome (DSPS) where sleep occurs in the morning and often continues to beyond midday and free running disorder (Fig. 4.5).

Actigraphy has been used in patient groups whose sleep habits are difficult to monitor, such as children and the elderly (Kushida et al. 2005). Other uses of actigraphy include assessing shift work disorder, calculating sleep times in patients with insomnia or hypersomnia and assessing treatment responses in patients with circadian rhythm

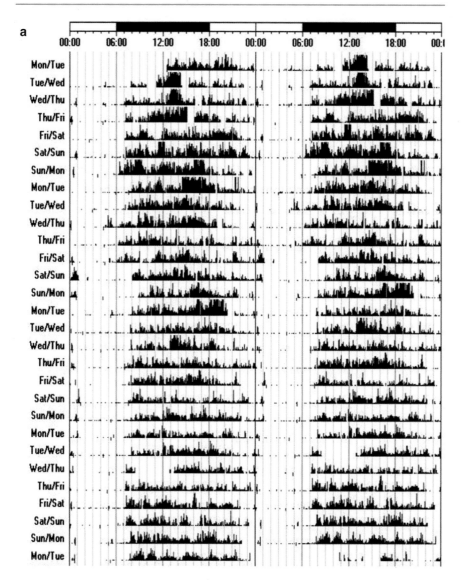

Fig. 4.5 Wrist actigraphy. (Images courtesy of Samantha Briscoe) (**a**) Four weeks of wrist actigraphy in a patient with a normal sleep pattern. (**b**) Four weeks of wrist actigraphy in a patient with free running disorder (also known as non 24-hour sleep wake syndrome). The normal human body clock is longer than 24 hours, on average 24.5 hours. Normally synchronization to 24 hours occurs through a process of entrainment using time cues (zeitgebers) such as light, clocks and routines. In free running disorder there is failure of entrainment. It occurs in patients who are visually impaired and in patients with psychiatric disorders

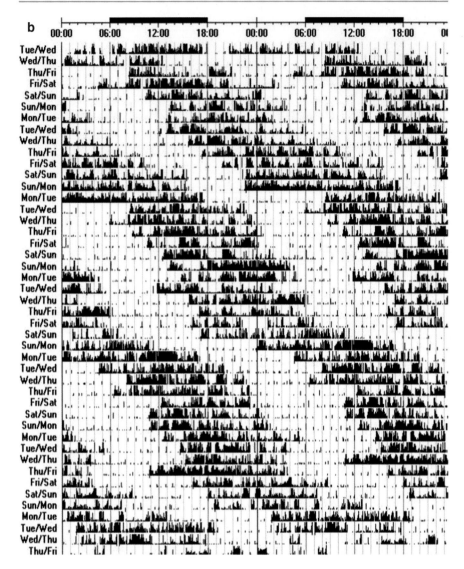

Fig. 4.5 (continued)

disorders or insomnia. Ankle actigraphy is also used to record periodic limb movements in sleep and may be helpful in assessing treatment response (Sforza et al. 2005).

4.6.2 Advantages

Actigraphy can record movement over several weeks allowing for the patient's sleep pattern to be inferred. Actigraphy is lightweight and not invasive, making it useful in difficult patient populations such as children, the elderly and patients with mental illness. It is also inexpensive. More recent devices allow for recording of light of different spectra providing information about the patient's light exposure.

4.6.3   Disadvantages

Actigraphy does not distinguish between sleep and wake states; it simply uses the absence of movement to infer the subject is asleep. If the patient is restless or moving in sleep, this may be reported as wake, thus providing inaccurate results. It cannot distinguish periodic limb movements in sleep and limb movements related to other causes such as sleep apnoea.

4.6.4   Reliability

It has been demonstrated that actigraphy significantly correlates with PSG-determined parameters such as total sleep time and wake after sleep onset in normal healthy subjects (De Souza et al. 2003), in a general sleep disorders population (Kushida et al. 2001), in sleep-disordered breathing patients (Hedner et al. 2004) and in patients with insomnia (Lichstein et al. 2006). The sensitivity of actigraphy to detect sleep is regarded as high, whilst the specificity to detect wake is low (Kushida et al. 2001; Blackwell et al. 2008; Blood et al. 1997).

4.7   Other Tests

Blood tests are important in excluding other causes of tiredness or sleepiness. Tiredness can be due to anaemia, hypothyroidism, liver disease and kidney dysfunction. Blood tests used to search for causes of restless leg syndrome (RLS) include iron studies, ferritin, vitamin B12, renal studies and serum glucose or glycosylated haemoglobin.

Serum HLA typing for HLA DQ B*0106 is not usually helpful for the diagnosis of narcolepsy as it can be found in the general population. However it may have a use in discerning cataplexy from pseudo-cataplexy. Almost all patients who have narcolepsy with cataplexy are HLA DQ B*0106 positive.

Analysis of cerebrospinal fluid (CSF) may be helpful in the assessment of patients with suspected narcolepsy. Patients with narcolepsy with cataplexy have absent levels of the neurochemical hypocretin in their cerebrospinal fluid (Mignot et al. 2002). In patients who have narcolepsy without cataplexy, the CSF hypocretin levels are often low to normal compared to healthy individuals. Hypocretin (also termed orexin) is a neurochemical produced by hypocretin cells located exclusively in the lateral hypothalamus and is involved in sleep regulation and REM sleep stability. In narcolepsy with cataplexy, there is death of the hypocretin-producing cells resulting in no measurable hypocretin in the cerebrospinal fluid. Confirming absent

CSF hypocretin levels by lumbar puncture can be useful in patients where there is a clinical suspicion of narcolepsy with cataplexy, but their sleep studies are confounded by medications or psychiatric disorders.

References

American Academy of Sleep Medicine (2005) International classification of sleep disorders – second edition (ICSD-2), p 298. ©2005 American Academy of Sleep Medicine, ISBN 0965722023 ISBN 978–0965722025.

Berry RB, Brooks R, Gamaldo CE, Harding SM, Lloyd RM, Marcus CL, Vaughn BV, for the American Academy of Sleep Medicine. The AASM manual for the scoring of sleep and associated events. Rules, terminology and technical specifications, version 2.0.3. Darien, IL: American Academy of Sleep Medicine; 2014. www.aasmnet.org

Blackwell T, Redline S, Ancoli-Israel S, Scheider JL, Surovec S, Johnson NL, Cauley JA, Stone KL, for the Study of Osteoporotic Fractures Research Group. Comparison of sleep parameters from actigraphy and polysomnography in older women: the SOF study. Sleep. 2008;31:283–91.

Blood ML, Sack RL, Percy DC, Pen JC. A comparison of sleep detection by wrist actigraphy, behavioural response and polysomnography. Sleep. 1997;20:388–95.

Briscoe S, Hardy E, Pengo MF, Kosky C, Williams AJ, Hart N, Steier J. Comparison of 7 versus 14 days wrist actigraphy monitoring in a sleep disorders clinic population. Chronobiol Int. 2014;31(3):356–62.

Chiner E, Signes-Costa J, Arriero JM, Marco J, Fuentes I, Sergado A. Nocturnal oximetry for the diagnosis of sleep apnoea hypopnea syndrome: a method to reduce the number of polysomnographies? Thorax. 1999;54:968–71.

Collop NA, Anderson WM, Boehlecke B, Claman D, Goldberg R, Gottlieb DJ, Hudgel D, Sateia M, Schwab R, Portable Monitoring Task Force of the American Academy of Sleep Medicine. Clinical guidelines for the use of unattended portable monitors in the diagnosis of obstructive sleep apnea in adult patients. J Clin Sleep Med. 2007;3(7):737.

De Souza L, Benedito-Silva AA, Pires MLN, Poyares D, Tufik S, Calil HM. Further validation of actigraphy for sleep studies. Sleep. 2003;26:81–5.

Drakatos P, Kosky CA, Higgins SE, Muza RT, Williams AJ, Leschziner GD. First rapid eye movement sleep periods and sleep-onset rapid eye movement periods in sleep-stage sequencing of hypersomnias. Sleep Med. 2013;14(9):897–901.

Ferber R, Millman R, Coppola M, Fleetham J, Murray CF, Iber C, Mccall V, Nino-Murcia G, Pressman M, Sanders M. Portable recording in the assessment of obstructive sleep apnea. ASDA standards of practice. Sleep. 1994;17(4):378.

Hedner J, Pillar G, Pittman SD, Zou D, Grote L, White DP. A novel adaptive wrist actigraphy algorithm for sleep-wake assessment in sleep apnea patients. Sleep. 2004;27:1560–6.

Jagannath A, Peirson SN, Foster RG. Sleep and circadian rhythm disruption in neuropsychiatric illness. Curr Opin Neurobiol. 2013;23(5):888–94.

Kingshott RN, Douglas NJ. The effect of in laboratory polysomnography on sleep and objective daytime sleepiness. Sleep. 2000;23(8):1–5.

Krishnaswamy UM, Higgins SE, Kosky CA, deLacy S, Williams AJ. Diagnosis of PLMD from increased pulse rate variability on overnight oximetry. Nat Sci Sleep. 2010;2:1–8.

Kushida CA, Chang A, Gadkary C, Guilleminault C, Carillo O, Dement WC. Comparison of actigraphic, polysomnographic, and subjective assessment of sleep parameters in sleep-disordered patients. Sleep Med. 2001;2:389–96.

Kushida CA, Littner MR, Morgenthaler T, Alessi CA, Bailey D, Coleman J, Friedman L, Hirshkowitz M, Kapen S, Kramer M, Lee-Chiong T, Loube DL, Owens J, Pancer JP, Wise M. Practice parameters for the indications for polysomnography and related procedures: an update for 2005. Sleep. 2015;28:499–521.

Lichstein KL, Stone KC, Donaldson J, Nau SD, Soeffing JP, Murray D, Lester BA, Aquillard N. Actigraphy validation with insomnia. Sleep. 2006;29:232–9.

Ling IT, James AL, Hillman DR. Interrelationships between body mass, oxygen desaturation and apnea-hypopnea indices in a sleep clinic population. Sleep. 2012;35(1):89:96.

Littner MR, Kushida C, Wise M, Davila DG, Morgenthaler T, Lee-Chiong T, Hirshkowitz M, Daniel LL, Bailey D, Berry RB, Kapen S, Kramer M, Standards of Practice Committee of the American Academy of Sleep Medicine. Practice parameters for the clinical use of the multiple sleep latency test and maintenance of wakefulness test. Sleep. 2005;28(1):113–21.

Meyer TJ, Eveloff SE, Kline LR, Millman RP. One negative polysomnogram does not exclude obstructive sleep apnea. Chest. 1993;103(3):756.

Mignot E, Lammers GJ, Ripley B, Okun M, Nevsimalova S, Overeem S, Vankova J, Black J, Harsh J, Bassetti C, Schrader H, Nishino S. The role of cerebrospinal fluid hypocretin measurement in the diagnosis of narcolepsy and other hypersomnias. Arch Neurol. 2002;59(10):1553–62.

Morgenthaler T, Alessi MD, Freidman L, Owens J, Kapur V, Boehlecke B, Brown T, Chesson A, Coleman J, Lee-Chiong T, Pancer J, Swick TJ. Practice parameters for the use of actigraphy in the assessment of sleep and sleep disorders: an update for 2007. Sleep. 2017;30:519–29.

Rosen CL, Auckley D, Benca R, Foldvary-Schaefer N, Iber C, Kapur V, Rueschman M, Zee P, Redline S. A multisite randomized trial of portable sleep studies and positive airway pressure autotitration versus laboratory-based polysomnography for the diagnosis and treatment of obstructive sleep apnea: the HomePAP study. Sleep. 2012;35(6):757–67.

Sériès F, Kimoff R, Morrison D, et al. Prospective evaluation of nocturnal oximetry for detection of sleep-related breathing disturbances in patients with chronic heart failure. Chest. 2005;127(5):1507–14.

Sforza E, Johannes M, Claudio B. The PAM-RL ambulatory device for detection of periodic leg movements: a validation study. Sleep Med. 2005;6(5):407–13.

Vernet C, Arnulf I. Idiopathic hypersomnia with and without long sleep time: a controlled series of 75 patients. Sleep. 2009;32(6):753–9.

Wallberg L, De Lacy S, Murphy P, Muza R, Kosky C, Reis PJ, Williams AJ. The utility of 2-night recording of home overnight pulse oximetry in the evaluation of patients with possible obstructive sleep apnoea. J Sleep Res. 2010;19:A1046.

Wulff K, Dijk DJ, Middleton B, Foster RG, Joyce EM. Sleep and circadian rhythm disruption in schizophrenia. Br J Psychiatry. 2012;200(4):308–16.

Zamarrón C, Gude F, Barcala J, Rodriguez JR, Romero PV. Utility of oxygen saturation and heart rate spectral analysis obtained from pulse oximetric recordings in the diagnosis of sleep apnea syndrome. Chest. 2003;123(5):1567–76.

Zandra A, Pilon M, Montplaisir J. Polysomnographic diagnosis of sleepwalking; effects of sleep deprivation. Ann Neurol. 2008;63(4):513–9.

Pharmacology of Psychiatric Drugs and Their Effects on Sleep

5

Sue Wilson

5.1 Introduction

This chapter provides an overview of psychotropic drugs encountered in psychiatry and includes the effects on sleep of those frequently prescribed for depression, anxiety, psychosis, dementia and ADHD, with a small section about recreational drugs. Drugs which treat, exacerbate or provoke sleep disorders are covered in the last section.

Most drugs which affect the brain do so by affecting neurotransmitter function in the brain, which they can do by:

- Simulating the action of a brain neurotransmitter on the receptor (agonists, partial agonists)
- Blocking its action on postsynaptic receptors (antagonists)
- Changing the receptor's sensitivity (allosteric modulators)
- Increasing the amount of neurotransmitter present in the synapse, either by increasing the release of it into the synaptic cleft, blocking its transportation out of the cleft or preventing the action of enzymes which break it down

The brain's arousal is maintained by parallel neurotransmitter systems whose cell bodies are located in brainstem or midbrain centres, with projections to the thalamus and forebrain. These activating neurotransmitters are noradrenaline, serotonin, acetylcholine, dopamine, histamine as well as the orexin system with cell bodies in the hypothalamus which promotes wakefulness through regulating arousal pathways (and inhibiting sedating ones). For all these arousing neurotransmitters, waking can be promoted by increasing their function, and sleep or sedation by decreasing their function in the brain.

S. Wilson
Division of Brain Sciences, Centre for Psychiatry, Imperial College London, London, UK
e-mail: sue.wilson@imperial.ac.uk

© Springer-Verlag GmbH Germany, part of Springer Nature 2018
H. Selsick (ed.), *Sleep Disorders in Psychiatric Patients*,
https://doi.org/10.1007/978-3-642-54836-9_5

The promotion of sleep is regulated by a number of other neurotransmitters; primary amongst these is gamma-aminobutyric acid (GABA), the main inhibitory neurotransmitter in the brain. The majority of brain cells are inhibited by GABA, so increasing its function reduces arousal and produces sleep and eventually anaesthesia. There are many subsets of GABA neurons distributed throughout the brain, but a particular cluster in the hypothalamus (ventrolateral preoptic nucleus) can be considered to be the sleep 'switch' (Saper et al. 2005). These neurons switch off brain arousal systems at the level of the cell bodies and therefore promote sleep. GABA receptors in the cortex can also promote sedation and sleep by inhibiting the target neurons of the arousal system. Most drugs used in insomnia, and benzodiazepines used in anxiety, act by increasing the effects of GABA at the GABA-A receptor (allosteric modulation).

5.2   Drugs for Depression

Many of these drugs are used not only to treat depression but also anxiety disorders, and most have profound effects on sleep architecture, particularly on rapid eye movement (REM) sleep; some also affect daytime sleepiness. Both REM effects and daytime sedation effects appear to be similar in depressed patients and healthy volunteers and therefore can be thought of as markers of brain pharmacological action, but there are also effects on non-REM (NREM) sleep and subjective sleep, which are different in the patient population and appear to relate to therapeutic action (Wilson and Argyropoulos 2005).

These effects on sleep are strongly associated with their effects on neurotransmitter systems in the brain, particularly their property of increasing synaptic levels of monoamines. The mechanism common to the most widely used antidepressants is that of inhibition of reuptake of serotonin (serotonin reuptake inhibitors (SRIs), e.g. fluoxetine), noradrenaline (noradrenaline reuptake inhibitors, e.g. reboxetine) and drugs which inhibit reuptake of both (dual reuptake inhibitors, e.g. amitriptyline, venlafaxine) into the presynaptic neuron. Monoamine oxidase inhibitors (MAOIs) also increase the level of synaptic serotonin and noradrenaline (and to a lesser extent dopamine) by preventing breakdown by the enzyme. Other drugs like mirtazapine act on the autoreceptors responsible for homeostatic maintenance of monoamine levels, blocking their negative feedback action and so increasing synaptic levels of noradrenaline and serotonin.

As well as their main action to increase monoamine levels, many antidepressants have (usually antagonist) effects on a variety of brain neurotransmitters including acetylcholine via cholinergic muscarinic receptors, noradrenaline via alpha-1 and alpha-2 adrenoceptors, histamine via H1 receptors and serotonin via 5-HT1A and 5-HT2 receptors.

5.3   Serotonin Reuptake Inhibitors and Dual Reuptake Inhibitors

There are two major REM sleep effects described with all SRIs and dual reuptake inhibitors such as venlafaxine. These effects are dose related and common to patients and healthy volunteers. They consist of:

- Reduction in the overall amount of REM sleep over the night
- Delay of the first entry into REM sleep (increased REM onset latency, ROL)

which together can be called REM suppression (Wilson and Argyropoulos 2005). This is usually within the first few days of treatment, (i.e. before therapeutic effects are manifest), and the size of the effect is similar with all SRIs except fluoxetine, where the changes are generally smaller and do not reach a maximum so quickly (Feige et al. 2002). The decrease in REM amount becomes less evident after chronic treatment, but REM onset latency remains long throughout treatment. This REM suppression after SRIs and venlafaxine is probably caused by increased levels of synaptic serotonin, and it is probable that this stimulates serotonin receptors of the 5-HT1A type in the brainstem REM-initiating areas, which in turn inhibits the initiation of REM sleep (Monaca et al. 2003).

Acute changes in NREM sleep and sleep maintenance following SRI or venlafaxine administration are also similar in volunteers and depressed patients and consist of:

- Increased light (stage 1) sleep
- Increased waking during the night

In general, this arousing effect is larger in normal volunteers, but depressed patients start out with very disrupted sleep, and further deterioration is therefore less obvious. These sleep disturbances diminish over time, with most studies in depressed patients showing no difference from baseline after a few days of treatment. The exception to this is fluoxetine, which tends to continue disrupting sleep continuity, and many doctors use a hypnotic to minimise the insomnia and distress that these drugs can induce. Recently, a study has compared the therapeutic response to fluoxetine with and without cotreatment with the new hypnotic eszopiclone. They found that depression scores improved significantly more in the group given the hypnotic and that this effect was not simply due to their having better scores on the sleep items on the depression scales (Fava et al. 2006).

The dual serotonin/noradrenaline reuptake inhibitor duloxetine has smaller effects on REM and sleep continuity than venlafaxine, which may reflect its lower selectivity for serotonin transporters.

5.4   Older Dual Reuptake Inhibitors

These are usually of tricyclic structure, and, as well as being reuptake inhibitors, they have many other, usually unwanted, properties such as antihistaminergic, anticholinergic and antiadrenergic effects, all of which may impact on arousal and sleep. Their REM effects in general are similar to those of SRIs; clomipramine and imipramine target the serotonin transporter preferentially and are the most REM-suppressing.

They also differ from each other in their effects on sleep initiation and maintenance:

- Clomipramine, desipramine (a selective noradrenaline uptake blocker) and imipramine tend to disrupt sleep on the first night, with increased amounts of waking during sleep. After a few days, this effect is no longer present in patients but continues in normal volunteers who were good sleepers at baseline.
- Amitriptyline and dothiepin improve sleep acutely in normal volunteers, but not in depressed patients. After a few days of treatment, most studies show no difference in sleep continuity from baseline.

These differences are probably explained by the fact that as well as inhibiting reuptake, the latter drugs are also potent antihistamines and antagonists at the serotonin 5-HT2 receptor—other 5-HT2 receptor antagonists have effects on sleep—see below. These sleep-promoting effects are occasionally useful in the depressed patient with insomnia.

There is no evidence for the widespread use of low-dose amitriptyline for non-depression-related insomnia, particularly in primary care. At doses below 50 mg per day, amitriptyline is primarily an antihistamine. There are no controlled studies of hypnotic efficacy of low-dose amitriptyline in insomnia. Drugs with tricyclic structure are more likely to be lethal than licensed hypnotics in overdose (Nutt 2005), and sometimes their side effects can be troublesome; therefore it has been recommended that these only be used in insomnia when there is coexistent mood disorder and at antidepressant doses (Wilson et al. 2010).

5.5   Monoamine Oxidase Inhibitors (MAOIs)

Suppression of REM sleep by the older, irreversible MAOIs is the most marked of all the antidepressants. Total suppression of REM sleep has been described in at least two studies of depressed patients after about a week of treatment at doses from 45 to 75 mg/day of the most popular MAOI, phenelzine. An important research finding is that the REM suppression by phenelzine is reversed by rapid tryptophan depletion, implying that its REM effects are via increased serotonin function (Landolt et al. 2003).

In addition to these actions on REM, phenelzine and tranylcypromine decrease total sleep time and fragment sleep both acutely and chronically, presumably because they increase serotonin and noradrenaline availability (Landolt et al. 2001).

5.5.1 Rebound Effects of REM-Suppressing Antidepressants

REM sleep rebound (i.e. shortened REM onset latency and increased total REM sleep) occurs after stopping drugs which suppress REM. For most SRIs and dual reuptake inhibitors, this will usually occur within 3–5 days (fluoxetine 10 days), and for MAOIs up to 2–3 weeks. This is important for diagnostic tests for sleep disorders like narcolepsy where early onset of REM sleep is key; if the patient is taking drugs for depression, or has recently stopped them, this is likely to invalidate these tests.

5.6 Other Antidepressants

- Vortioxetine has similar effects to SRIs.
- Trazodone is an antagonist at 5-HT2 receptors. It increases deep non-REM sleep and reduces intra-sleep waking in depression, insomnia and healthy volunteers (Mouret et al. 1988; Paterson et al. 2007, 2009) but has little impact on REM sleep. Sleep-disturbing effects of SRIs are thought to be mediated by increased impact of serotonin on this receptor, and some psychiatrists use a small dose of trazodone to alleviate troubling SRI-induced insomnia (Kaynak et al. 2004).
- Mirtazapine is also a 5-HT2 antagonist and also increases noradrenergic and serotonergic transmission—it improved subjective sleep in depression compared with venlafaxine (Benkert et al. 2006) and clinically seems to ameliorate insomnia-related problems in depression. It has no effect on REM sleep.
- Agomelatine is a melatonin agonist and 5-HT2 antagonist. It is reported to improve subjective sleep in depressed patients, although it has very little effect on sleep architecture (Sharpley et al. 2011).
- Trimipramine (which has tricyclic structure but is not a reuptake inhibitor) is a potent blocker of the 5-HT2 receptor and is strongly sleep promoting, with decreased sleep onset latency, higher sleep efficiency and longer sleep times reported in acute studies of normal volunteers, depression and insomnia (Riemann et al. 2002), and clinical experience suggests the subjective improvement in sleep continuity may be sustained into chronic treatment in depression. Its dopamine receptor blocking actions however mean it is not widely used because of D2 receptor-related risks such as tardive dyskinesia. There are no effects on REM sleep.
- Reboxetine is a noradrenaline uptake blocker with no direct action on serotonergic transport. It is very selective and has little action at other brain receptors. It suppresses REM sleep with the same pattern as dual reuptake inhibitors but less

markedly. It seems to have no significant effect on sleep continuity. It is sometimes used in narcolepsy, with both anticataplectic and arousing actions due to increased noradrenergic function (Larrosa et al. 2001).

5.6.1 Daytime Sedation

Many antidepressants have effects on vigilance levels or psychomotor function that lead to impairment of performance on daytime functioning such as driving. It is mainly the older drugs such as tricyclic antidepressants that affect central muscarinic acetyl-choline or H1 histamine receptors which produce these effects. However, sedative side effects have been reported with nearly all antidepressants, and a wise precaution would be to warn patients at the time of first prescription not to drive until an adequate period has elapsed in which they can assess its sedative action (i.e. 1–2 weeks).

5.7 Drugs for Psychosis

Most of these drugs, as well as blocking dopamine D2 receptors, can affect a variety of other brain receptors to different degrees. In addition to blocking dopamine D2 receptors, they also have receptor actions on serotonin (5-HT1A partial agonism, 5-HT2A antagonism), noradrenaline (alpha-1 antagonism), histamine (H1 antagonism) and muscarinic (ACh antagonism). Therefore, their effects on sleep are also varied.

In the few studies in healthy volunteers, drugs with D2 and 5-HT2A antagonism decrease waking during sleep and prolong sleep. Olanzapine and ziprasidone also increase slow-wave sleep.

The typical antipsychotics haloperidol and flupentixol and the atypical antipsychotics olanzapine, risperidone and clozapine tend to decrease sleep onset latency and improve sleep maintenance in schizophrenia patients (Monti and Monti 2004).

Subjective sleep improvements have been reported after most antipsychotics, particularly chlorpromazine, risperidone, olanzapine and quetiapine.

5.8 Wake-Promoting Drugs

Amphetamine-like stimulants used in ADHD and narcolepsy (e.g. methylphenidate, lisdexamfetamine) increase wakefulness by blocking dopamine and noradrenaline reuptake, by stimulating dopamine release or by both mechanisms. Modafinil probably increases wakefulness through activation of dopaminergic systems by dopamine reuptake inhibition. Caffeine inhibits adenosine receptors, which in turn can produce activation via interaction with GABAergic and dopaminergic neurotransmission. These drugs are detrimental to sleep, increasing sleep onset latency and waking during sleep; patients who take them, and their doctors, should take care to time the dosing so that stimulant effects do not impinge on desired sleep.

5.9 Drugs for Bipolar Disorder

The mechanism of action of these drugs is not well worked out, but they appear to have their actions either by affecting cell signalling via enzyme interactions (lithium) or by modulation of glutamate by blocking sodium and calcium ion channels (valproate and carbamazepine).

- Lithium and carbamazepine have a fairly neutral or a slightly positive impact on sleep continuity, and both of these tend to increase slow-wave sleep (Friston et al. 1989; Gann et al. 1994).
- Valproate and levetiracetam do not appear to change sleep but may cause daytime sleepiness in higher doses (Harding et al. 1985; Bell et al. 2002);
- There have only been a few studies with lamotrigine, but so far there is no indication that it changes sleep (Jain and Glauser 2014).

5.10 Drugs for Anxiety Disorders

Some of these which also treat depression have been covered above.

Short-term treatment of anxiety often includes benzodiazepine receptor agonist drugs, which modulate the GABA-A receptor to increase the effects of GABA in the brain (positive allosteric modulators). GABA is the major inhibitory neurotransmitter in the CNS and increasing its function has anticonvulsant, sedative, anxiolytic and muscle-relaxant effects, the duration of which depends on half-life of the agent used. For daytime anxiety, longer-acting benzodiazepines are used, such as diazepam, lorazepam, clonazepam and oxazepam. These are likely to cause sleepiness, unsteadiness and difficulties with memory—they mainly affect the acquiring of memorable information. All will increase beta activity in the EEG at night, and they also increase sleep spindles. At higher doses they may decrease slow-wave sleep.

Gabapentin and pregabalin are very similar drugs, but pregabalin is more readily absorbed. In spite of their name, they have their action not through the GABA receptor but via an ion channel and probably affect glutamate signalling. They both tend to increase slow-wave sleep and have been shown to improve sleep continuity and subjective sleep (Garcia-Borreguero et al. 2014).

Buspirone is a serotonin 1A receptor partial agonist which improves sleep continuity modestly, and delays and suppresses REM sleep like the serotonin reuptake inhibitors (Wilson et al. 2005), probably because these receptors are situated in some of the REM-controlling brainstem nuclei.

5.11 Drugs for Dementia

Most of these (donepezil, rivastigmine, galantamine) act by inhibiting the cholinesterase enzymes and thus increasing cholinergic function in the brain. Because REM sleep is highly regulated by cholinergic neurons in the pons, these drugs tend to bring REM sleep forward in the night and increase it (Schredl et al. 2006, 2000; Riemann et al. 1994), although this effect would appear to be short-lived. Patients taking these drugs, and also those taking the nicotinic receptor partial agonist varenicline for smoking cessation, report vivid dreaming and sometimes nightmares.

There are no reports of the effects on sleep structure by the NMDA antagonist memantine; however there has been a report that symptoms of REM behaviour disorder in dementia with Lewy bodies are ameliorated by this drug (Larsson et al. 2010).

5.12   Other Drugs

5.12.1 Sodium Oxybate

The agent for treatment of cataplexy in narcolepsy, sodium oxybate, has marked interesting effects on subjective sleep and sleep architecture. It is the sodium salt of gamma-hydroxybutyric acid (GHB), which probably acts mainly through GABA-B receptors in the brain but may have a neurotransmitter system of its own (GHB receptors). It may also be metabolised to GABA, so it may directly affect GABA-A receptors. This drug is abused for its euphoriant, intoxicating and growth-hormone-promoting effects. Its half-life in plasma is very short, but its central effects are somewhat longer lasting.

Its effects on sleep are to shorten sleep latency, reduce waking and markedly increase slow-wave sleep (Moldofsky et al. 2010). In narcolepsy, it appears to reduce the fragmented occurrence of REM sleep, decreasing the number of REM episodes and lengthening them (Plazzi et al. 2014).

5.12.2 Alcohol

In healthy good sleepers who are light social drinkers, the effects of going to bed with a blood alcohol concentration (BAC) of about 0.03% (e.g. after about two drinks) on sleep architecture are small. If the BAC is 0.1% (e.g. after five or six drinks), there is a larger effect, with sleep onset latency, light stage 1 sleep and awakenings reduced and slow-wave sleep increased in the first half of the night and decreased in the second half (Feige et al. 2006). In this same study, subjects were recorded with alcohol for three consecutive nights and then for the next two nights without alcohol. There was no rebound effect on withdrawal, and the authors remarked that this was probably because the rebound happens later on the drinking night.

Chronic alcoholics have decreased slow-wave sleep and increased intra-sleep waking during sleep in early abstinence.

5.12.3 Opiates

Sleep after oral morphine in normal subjects has decreased slow-wave sleep, and, when it is given intravenously, there is also REM suppression. Methadone, although it has similar effects to oral morphine on opiate receptors, seems to improve sleep. During withdrawal from heroin, there is major sleep disruption with reduced total sleep and increased sleep onset latency. This resolves within 3–7 days. However, in studies after methadone withdrawal, insomnia appears to last for much longer and can be present 6–8 weeks after the last methadone dose (Gossop and Bradley 1984).

5.12.4 Ecstasy (3,4-Methylenedioxy-*N*-methylamphetamine, MDMA)

There is no acute study of sleep after MDMA use. It is used in situations where people want to be awake, but surveys have shown that sleep may be more fragmented in MDMA-only users: however the effects of disrupted circadian rhythm due to being awake all night were not controlled for (Carhart-Harris et al. 2009). There has been a PSG study after another drug with similar effects called Eve (3, 4 methylenedioxyethamphetamine) (Gouzoulis et al. 1992). In this study, subjects were dosed at 11 p.m. and went to sleep normally. They woke after 1–2 h and stayed awake for about 3 h. Subsequent sleep showed total REM suppression—this would be expected, as it releases serotonin and increased serotonin function suppresses REM sleep.

5.12.5 Cannabis

Many people say they use cannabis in the evening to help them sleep. This effect may be mediated through enhanced relaxation at bedtime, as there are few objective effects on sleep. Cannabis contains many chemical compounds, but the main two psychoactive ones are tetrahydrocannabinol (THC) and cannabidiol (CBD). THC appears to have no objectively measured effects on sleep in healthy volunteers but increases sleepiness on awakening in the morning after high doses. On the other hand, CBD produces more wakefulness during sleep after high doses and less morning sleepiness (Nicholson et al. 2004). These effects may counteract each other, but relative THC/CBD proportions in cannabis preparations vary as do individuals' reactions to the drug. There is some evidence that cannabis receptors are involved in pain perception, and in clinical trials of a nasal spray containing THC and cannabidiol for the relief of chronic pain in various long-term illnesses, there was a preliminary improvement in sleep reported by the patients (Russo et al. 2007).

Table 5.1 Sleep disorders and the drugs which may trigger or exacerbate them

Insomnia
Excessive daytime sleepiness
Non-REM parasomnia (e.g. sleepwalking)
REM behaviour disorder
Nightmares, increased vividness or unpleasantness of dreams
Restless legs syndrome
Bruxism

5.13 Impact of These Psychotropic Medications on Sleep Disorders

Some of these powerful medications may improve sleep disorders, but some may cause or exacerbate them. Table 5.1 summarises these effects.

All drugs which affect neurotransmitters in the brain are likely to affect sleep, be it just an alteration in sleep structure not perceived by the patient, subjective sleep disturbance or improvement or provocation or exacerbation of a sleep disorder. We need to be aware of these effects even if not working in psychiatry, as a large proportion of the population are taking these drugs and their sleep effects may impact on other disorders.

References

Bell C, Vanderlinden H, Hiersemenzel R, Otoul C, Nutt D, Wilson S. The effects of levetiracetam on objective and subjective sleep parameters in healthy volunteers and patients with partial epilepsy. J Sleep Res. 2002;11:255–63.

Benkert O, Szegedi A, Philipp M, Kohnen R, Heinrich C, Heukels A, van der Vegte-Senden M, Baker RA, Simmons JH, Schutte AJ. Mirtazapine orally disintegrating tablets versus venlafaxine extended release: a double-blind, randomized multicenter trial comparing the onset of antidepressant response inpatients with major depressive disorder. J Clin Psychopharmacol. 2006;26:75–8.

Carhart-Harris RL, Nutt DJ, Munafo M, Wilson SJ. Current and former ecstasy users report different sleep to matched controls: a web-based questionnaire study. J Psychopharmacol. 2009;23:249–57.

Fava M, McCall WV, Krystal A, Wessel T, Rubens R, Caron J, Amato D, Roth T. Eszopiclone co-administered with fluoxetine in patients with insomnia coexisting with major depressive disorder. Biol Psychiatry. 2006;59:1052–60.

Feige B, Voderholzer U, Riemann D, Dittmann R, Hohagen F, Berger M. Fluoxetine and sleep EEG: effects of a single dose, subchronic treatment, and discontinuation in healthy subjects. Neuropsychopharmacology. 2002;26:246–58.

Feige B, Gann H, Brueck R, Hornyak M, Litsch S, Hohagen F, Riemann D. Effects of alcohol on polysomnographically recorded sleep in healthy subjects. Alcohol Clin Exp Res. 2006;30:1527–37.

Friston KJ, Sharpley AL, Solomon RA, Cowen PJ. Lithium increases slow wave sleep: possible mediation by brain 5-HT-2 receptors. Psychopharmacology. 1989;98:139–40.

Gann H, Riemann D, Hohagen F, Muller WE, Berger M. The influence of carbamazepine on sleep-EEG and the clonidine test in healthy subjects: results of a preliminary study. Soc Biol Psychiatry. 1994;35:893–6.

Garcia-Borreguero D, Patrick J, DuBrava S, Becker PM, Lankford A, Chen C, Miceli J, Knapp L, Allen RP. Pregabalin versus pramipexole: effects on sleep disturbance in restless legs syndrome. Sleep. 2014;37:635–43.

Gossop M, Bradley B. Insomnia among addicts during supervised withdrawal from opiates: a comparison of oral methadone and electrostimulation. Drug Alcohol Dep. 1984;13:191–8.

Gouzoulis E, Steiger A, Ensslin M, Kovar A, Hermle L. Sleep EEG effects of 3,4-methylenedio xyethamphetamine (MDE; "eve") in healthy volunteers. Biol Psychiatry. 1992;32:1108–17.

Harding GFA, Alford CA, Powell TE. The effects of sodium valproate on sleep, reaction times, and visual evoked potential in normal subjects. Epilepsia. 1985;26:597–601.

Jain SV, Glauser TA. Effects of epilepsy treatments on sleep architecture and daytime sleepiness: an evidence-based review of objective sleep metrics. Epilepsia. 2014;55:26–37.

Kaynak H, Kaynak D, Gozukirmizi E, et al. The effects of trazodone on sleep in patients treated with stimulant antidepressants. Sleep Med. 2004;5:15–20.

Landolt HP, Raimo EB, Schnierow BJ, Kelsoe JR, Rapaport MH, Gillin JC. Sleep and sleep electroencephalogram in depressed patients treated with phenelzine. Arch Gen Psychiatry. 2001;58:268–76.

Landolt HP, Kelsoe JR, Rapaport MH, Gillin JC. Rapid tryptophan depletion reverses phenelzine-induced suppression of REM sleep. J Sleep Res. 2003;12:13–8.

Larrosa O, de la Llave Y, Bario S, Granizo JJ, Garcia-Borreguero D. Stimulant and anticataplectic effects of reboxetine in patients with narcolepsy: a pilot study. Sleep. 2001;24:282–5.

Larsson V, Aarsland D, Ballard C, Minthon L, Londos E. The effect of memantine on sleep behaviour in dementia with Lewy bodies and Parkinson's disease dementia. Int J Geriatr Psychiatry. 2010;25:1030–8.

Moldofsky H, Inhaber NH, Guinta DR, Alvarez-Horine SB. Effects of sodium oxybate on sleep physiology and sleep/wake-related symptoms in patients with fibromyalgia syndrome: a double-blind, randomized, placebo-controlled study. J Rheumatol. 2010;37:2156–66.

Monaca C, Boutrel B, Hen R, Hamon M, Adrien J. 5-HT 1A/1B receptor-mediated effects of the selective serotonin reuptake inhibitor, citalopram, on sleep: studies in 5-HT 1A and 5-HT 1B knockout mice. Neuropsychopharmacology. 2003;28:850–6.

Monti JM, Monti D. Sleep in schizophrenia patients and the effects of antipsychotic drugs. Sleep Med Rev. 2004;8:133–48.

Mouret J, Lemoine P, Minuit MP, Benkalfat C, Renardet M. Effects of trazodone on the sleep of depressed patients. Psychopharmacology. 1988;95:S37–43.

Nicholson AN, Turner C, Stone BM, Robson PJ. Effect of delta-9-tetrahydrocannabinol and cannabidiol on nocturnal sleep and early-morning behavior in young adults. J Clin Psychopharmacol. 2004;24:305–13.

Nutt DJ. Death by tricyclic: the real antidepressant scandal? J Psychopharmacol. 2005;19(2):123–4.

Paterson LM, Wilson SJ, Nutt DJ, Hutson PH, Wilson SJ. A translational, caffeine-induced model of onset insomnia in rats and healthy volunteers. Psychopharmacology. 2007;191:943–50.

Paterson LM, Nutt DJ, Durant C, Wilson SJ. Efficacy of trazodone in primary insomnia: a double-blind randomised placebo-controlled polysomnographic study. J Psychopharmacol. 2009;23:A32.

Plazzi G, Pizza F, Vandi S, Arico D, Bruni O, Dauvilliers Y, Ferri R. Impact of acute administration of sodium oxybate on nocturnal sleep polysomnography and on multiple sleep latency test in narcolepsy with cataplexy. Sleep Med. 2014;15:1046–54.

Riemann D, Gann H, Dressing H, Muller WE, Aldenhoff JB. Influence of the cholinesterase inhibitor galanthamine hydrobromide on normal sleep. Psychiatry Res. 1994;51:253–67.

Riemann D, Voderholzer U, Cohrs S, Rodenbeck A, Hajak G, Ruther E, Wiegand MH, Laakmann G, Baghai T, Fischer W, Hoffmann M, Hohagen F, Mayer G, Berger M. Trimipramine in primary insomnia: results of a polysomnographic double-blind controlled study. Pharmacopsychiatry. 2002;35:165–74.

Russo EB, Guy GW, Robson PJ, Baghai T, Fischer W, Hoffmann M, Hohagen F, Mayer G, Berger M. Cannabis, pain, and sleep: lessons from therapeutic clinical trials of Sativex, a cannabis-based medicine. Chem Biodivers. 2007;4:1729–43.

Saper CB, Scammell TE, Lu J. Hypothalamic regulation of sleep and circadian rhythms. Nature. 2005;437:1257–63.

Schredl M, Weber B, Braus D, et al. The effect of rivastigmine on sleep in elderly healthy subjects. Exp Gerontol. 2000;35:243–9.

Schredl M, Hornung O, Regen F, et al. The effect of donepezil on sleep in elderly, healthy persons: a double-blind placebo-controlled study. Pharmacopsychiatry. 2006;39:205–8.

Sharpley AL, Rawlings NB, Brain S, McTavish SF, Cowen PJ. Does agomelatine block 5-HT2C receptors in humans? Psychopharmacology. 2011;213:653–5.

Wilson S, Argyropoulos S. Antidepressants and sleep: a qualitative review of the literature. Drugs. 2005;65:927–47.

Wilson SJ, Bailey JE, Rich AS, et al. The use of sleep measures to compare a new 5HT1A agonist with buspirone in humans. J Psychopharmacol. 2005;19:609–13.

Wilson SJ, Nutt DJ, Alford C, et al. British Association for Psychopharmacology consensus statement on evidence-based treatment of insomnia, parasomnias and circadian rhythm disorders. J Psychopharmacol. 2010;24:1577–601.

Part 2

Insomnia

Insomnia: Epidemiology, Subtypes, and Relationship to Psychiatric Disorders

6

Jonathan A. E. Fleming

6.1 Epidemiology

Insomnia, as defined by the Diagnostic and Statistical Manual of Mental Disorders V (DSM-V) (American Psychiatric Association 2013), is a complaint of dissatisfaction with sleep quantity or quality that is associated with difficulty initiating and/or maintaining sleep. It is an occasional complaint even among the best sleepers but is considered a disorder when it occurs frequently (at least three nights per week), persists (for at least 3 months), and causes clinically significant distress in important areas of functioning.

Many epidemiological studies have been conducted to document the prevalence of insomnia and have reported widely varying rates from 5% to 50% of the populations surveyed (Ohayon 2002). These rates shrink as stringency—frequency of complaint, chronicity, associated impairments, and diagnostic criteria—is applied: population estimates consistently show that about one third of adults report insomnia symptoms alone; between 10% and 15% have daytime impairment from disrupted sleep and between 6% and 10% meet criteria for DSM-V-defined insomnia disorder (ID) (American Psychiatric Association 2013).

These epidemiological studies have significantly influenced criterion-based diagnostic systems (Ohayon et al. 2012) such as the DSM-V, its three predecessors, and the International Classification of Sleep Disorders (AASM 2005). In clinical practice, distinguishing between insomnia symptoms alone, insomnia with or without daytime impairment, and ID is necessary for both accurate diagnosis and appropriate treatment.

Six sociodemographic variables are known to affect the prevalence of insomnia: gender, age, marital status, education, occupational status, and income. Females report

J. A. E. Fleming
Department of Psychiatry, Faculty of Medicine, University of British Columbia,
Vancouver, BC, Canada
e-mail: j.fleming@ubc.ca

© Springer-Verlag GmbH Germany, part of Springer Nature 2018
H. Selsick (ed.), *Sleep Disorders in Psychiatric Patients*,
https://doi.org/10.1007/978-3-642-54836-9_6

more insomnia symptoms, associated daytime impairments, and dissatisfaction with sleep than males, and they are twice as likely as males to meet criteria for insomnia diagnoses (Ohayon 2002).

Both community (Maggi et al. 1998) and large population-based epidemiologic studies (Ohayon 2002) show that impaired sleep performance is common in the elderly; 15–45% of noninstitutionalized elderly report difficulties initiating sleep, 20–65% report disrupted sleep, and 15–45% report early-morning awakening. However, in a 3-year follow-up of over 9000 community-dwelling adults over age 65 (Foley et al. 1999), about 50% of those with chronic insomnia at baseline no longer had symptoms, and this improvement in sleep was associated with an improvement in overall health suggesting—as have other studies (Ohayon et al. 2004; Foley et al. 1995)—that it is the accompaniments of aging (loss of physical function and co-morbid illness) that affects sleep and sleep performance in the elderly.

Supportive relationships can provide protection from aversive life events, and their disruption can place individuals—particularly older males—at an increased risk for impairing and distressing psychological and sleep-related symptoms (Kamiya et al. 2013). A number of studies (Kamiya et al. 2013; Ohayon et al. 1997a, b) have noted a higher prevalence of insomnia complaints in the separated, divorced, or widowed with this effect being more pronounced in females (Ohayon et al. 1997a).

Education, occupation, and income are interlinked; education affects occupation which, in turn, affects income. The prevalence of insomnia is higher in individuals with lower education (Bixler et al. 1979; Ancoli-Israel and Roth 1999; Kim et al. 2000) and incomes (Ohayon et al. 1997b; Bixler et al. 1979; Newman et al. 1997), but this association may be misleading (Ohayon 2002), and studies utilizing multivariate analyses have not linked lower income and education levels as independent risk factors for insomnia symptoms (Ohayon et al. 1997a; Bixler et al. 1979). Other studies have failed to demonstrate an association with education (Breslau et al. 1996; Henderson et al. 1995) or incomes (Ancoli-Israel and Roth 1999), suggesting that other factors are involved. Ohayon et al. (2002) suggest that an index which takes into account age, education, household income, and size of the household would provide a better indication of the importance of poverty in insomnia.

Utilizing data from 2007 to 2008, National Health and Nutrition Examination Survey, Grandner et al. (2013) demonstrated that food security—categorized as full, marginal, low, and very low food security—was associated with an increased prevalence of all measured sleep symptoms. They suggest that food insecurity is a unique stressor, affecting sleep over and above the effects of any measured sociodemographic or socioeconomic variable including poor physical and/or mental health.

6.2   Insomnia Subtypes

Traditionally, insomnia has been subtyped by one or more of the cardinal sleep symptoms noted in the DSM-V: sleep onset insomnia (or initial insomnia), sleep-maintenance insomnia (or middle insomnia), late insomnia (early-morning awakening with an inability to return to sleep), and non-restorative sleep (NRS), although these symptoms lack stability over time (4 months) (Hohagen et al. 1994).

Difficulty maintaining sleep is the most common single symptom of insomnia (approximately 50–70%), followed by difficulty initiating sleep (35–60%), and late insomnia (5–9%) with a combination of these symptoms being the most common presentation of patients with insomnia (Ohayon 2002; Morin et al. 2006, 2011; Roth et al. 2006). NRS, a criterion symptom for primary insomnia in the DSM-IV text revision (American Psychiatric Association 2000) and DSM-V (American Psychiatric Association 2013), is associated with significant daytime dysfunction as well as medical and psychiatric disorders (Wilkinson and Shapiro 2012). Defined by the DSM-V, as a complaint of poor sleep quality despite adequate duration that leaves the sleeper unrested upon awakening—NRS can accompany difficulty initiating or maintaining sleep, or less frequently it can occur in isolation. Like insomnia, its prevalence in populations depends on its definition with rates varying from 1.4% to 35% (Zhang et al. 2012).

Early physiological studies of core body temperature, skin resistance, heart rate, etc. (Monroe 1967; Bonnet and Arand 2010) led to the conceptualization of insomnia as a disorder of cognitive-emotional and physiological hyperarousal. Vgontzas et al. (2001, 2009) demonstrated that insomniacs with objective short sleep duration had increased catecholamine and cortisol levels, but those with insomnia complaints and objectively normal sleep duration did not. These findings led to the hypothesis that insomnia could be of two types: one associated with physiological hyperarousal and activation of the stress system and the other not. Further studies of insomnia with objective short sleep duration have been associated with a number of significant clinical states (Vgontzas and Fernandez-Mendoza 2013) including chronicity of insomnia (Fernandez-Mendoza et al. 2012), hypertension risk (Vgontzas et al. 2009), metabolic syndrome (Troxel et al. 2010), and neurocognitive impairment (Fernandez-Mendoza et al. 2010). Notably, in a large epidemiological study, 95.3% of individuals living in Europe who reported bedtime hyperarousal with a racing, worrisome mind also had a mental disorder (Ohayon and Roth 2001).

Frequently there is a significant disparity between subjective sleep estimation and objectively measured sleep performance (Dement et al. 1984). In a secondary data analysis of six clinical trials, Troxel et al. (2012) demonstrated, in a predominantly female, Caucasian, moderately depressed sample, that insomnia complaints and objective sleep disruption (sleep latency >30 min, wakefulness after sleep onset >30 min, or total sleep time ≤6 h)—individually and in combination—were associated with a significantly increased risk of non-remission of depression treated either pharmacologically or by evidence-based psychotherapy. In a discussion of their findings, they propose that the combination of an objective marker of sleep disturbance (an overnight sleep study) with a significant subjective insomnia complaint may represent a more biologically severe phenotype of insomnia.

Recent research suggests that NRS should be considered an additional insomnia subtype, although it can occur in the absence of insomnia symptoms (Wilkinson and Shapiro 2012; Stone et al. 2008). Unlike other insomnia symptoms, NRS is more common in young adults (Ohayon and Roth 2001) and affects daytime functioning more than other insomnia subtypes (Roth et al. 2006), and—in about one third of cases—there is a chronic course (Zhang et al. 2012).

Recognizing that previous epidemiologic studies did not isolate NRS separately from nocturnal insomnia symptoms (NIS) and that NRS is a core symptom of several disorders associated with increased inflammatory responses, Zhang et al. (2013) examined sociodemographic correlates, medical and sleep comorbidities, C-reactive protein, and functional impairment associated with NRS and NIS in a representative American sample. They report 1-month prevalence estimates of 18.1% for any insomnia symptoms, 7.9% for NIS only, 5.4% for NRS only, and 4.8% for those with both NIS and NRS. Confirming previous epidemiological studies, they found that females, non-Hispanic whites, the impoverished, and those with lower educational levels were more likely to report insomnia symptoms than controls. They noted substantial differences in age, socioeconomic status, education level, and ethnicity in those with NIS only compared to those with NRS only—the prevalence of NRS decreased with age was highest in non-Hispanic whites and was not increased by lower education levels or socioeconomic status. Because of the close associations of NRS with medical conditions and depression revealed in this study, the authors argue for a further subtyping by stratification of NRS into NRS secondary to medical conditions, NRS secondary to psychiatric conditions, and NRS alone.

6.3   Relationship to Psychiatric Disorders

Disturbed sleep is common in acute, major psychiatric disorders and is commonly viewed as a syndromal symptom of those disorders and incorporated into their diagnostic criteria (Krystal 2012). However, the interrelationship between sleep and psychiatric disorders is complex. It can be bidirectional—protracted disrupted sleep causing mood (Sivertsen et al. 2012) disorders and mood disorders being ameliorated by improving sleep (Fava et al. 2006; Manber et al. 2008).

The relationship between the cardinal symptoms of sleep disruption (initial, maintenance, late insomnia, and NRS as opposed to changes in sleep structure or stages) and psychiatric disorders has been studied using both subjective and objective measures, particularly in major depressive disorder (MDD), bipolar affective disorder (BAD), schizophrenia (SCZ), generalized anxiety disorder (GAD), and posttraumatic stress disorder (PTSD) (Table 6.1).

Table 6.1 Sleep changes in mood disorders (Peterson and Benca 2008)

Patient's complaint	Sleep study finding
"I can't fall asleep"	Prolonged latency to stages 1 (N1) and 2 (N2) sleep
"I wake up through the night"	Increased arousals and awakenings through the night
"I wake up early"	Early awakening without return to consolidated sleep
"My sleep is too short"	Reduced total sleep time
"My sleep is shallow and unrefreshing"	Increased stage I (N1) Decreased stages 3 and 4 (N3)
"My dreams are disturbing"	Awakening from REM sleep with difficulty returning to sleep Multiple REM sleep abnormalities including increased REM sleep time, increased eye movements in REM, etc.

6.4   Major Depressive Disorder

Patients with mood disorders complain of sleep disturbances before, during, and after remission of the mood episode, with 65–75% of adults, adolescents, or children with depression complaining of insomnia or, more rarely, hypersomnia (Perlis et al. 1997; Liu et al. 2007). In addition to disrupted and non-restorative sleep during the mood episode, patients are more likely to complain of increased awakenings, disturbing dreams, and decreased sleep time. These subjective complaints have been documented by numerous polysomnographic research studies, and these objective measures can distinguish between subjects with mood disorders, insomnia, and controls (Gillin et al. 1979).

6.5   Bipolar Affective Disorder

Both affective and cognitive stimuli affect sleep initiation (Schmidt and Van der Linden 2013) and happy stimuli delay sleep onset in bipolar patients (Talbot et al. 2009). Actigraphy studies confirm that bipolar patients have prolonged sleep latencies and differ significantly from healthy controls in their lifetime sleeping habits and their subjective sleep experience (Ritter et al. 2012). The ubiquitous sleep disruption associated with mania is a decreased need for sleep characterized by more difficulty initiating sleep than maintaining it (Krystal 2012; Mullin et al. 2011).

Significant insomnia is the most commonly reported residual symptom during remission of mood episodes in patients with major depression (Peterson and Benca 2008) or bipolar disorder (Harvey et al. 2005). In addition to increasing the risk of recurrence, residual insomnia is also associated with concentration difficulties, decreased functioning, suicidal ideation, suicide attempts, and completed suicide (Krystal 2012).

6.6   Schizophrenia

Sleep studies in patients with schizophrenia show that they take longer to fall asleep and have increased wake time during the night, a decreased total sleep time, as well as changes in normal sleep architecture (Krystal 2012). As with mood disorders, disturbed sleep may precede the more florid symptoms of schizophrenia (hallucinations and delusions) by many months. Severe insomnia is one of the prodromal signs associated both with impending psychotic exacerbation (Fitzgerald 2001) and relapse following the discontinuation of antipsychotic medication in chronic schizophrenia (Benson 2008).

The subjective sleep experiences of patients with schizophrenia have been confirmed by a large meta-analysis of drug-free patients with schizophrenia (Chouinard et al. 2004), and a recent actigraphy study confirmed circadian rhythm disturbances in half of the subjects, with all subjects having some form of sleep disturbance (Wulff et al. 2012).

6.7   Anxiety Disorders

Insomnia is the most prominent sleep complaint reported by patients with anxiety disorders. Ohayon and Roth (Ohayon and Roth 2001) noted that 61% of panic disorder patients and 44% of patients with generalized anxiety disorder had insomnia, and in a large meta-analysis of sleep studies, Benca and colleagues confirmed consistently increased sleep latencies and decreased sleep efficiency in these patients (Benca et al. 1992).

Panic attacks can occur during sleep and subsequently may affect sleep performance (Craske and Tsao 2005): up to 68% of patients with panic disorder report difficulties falling asleep and 77% of patients with panic disorder endorse difficulties maintaining sleep (Papadimitriou and Linkowski 2005).

Sleep is commonly disturbed after acute trauma. In one study, complaints of insomnia and excessive daytime sleepiness 1 month after a motor vehicle accident predicted the diagnosis of posttraumatic stress disorder (PTSD) at 3 months. Interestingly, in this study, sleep complaints were not supported objectively by actigraphy (Klein et al. 2003). This suggests that altered sleep perception—rather than sleep disturbance—may result in complaints of poor sleep in PTSD. Sleep study findings in chronic PTSD are variable, with both normal or reduced sleep efficiency and normal or increased nocturnal awakenings being reported (Abad and Guilleminault 2005). Regardless, following trauma exposure, pre-existing complaints of poor sleep increase the risk of PTSD and other stress-related psychiatric disorders (Breslau et al. 1996), and there is growing evidence that individual differences in sleep or in REM sleep may be markers of vulnerability to poor psychiatric outcomes following that exposure (Germain 2013).

6.8   Personality Disorders

None of the DSM-V-defined personality disorders have sleep disturbances as a criterion symptom, but, compared with good sleepers, patients with insomnia have more signs of neuroticism (Calkins et al. 2013) and traits associated with perfectionism—factors that may play a role in the generation and maintenance of insomnia complaints (van de Laar et al. 2010). Disturbed sleep is seen in patients with personality disorders but has been noted and studied particularly in patients with borderline personality disorder. These patients are high users of sleep-promoting medicines (Plante et al. 2009), and their subjective sleep disturbances are significantly related to expression of borderline symptoms (e.g., emotional dysregulation) (Selby 2013) and outcome (Plante et al. 2013).

In conclusion, the epidemiological studies of both generally disturbed sleep and specific symptoms of insomnia have helped shape the current diagnostic criteria for sleep disorders and focused attention on potential mechanisms that may initiate, exacerbate, or prolong significant psychiatric disorders. This may lead to effective interventions that normalize and protect sleep, thereby reducing sleep-related distress and impairment.

References

AASM (American Academy of Sleep Medicine). International classification of sleep disorders (ICSD-2). 2nd ed. Westchester, IL: American Academy of Sleep Medicine (ICSD-2); 2005.

Abad VC, Guilleminault C. Sleep and psychiatry. 1. Dialogues Clin Neurosci. 2005;7:291–303.

American Psychiatric Association. Diagnostic and statistical manual of mental disorders, fourth edition-TR. Arlington, VA: American Psychiatric Association; 2000.

American Psychiatric Association. Diagnostic and statistical manual of mental disorders. 5th ed. Arlington, VA: American Psychiatric Association; 2013.

Ancoli-Israel S, Roth T. Characteristics of insomnia in the United States: results of the 1991 National Sleep Foundation Survey I. Sleep. 1999;22(Suppl. 2):S347–53.

Benca RM, Obermeyer WH, Thisted RA, et al. Sleep and psychiatric disorders. A meta-analysis. Arch Gen Psychiatry. 1992;49:651–68.

Benson KL. Sleep in schizophrenia. Sleep Med Clin. 2008;3:251–60.

Bixler EO, Kales A, Soldatos CR, Kales JD, Healey S. Prevalence of sleep disorders in the Los Angeles metropolitan area. Am J Psychiatry. 1979;136:1257–62.

Bonnet MH, Arand DL. Hyperarousal and insomnia: state of the science. Sleep Med Rev. 2010;14:9–15.

Breslau N, Roth T, Rosenthal L, Andreski P. Sleep disturbance and psychiatric disorders: a longitudinal study of young adults. Biol Psychiatry. 1996;39:411–8.

Calkins AW, Hearon BA, Capozzoli MC, Otto MW. Psychosocial predictors of sleep dysfunction: the role of anxiety sensitivity, dysfunctional beliefs, and neuroticism. Behav Sleep Med. 2013;11:133–43.

Chouinard S, Poulin J, Stip E, Godbout R. Sleep in untreated patients with schizophrenia: a meta-analysis. Schizophr Bull. 2004;30:957–67.

Craske MG, Tsao JC. Assessment and treatment of nocturnal panic attacks. Sleep Med Rev. 2005;9:173–84.

Dement W, Seidel W, Carskadon M. Issues in the diagnosis and treatment of insomnia. Psychopharmacology Suppl. 1984;1:11–43.

Fava M, McCall WV, Krystal A, et al. Eszopiclone co-administered with fluoxetine in patients with insomnia coexisting with major depressive disorder. Biol Psychiatry. 2006;59:1052–60.

Fernandez-Mendoza J, Calhoun S, Bixler EO, et al. Insomnia with objective short sleep duration is associated with deficits in neuropsychological performance: a general population study. Sleep. 2010;33:459–65.

Fernandez-Mendoza J, Vgontzas AN, Bixler EO, et al. Clinical and polysomnographic predictors of the natural history of poor sleep in the general population. Sleep. 2012;35:689–97.

Fitzgerald PB. The role of early warning symptoms in the detection and prevention of relapse in schizophrenia. Aust N Z J Psychiatry. 2001;35:758–64.

Foley DJ, Monjan AA, Brown SL, Simonsick EM, Wallace RB, Blazer DG. Sleep complaints among elderly persons: an epidemiologic study of three communities. Sleep. 1995;18:425–32.

Foley DJ, Monjan A, Simonsick EM, Wallace RB, Blazer DG. Incidence and remission of insomnia among elderly adults: an epidemiologic study of 6,800 persons over three years. Sleep. 1999;22(suppl 2):S366–72.

Germain A. Sleep disturbances as the hallmark of PTSD: where are we now? Am J Psychiatry. 2013;170:372–82.

Gillin JC, Duncan WC, Pettigrew KD, et al. Successful separation of depressed, normal and insomniac subjects by EEG sleep data. Arch Gen Psychiatry. 1979;6:85–90.

Grandner MA, Petrov ME, Rattanaumpawan P, Jackson N, Platt A, Patel NP. Sleep symptoms, race/ethnicity, and socioeconomic position. J Clin Sleep Med. 2013;9:897–905.

Harvey AG, Schmidt DA, Scarna A, et al. Sleep-related functioning in euthymic patients with bipolar disorder, patients with insomnia, and subjects without sleep problems. Am J Psychiatry. 2005;162(1):50–7.

Henderson S, Jorm AF, Scott LR, Mackinnon AJ, Korten AE. Insomnia in the elderly: its prevalence and correlates in the general population. Med J Aust. 1995;162:22–4.

Hohagen F, Käppler C, Schramm E, Riemann D, Weyerer S, Berger M. Sleep onset insomnia, sleep maintaining insomnia and insomnia with early morning awakening—temporal stability of subtypes in a longitudinal study on general practice attenders. Sleep. 1994;17:551–4.

Kamiya Y, Doyle M, Henretta JC, Timonen V. Depressive symptoms among older adults: the impact of early and later life circumstances and marital status. Aging Ment Health. 2013;17:349–57.

Kim K, Uchiyama M, Okawa M, Liu X, Ogihara R. An epidemiological study of insomnia among the Japanese general population. Sleep. 2000;23:41–7.

Klein E, Koren D, Arnon I, Lavie P. Sleep complaints are not corroboratedby objective sleep measures in post-traumatic stress disorder: a 1-year prospective study in survivors of motor vehicle crashes. J Sleep Res. 2003;12:35–41.

Krystal AD. Psychiatric disorders and sleep. Neurol Clin. 2012;30:1389–413.

van de Laar M, Verbeek I, Pevernagie D, Aldenkamp A, Overeem S. The role of personality traits in insomnia. Sleep Med Rev. 2010;14:61–8.

Liu X, Buysse DJ, Gentzler AL, et al. Insomnia and hypersomnia associated with depressive phenomenology and comorbidity in childhood depression. Sleep. 2007;30(1):83–90.

Maggi S, Langlois JA, Minicuci N, Grigoletto F, Pavan M, Foley DJ, Enzi G. Sleep complaints in community-dwelling older persons: prevalence, associated factors, and reported causes. J Am Geriatr Soc. 1998;46:161–8.

Manber R, Edinger JD, Gress JL, et al. Cognitive behavioral therapy for insomnia enhances depression outcome in patients with comorbid major depressive disorder and insomnia. Sleep. 2008;31:489–95.

Monroe LJ. Psychological and physiological differences between good and poor sleepers. J Abnorm Psychol. 1967;72:255–64.

Morin CM, LeBlanc M, Daley M, Gregoire JP, Merette C. Epidemiology of insomnia: prevalence, self-help treatments, consultations, and determinants of help seeking behaviors. Sleep Med. 2006;7:123–30.

Morin CM, LeBlanc M, Bélanger L, Ivers H, Mérette C, Savard J. Prevalence of insomnia and its treatment in Canada. Can J Psychiatr. 2011;56:540–8.

Mullin BC, Harvey AG, Hinshaw SP. A preliminary study of sleep in adolescents with bipolar disorder, ADHD, and non-patient controls. Bipolar Disord. 2011;13(4):425–32.

Newman AB, Enright PL, Manolio TA, Haponik EF, Wahl PW. Sleep disturbance, psychosocial correlates, and cardiovascular disease in 5201 older adults: the Cardiovascular Health Study. J Am Geriatr Soc. 1997;45:1–7.

Ohayon MM. Epidemiology of insomnia: what we know and what we still need to learn. Sleep Med Rev. 2002;6:97–111.

Ohayon MM, Roth T. What are the contributing factors for insomnia in the general population? J Psychosom Res. 2001;51:745–55.

Ohayon MM, Caulet M, Guilleminault C. Complaints about nocturnal sleep: how a general population perceives its sleep, and how this relates to the complaint of insomnia. Sleep. 1997a;20:715–23.

Ohayon MM, Caulet M, Priest RG, Guilleminault C. DSM-IV and ICSD-90 insomnia symptoms and sleep dissatisfaction. Br J Psychiatry. 1997b;171:382–8.

Ohayon MM, Carskadon MA, Guilleminault C, Vitiello MV. Meta-analysis of quantitative sleep parameters from childhood to old age in healthy individuals: developing normative sleep values across the human lifespan. Sleep. 2004;27:1255–73.

Ohayon MM, Riemann D, Morin C, Reynolds CF III. Hierarchy of insomnia criteria based on daytime consequences. Sleep Med. 2012;13:52–7.

Papadimitriou GN, Linkowski P. Sleep disturbance in anxiety disorders. Int Rev Psychiatry. 2005;17:229–36.

Perlis ML, Giles DE, Buysse DJ, et al. Self-reported sleep disturbance as a prodromal symptom in recurrent depression. J Affect Disord. 1997;42(2–3):209–12.

Peterson MJ, Benca RM. Sleep in mood disorders. Sleep Med Clin. 2008;3:231–49.

Plante DT, Zanarini MC, Frankenburg FR, Fitzmaurice GM. Sedative-hypnotic use in patients with borderline personality disorder and axis II comparison subjects. J Personal Disord. 2009;23:563–71.

Plante DT, Frankenburg FR, Fitzmaurice GM, Zanarini MC. Relationship between sleep disturbance and recovery in patients with borderline personality disorder. J Psychosom Res. 2013;74(4):278–82.

Ritter PS, Marx C, Lewtschenko N, Pfeiffer S, Leopold K, Bauer M, Pfennig AJ. The characteristics of sleep in patients with manifest bipolar disorder, subjects at high risk of developing the disease and healthy controls. Neural Transmission. 2012;119:1173–84.

Roth T, Jaeger S, Jin R, Kalsekar A, Stang PE, Kessler RC. Sleep problems, comorbid mental disorders, and role functioning in the national comorbidity survey replication. Biol Psychiatry. 2006;60:1364–71.

Schmidt RE, Van der Linden M. Feeling too regretful to fall asleep: experimental activation of regret delays sleep onset. Cogn Ther Res. 2013;37:872–80.

Selby EA. Chronic sleep disturbances and borderline personality disorder symptoms. J Consult Clin Psychol. 2013;81:941–7.

Sivertsen B, Salo P, Mykletun A, Hysing M, Pallesen S, Krokstad S, Nordhus IH, Øverland S. The bidirectional association between depression and insomnia: the HUNT study. Psychosom Med. 2012;74:758–65.

Stone KC, Taylor DJ, McCrae CS, Kalsekar A, Lichstein KL. Nonrestorative sleep. Sleep Med Rev. 2008;12:275–88.

Talbot LS, Hairston IS, Eidelman P, Gruber J, Harvey AG. The effect of mood on sleep onset latency and REM sleep in interepisode bipolar disorder. J Abnorm Psychol. 2009 Aug;118:448–58.

Troxel WM, Buysse DJ, Matthews KA, et al. Sleep symptoms predict the development of the metabolic syndrome. Sleep. 2010;33(12):1633–40.

Troxel WM, Kupfer DJ, Reynolds CF III, Frank E, Thase ME, Miewald JM, Buysse DJ. Insomnia and objectively measured sleep disturbances predict treatment outcome in depressed patients treated with psychotherapy or psychotherapy-pharmacotherapy combinations. J Clin Psychiatry. 2012;73:478–85.

Vgontzas AN, Fernandez-Mendoza J. Objective measures are useful in subtyping chronic insomnia. Sleep. 2013;36:1125–6.

Vgontzas AN, Bixler EO, Lin HM, et al. Chronic insomnia is associated with nyctohemeral activation of the hypothalamic-pituitary-adrenal axis: clinical implications. J Clin Endocrinol Metab. 2001;86:3787–94.

Vgontzas AN, Liao D, Bixler EO, Chrousos GP, Vela-Bueno A. Insomnia with objective short sleep duration is associated with a high risk for hypertension. Sleep. 2009;32:491–7.

Wilkinson K, Shapiro C. Non-restorative sleep: symptom or unique diagnostic entity? Sleep Med. 2012;13:561–9.

Wulff K, Dijk DJ, Middleton B, Foster RG, Joyce EM. Sleep and circadian rhythm disruption in schizophrenia. Br J Psychiatry. 2012;200:308–16.

Zhang J, Lam SP, Li SX, Li AM, Wing YK. The longitudinal course and impact of non-restorative sleep: a five-year community-based follow-up study. Sleep Med. 2012;13:570–6.

Zhang J, Lamers F, Hickie IB, He JP, Feig E, Merikangas KR. Differentiating nonrestorative sleep from nocturnal insomnia symptoms: demographic, clinical, inflammatory, and functional correlates. Sleep. 2013;36:671–9.

Insomnia Assessment

7

Hugh Selsick

7.1 Introduction

The assessment of insomnia is not markedly different from the assessment of sleep disorders in general, and a good insomnia history will necessarily include a good sleep history, psychiatric history and medical history. However, it is also possible to take a brief history that will ascertain the cardinal features of the disorder and allow one to formulate a management plan. In this chapter I will examine the aspects of history taking that are specifically important in insomnia patients, when to order investigations, what investigations are useful and the limitations of those investigations. I will conclude with a suggested formula for conceptualizing the patient's insomnia and organizing the information you have gleaned so that the appropriate treatments can be selected.

7.2 Taking an Insomnia History

When taking an insomnia history, it can be helpful to bear in mind the 'Three P' theory of disease: predisposing, precipitating and perpetuating factors. In this model each patient has certain inherent factors that predispose them to getting insomnia. Certain personality traits, socio-economic variables, medical conditions and psychiatric disorders can increase the susceptibility to insomnia. Many of these predisposing variables will be beyond the ability of the clinician to modify. However, many people with a high predisposition to developing insomnia will never get it; therefore there must be some precipitating factor which initiates the illness. Unlike most other sleep disorders, insomnia may have a very definite onset and clear precipitant, and many patients will be able to identify specific events that caused the insomnia.

H. Selsick
Insomnia Clinic, Royal London Hospital for Integrated Medicine, London, UK
e-mail: hugh@selsick.net

© Springer-Verlag GmbH Germany, part of Springer Nature 2018
H. Selsick (ed.), *Sleep Disorders in Psychiatric Patients*,
https://doi.org/10.1007/978-3-642-54836-9_7

Clearly, if that precipitant is still present, then this should be explored and, if possible, addressed. However, in chronic insomnia patients, it is commonly the case that the precipitant will have resolved by the time the patient presents to a clinician, yet the insomnia persists, and so there must be separate perpetuating factors driving their insomnia. To a large extent, it is these perpetuating factors that need to be teased out by the history.

7.2.1 Main Complaint

A common perception is that insomnia describes difficulty getting to sleep and so patients who have no problems with sleep initiation, but struggle with sleep maintenance or early morning waking, may not report that they have insomnia. It is also important to remember that patients' broad descriptions of their problems may not always correspond with the picture elicited when a more detailed history is taken. For example, it is not uncommon for patients to say 'I don't sleep' or 'I haven't slept in years'. Often this is a figure of speech, and what they mean is that they sleep badly or don't get enough sleep. However, it is important when hearing this statement to explore it further. Some patients with severe paradoxical insomnia will report never getting any sleep at all, and this presents a different set of challenges.

It is important to explore what the patient perceives to be the precipitating factors and whether these factors are still present and relevant to the insomnia. Another useful—and underutilized—question is simply to ask the patient why they think they cannot sleep. This will often elicit a great deal of useful information about environmental factors, anxieties and dysfunctional sleep perceptions and behaviours. Many patients will express fears that their insomnia is a sign of a serious underlying physical problem. It will also reveal some, though rarely all, of the perpetuating factors.

7.2.2 Typical Night

Here one is looking at two areas. The first is a numerical/temporal description of the sleep pattern, i.e. what time the patient goes to bed, how long it takes to fall asleep, etc. The other is the person's bedtime habits and routines, how they use the bedroom and the bed environment. At this point it is also useful to ask if they sleep alone or if there is a bed partner and, if so, what the partner's bedtime routine is, whether they snore, etc.

One wants to ascertain:

- What time the patient goes to bed
- How long it takes to fall asleep—sleep onset latency (SOL)
- How many times they wake during the night and what wakes them
- How long they think they are awake for during the night; this includes time spent awake in the bed in the morning before rising—wakefulness after sleep onset (WASO)

- What time they wake in the morning and if this is spontaneous or to an alarm
- What time their alarm is set for if they are not woken by their alarm
- What time they get up
- How long they think they slept in total—total sleep time (TST)

From these figures one can calculate a number of important sleep parameters:

- The difference between the rising time and the bed time gives you the time in bed (TIB).
- TIB − SOL − WASO = TST. One can thus calculate the total sleep time from the other figures, and it will often give a very different figure from the patient's self-reported TST. It can be useful to explore why this is. Often it is because the patient gives the worst case scenario for each of the above parameters rather than the typical or average figures.
- TST/TIB × 100 gives you the sleep efficiency (SE).

At the same time, one should determine:

- What the patient does when they first go to bed, e.g. do they read, watch TV, play on their phone, listen to music or try to go to sleep immediately on going to bed?
- What the patient does if they have difficulty falling asleep or if they wake up during the night. Do they stay in bed, get up, take a sleeping pill, turn on the TV, etc.?
- What environmental factors there are that may affect sleep. Is there intrusive light or noise? Does their partner snore or keep different bed and rising times? Is the room cool or warm?

An additional tool that will, of course, be useful is a sleep diary. An example of a sleep diary is found in Appendix C. This will allow one to get a longitudinal view of the sleep pattern and of the night to night variability of the various sleep parameters. However, a diary should not be a substitute for the history. Although the diary gives very useful quantitative information, it is not able to capture the qualitative data. Hearing the verbal description of the typical night gives you important information about the patient's emotions, thought processes and anxieties during the night. It helps you to understand the degree of distress their symptoms cause them and to recognize any dysfunctional thoughts and habits they have with regard to their sleep. Sometimes a seemingly insignificant comment, if picked up and pursued, can lead to profound insights into the patient's condition, and it is also important to patients that they are able to tell their story.

7.2.3 Daytime Symptoms

This is too often forgotten in insomnia assessments. Short sleep in the absence of daytime symptoms does not meet the criteria for insomnia. The pervasive idea that we are meant to sleep for 8 h means that those with a shorter sleep need may assume there is a problem with their sleep despite feeling well during the day. One should therefore ascertain whether the patient experiences fatigue, cognitive difficulties, mood changes or occupational dysfunction.

It is also informative to differentiate between fatigue and sleepiness. Many, but not all, insomnia patients are 'tired but wired', i.e. tired but not sleepy. An Epworth Sleepiness Scale (ESS) (Appendix A) can be helpful in differentiating between fatigue and sleepiness as it asks the patient to focus on the likelihood of actually falling asleep. There is a perception amongst some clinicians that a patient with a normal or elevated Epworth score does not have insomnia and that another cause for their sleep disruption needs to be sought. While it is true that many insomnia patients have very low Epworth scores, it is by no means universal. Those patients who have a learned negative association with their bed and bedroom may well be sleepy during the day when they are not in their bedroom but find it difficult to initiate sleep when they are in the bedroom. In addition, many insomnia patients expend a great deal of effort trying to sleep at night. This effort actually reduces the likelihood of being able to sleep. During the day, when they are in situations where they are not trying to sleep, such as in a meeting, when watching TV or when reading, then the lack of effort allows their innate sleep drive to take over, and they fall asleep.

7.3   Other Sleep Disorders

Insomnia can be mimicked, or exacerbated, by a number of other sleep disorders. This is not only true of disorders such as restless legs or circadian rhythm disorders but is also true of sleep disorders more commonly associated with hypersomnolence such as obstructive sleep apnoea (OSS). Even if this is not the case in a particular patient, having insomnia is no bar to having other co-morbid sleep disorders. It is important therefore to screen for other sleep disorders when assessing insomnia. Given that most physicians have very little training in sleep medicine (Stores and Crawford 1998) it is highly likely that, when you take a sleep history, you will be the only person ever to do so! One should therefore screen for parasomnias, obstructive sleep apnoea, etc. However, one should pay particular attention to the circadian rhythm disorders, restless legs and periodic limb movements as these disorders often present as insomnia.

7.3.1   Circadian Rhythm Disorders

Insomnia is often the presenting complaint in patients with circadian rhythm disorders, particularly delayed sleep-wake phase disorder (DSWPD). Therefore, if patients have difficulty with sleep onset, one should ask what time of day they feel most tired and what time of day they feel most alert. In DSWPD they will typically feel worst in the morning with a gradual improvement in alertness leading to maximum alertness late at night. More rarely, advanced sleep-wake phase disorder (ASWPD) may be the underlying cause of early morning waking. (Note: terminal insomnia is a medical term that should be avoided in patient interactions and clinic letters: patients may misinterpret the term as meaning fatal insomnia, and early morning waking is a preferable term.) These patients typically wake very early in the morning and feel excessively sleepy in the early evening (American Academy of Sleep Medicine 2014). The Morningness-Eveningness Questionnaire (Horne and Ostberg 1976) (Appendix B) can be helpful in supporting the diagnosis. A non-24-h sleep-wake rhythm disorder will demonstrate a progressive delay (or rarely advance) of the sleep period (American Academy of Sleep Medicine 2014). Shift work disorder may present with insomnia symptoms, particularly during scheduled sleep times, and difficulty staying awake during work hours (American Academy of Sleep Medicine 2014).

A helpful way to differentiate between insomnia and a circadian rhythm disorder is to ask about the patient's sleep when the external constraints on their bed and rising times are removed, e.g. when on holiday. Circadian rhythm disorder patients will generally sleep well when allowed to sleep at the times dictated by their body clock and will therefore feel alert when awake. Insomnia patients will usually continue to experience poor sleep and daytime fatigue, even when they can choose their bed and rising times.

7.3.2 Restless Leg Syndrome

Restless legs will usually present as difficulty initiating sleep but may also cause difficulty with sleep maintenance. It is surprising how few patients volunteer the symptoms of restless legs until one explicitly asks about them. Restless legs can be exacerbated by antihistaminergic drugs. As antihistamines or antidepressants and antipsychotics with antihistaminergic properties are frequently prescribed for insomnia, if one hasn't detected the restless legs on history, there is a risk that the prescribed treatment could make the problem worse!

Similarly, periodic limb movements (PLMs) can mimic insomnia by causing sleep fragmentation. It is difficult to detect on history but should be suspected if the patient has even occasional restless leg symptoms, repeated leg twitches prior to sleep onset and signs of restless sleep on waking or reports of leg twitches during sleep from the bed partner. Because there is a circadian element, with the periodic limb movements being more severe in the first part of the night, some patients with PLMs will report having a better quality of sleep in the second half of the night or when sleeping during the day.

7.3.3 Medical Disorders

A full medical history is important, not only because one is looking for anything that may contribute to the insomnia but also because the presence of co-morbid medical conditions will inform your decisions on the safety of various treatments. For example, sleep scheduling, which can lead to a transient reduction in sleep time, may be contraindicated in epilepsy which may be sensitive to sleep loss. Similarly, one would be cautious about prescribing sedative antidepressants to treat insomnia in patients with cardiac disorders that might be affected by drugs with anticholinergic properties.

The medical history may also detect signs or risk factors of other sleep disorders. For example, nocturia, hypertension, type II diabetes and cardiac arrhythmias might raise one's index of suspicion for obstructive sleep apnoea, while chronic kidney disease or radiculopathies increase the likelihood of the patient having RLS or PLMs.

7.3.4   Psychiatric Disorders

The presence of psychiatric disorders can, of course, complicate the management of insomnia, but one should not fall into the trap of assuming that the insomnia is secondary to the psychiatric disorder. Particularly in the case of depression, it is often the case that the insomnia precedes the depression (Baglioni et al. 2011). For many patients, this is a fact which is important to acknowledge as they are often frustrated by the repeated attempts to treat their depression without tackling the insomnia. Indeed, one should not take a diagnosis of depression in a patient with insomnia at face value. It is not uncommon for euthymic patients with insomnia to be given a diagnosis of depression and treatment with antidepressants by primary care physicians. While it is true that insomnia can be a symptom of depression, one should look for the presence of other symptoms to determine if the diagnosis is valid.

7.3.5   Medications

In addition to determining what the current medication regime is, one is looking for any drugs that may be having an adverse impact on sleep, such as β-blockers or alerting antidepressants. One should enquire about the time that those medications are taken; it is not uncommon for patients (and doctors) to assume that all antidepressants are sedating and therefore to take alerting antidepressants at night. Ascertaining whether there have been any adverse drug reactions in the past is also essential.

7.3.6   Habits

A detailed assessment of the patient's caffeine, nicotine, alcohol and illicit or recreational drug use often yields information that can lead to simple and effective interventions. Caffeine is an effective stimulant with a half-life of 3.5 to 5 h and active metabolites that may extend the stimulant action of the caffeine (Nishino and Mignot 2017). Patients are often unaware that caffeine can therefore accumulate in the bloodstream with repeated dosing. Therefore one should ascertain how many

Table 7.1 Caffeine content of commonly consumed food and drinks

Beverage	Caffeine content (mg/ml of beverage or mg/g or food)
Coffee	0.2–2.1 mg/ml
Decaffeinated coffee	0.01 mg/ml
Black tea	0.2 mg/ml
Green tea	0.1 mg/ml
Decaffeinated tea	0.01–0.06 mg/ml
Cola	0.1–0.19 mg/ml
Energy drinks	0.11–0.68 mg/ml
Chocolate	0.2–0.7 mg/g
Cocoa or chocolate milk	0.01–0.07 mg/ml

Note: These values are approximate and will vary widely. Total caffeine consumption can be calculated by multiplying the concentration of the caffeine in each substance by the quantity of the substance consumed (Bazalakova and Benca 2017; Chin et al. 2008; Mitchell et al. 2014).

caffeinated substances they consume and at what time. As many patients are unaware that caffeine is found in green tea, some herbal teas, some soft drinks and sports drinks, etc., one should either ask them to describe everything they drink throughout the day or ask specific questions about all the common caffeinated foodstuffs (Table 7.1).

The stimulant effect of nicotine is under-recognized, and many patients will smoke immediately prior to bed in order to relax. The total amount and timing of nicotine-containing products should be ascertained. Similarly, patients may consume alcohol, marijuana or other sedative substances to aid their sleep. Once again the timing of these substances is as important as their quantity. For example, a patient who drinks throughout the day will require a very different approach from one who drinks at night only in order to induce sleep. The former patient is more likely to be dependent on alcohol and to be drinking for reasons other than insomnia, and their drinking may need to be addressed before the insomnia can be treated. The latter patient may be using alcohol to self-medicate for the insomnia, and providing alternative strategies to manage the insomnia may be the focus of their treatment.

7.4   Physical Examination and Investigations

Physical examination is rarely needed in the assessment of insomnia unless the history raises the possibility of specific conditions such as hyperthyroidism or obstructive sleep apnoea. Similarly, blood tests are rarely required unless one is concerned about poor kidney or liver function which may affect your choice and dose of medication. The exception to this is where you suspect the insomnia may be secondary to restless legs and periodic limb movements. In that case ferritin, folate, vitamin B12, kidney function and blood glucose tests are worth performing in order to look for any biochemical causes of the movement disorder. An electrocardiogram is warranted if one is considering treating the insomnia with drugs that can prolong the QTc interval.

Polysomnography (PSG) is not indicated for the routine assessment of insomnia, including insomnia in the context of other psychiatric disorders (Littner et al. 2003). PSGs are helpful if you suspect another underlying sleep disorder, particularly periodic limb movements or obstructive sleep apnoea. They may also be useful in patients who are very poor historians, and it is not possible to exclude other sleep disorders or quantify their sleep on the history alone. Finally, a PSG can be helpful in cases of paradoxical insomnia, especially if the patient believes they do not sleep at all. In these cases, the PSG fulfils two functions. Firstly, it allows the clinician to garner information about the patient's objective sleep time, albeit on a single night, which can be useful in planning behavioural treatments. Secondly, for some patients with paradoxical insomnia, it can be very therapeutic to see that they are in fact sleeping. However, it should be noted that some patients will be incensed by the evidence of their sleep state misperception and will not believe that the PSG they are seeing is their own and this may damage the therapeutic relationship. It may be helpful to explain to patients before their study how the PSG works, how different sleep stages are identified on the PSG, etc.

Actigraphy, which utilizes an accelerometer worn on the wrist to monitor movement and sleep-wake patterns, is also not routinely used for insomnia assessment (Schutte-rodin et al. 2017). Actigraphy may not be particularly accurate in the insomnia population though it is probably not any less accurate than sleep diaries (Tryon 2004). However, actigraphy may be useful if patients are unable to keep a sleep diary or you suspect that their sleep diary is not a good reflection of their sleep pattern. It is also a helpful investigation if one suspects that the patient has a circadian rhythm disorder.

7.5   Formulation of the Insomnia

A thorough history will give a rich picture of the patient's condition, the factors that contribute to their insomnia and the obstacles to improvement. In order to condense this information into a formulation that captures the most important factors and informs one's treatments, it can be helpful to conceptualize the factors affecting a patient's sleep using six categories as shown in Fig. 7.1.

7.5.1   Homeostatic Factors

This corresponds with Process S in the two-process model of sleep. It can be helpful to think about the homeostatic sleep drive as the fuel that drives our sleep. Put simply, during wakefulness we accumulate sleepiness, and we use that sleepiness to drive our sleep. In order to sleep well at night, we need to accumulate sufficient sleepiness during the day. A good history of the typical night and daytime behaviours will establish if this is happening. Patients who go to bed too early are likely

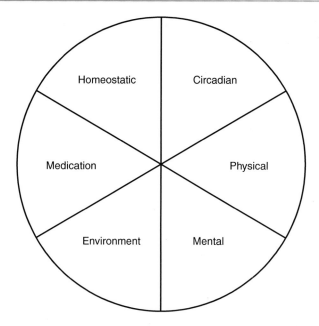

Fig. 7.1 Six factors contributing to insomnia

to be trying to sleep before they have accumulated sufficient sleepiness. Daytime naps (deliberate or unintended) use up some of the accumulated sleepiness and make it harder to initiate and maintain sleep at night. Irregular waking times mean that the patient is starting to accumulate sleepiness at a different time every morning, and so the time when they have enough sleepiness to initiate consolidated sleep will be different every night leading to chaotic sleep patterns. If these homeostatic factors are present, one should ensure the patient keeps a constant rising time, avoids napping and delays their bedtime until they have accumulated sufficient sleepiness. This is discussed in more detail in the chapter on cognitive behaviour therapy for insomnia.

7.5.2   Circadian Factors

This corresponds to Process C in the two-process model. This is obviously important in circadian rhythm disorders but also plays a role in insomnia. Our internal body clock drives our innate alertness drive. Broadly speaking, this innate drive progressively increases alertness throughout the day in order to offset the accumulating sleepiness. The alerting drive peaks at around 9 p.m. and then starts to drop. Once it has dropped sufficiently, it is no longer able to offset the sleepiness, and we fall asleep. The alertness drive reaches its nadir in the early hours of the morning. Once again, the description of a typical night will reveal whether the circadian cycle is being utilized optimally by the patient. Patients who try to initiate sleep too early in the evening will be trying to fall asleep when the alertness drive is too high. Conversely, patients who work night shifts may be trying to stay awake when the alertness drive is low but battle to sleep in the day when the alertness is increasing. As light is the most important factor (*zeitgeber*) synchronizing the body clock with the outside world, irregular waking hours and lack of exposure to daylight may weaken the circadian signal.

If these factors are playing a role, then one might concentrate on adjusting sleep times to better fit the circadian drive, strengthening the *zeitgebers* particularly by using light exposure, advising on optimal ways to schedule shifts and prescribing carefully timed melatonin.

7.5.3 Physical Factors

This refers to physical conditions that may impact on sleep. Physical factors that may adversely impact on sleep include restless legs, obstructive sleep apnoea, pain, hyperthyroidism, gastro-oesophageal reflux and asthma (which is often worse at night). On the other hand, exercise is a physical factor that can be beneficial to sleep. Clearly, if these factors are driving the insomnia, optimizing their treatment will be an important part of the treatment plan.

7.5.4 Mental Factors

These can be acute or chronic. Acute factors are time-limited and may vary from night to night, such as short-term stress, excitement, anger, contentment, etc. Chronic factors refer to longer term psychiatric illnesses and stable personality traits. It also includes learned anxiety about sleep itself and unhelpful cognitions around sleep. Many of the techniques in cognitive behaviour therapy for insomnia (and CBT in general) as well as relaxation techniques and mindfulness help patients to better manage these factors and, of course, psychiatric interventions are essential in improving the long-term mental factors.

7.5.5 Environmental Factors

Light, noise, room temperature, bed comfort, safety, etc. are obviously important. This is often the most difficult area for clinicians to alter. However, this category also includes whether the environment is being used in an appropriate way. Patients who use their beds and bedrooms for waking activities such as work, studying, eating or watching TV will come to associate the bed environment with wakefulness rather than sleep. Thus, for many patients with insomnia, the act of going to bed wakes them up. By banning these activities in the bedroom and avoiding spending any time in bed awake one can gradually change this conditioned association so that the bed becomes associated with sleep, and the act of going to bed induces sleep.

7.5.6 Medication

There are three aspects to the medication domain. The first is the impact of medications prescribed for other conditions such as hypertension, pain or psychiatric conditions. Many of these medications can have deleterious or beneficial effects on sleep. At times, the prescriber may have chosen the particular medication with its effects on sleep in mind, but more commonly any effects on sleep are unintended. Advising on alternative medications and judicious timing of medications allows one to minimize the impact of medications that adversely affect sleep and take advantage of any beneficial effects. The second aspect is the use of medications specifically prescribed for sleep which include hypnotics, medications to treat restless legs, melatonin and stimulant medications. One needs to determine how effective these treatments are, consider their side-effect/benefit ratio and record any concerns about inappropriate medication use. The third aspect to consider is the use of caffeine, nicotine, drugs and alcohol and their impact on sleep.

This system not only allows one to organize the information gathered in the history and investigations in a coherent and comprehensive manner but, if borne in mind while taking the history, acts as an effective aide-memoire to ensure that all areas of the history are covered. Finally, it encourages the clinician to formulate a holistic treatment plan for the insomnia that addresses as many of the contributory factors as possible.

References

American Academy of Sleep Medicine. International classification of sleep disorders. Darien, IL: American Academy of Sleep Medicine; 2014. https://doi.org/10.1111/febs.12678.

Baglioni C, Battagliese G, Feige B, Spiegelhalder K, Nissen C, Voderholzer U, et al. Insomnia as a predictor of depression: a meta-analytic evaluation of longitudinal epidemiological studies. J Affect Disord. 2011;135(1–3):10–9. https://doi.org/10.1016/j.jad.2011.01.011.

Bazalakova M, Benca RM. Wake-promoting medications: efficacy and adverse effects. In: Kryger MH, editor. Principles and practice of sleep medicine. Amsterdam: Elsevier; 2017. p. 462–479. e5. https://doi.org/10.1016/B978-0-323-24288-2.00044-1.

Chin JM, Merves ML, Goldberger B a, Sampson-Cone A, Cone EJ. Caffeine content of brewed teas. J Anal Toxicol. 2008;32(8):702–4. https://doi.org/10.1093/jat/32.8.702.

Horne J a, Ostberg O. A self-assessment questionnaire to determine morningness-eveningness in human circadian rhythms. Int J Chronobiol. 1976;4(2):97–110. https://doi.org/10.1177/0748730405285278.

Littner M, Hirshkowitz M, Kramer M, Kapen S, Anderson WM, Bailey D, et al. Standards of Practice Committee. Practice parameters for using polysomnography to evaluate insomnia: an update. Sleep. 2003;26(6):754–60. http://www.ncbi.nlm.nih.gov/pubmed/14572131

Mitchell DC, Knight CA, Hockenberry J, Teplansky R, Hartman TJ. Beverage caffeine intakes in the U.S. Food Chem Toxicol. 2014;63:136–42. https://doi.org/10.1016/j.fct.2013.10.042.

Nishino S, Mignot E. Wake-promoting medications: basic mechanisms and pharmacology. In: Kryger MH, editor. Principles and practice of sleep medicine. Amsterdam: Elsevier; 2017. p. 462–479.e5. https://doi.org/10.1016/B978-0-323-24288-2.00043-X.

Schutte-rodin S, Broch L, Ph D, Buysse D, Dorsey C, Ph D, Sateia M. Clinical guideline for the evaluation and management of chronic insomnia in adults. J Clin Sleep Med. 2017;13(5):307–49. http://www.aasmnet.org/Resources/clinicalguidelines/040515.pdf

Stores G, Crawford C. Medical student education in sleep and its disorders. J R Coll Phys Lond. 1998;32(2):149–53. http://www.ncbi.nlm.nih.gov/pubmed/9597633

Tryon WW. Issues of validity in actigraphic sleep assessment. Sleep. 2004;27(1):158–65. http://www.ncbi.nlm.nih.gov/pubmed/14998254

The Science and Art of Prescribing for Insomnia

8

Sue Wilson and Hugh Selsick

8.1 Introduction

The medical management of insomnia involves medications which either enhance the sleep-promoting mechanisms or inhibit the wakefulness-promoting mechanisms of the brain. A wide range of neurotransmitters are involved in sleep-wake regulation. There are therefore, in theory, multiple pathways by which we can enhance a patient's sleep. In practice, the licensed hypnotics focus on only a few of these pathways, but a clear understanding of the pharmacology of these drugs reveals a number of subtleties and allows for targeted and effective prescribing. Studies of the use of hypnotics in psychiatric patients are relatively limited, and one needs to utilize clinical acumen and a good understanding of the mechanisms of action of the drugs in addition to the research data.

This chapter will examine the underlying sleep mechanisms and the pharmacology of the drugs that promote sleep. In addition to the science of these medications, we will present an approach to prescribing these drugs in psychiatric patients as well as looking at when and how to stop prescribing.

8.2 Neurotransmitters of the Sleep-Wake Systems

The control of sleep and waking in the brain relies on a complex balance between arousing and sleep-inducing physiological systems. Current research suggests that arousal and wakefulness are promoted by parallel neurotransmitter systems whose

S. Wilson (✉)
Division of Brain Sciences, Centre for Psychiatry, Imperial College London, London, UK
e-mail: sue.wilson@imperial.ac.uk

H. Selsick
Insomnia Clinic, Royal London Hospital for Integrated Medicine, London, UK
e-mail: hugh@selsick.net

© Springer-Verlag GmbH Germany, part of Springer Nature 2018
H. Selsick (ed.), *Sleep Disorders in Psychiatric Patients*,
https://doi.org/10.1007/978-3-642-54836-9_8

Table 8.1 Neurotransmitter effects on sleep and wakefulness

Endogenous transmitter	Increasing function maintains wakefulness	Increasing function promotes sleep
GABA		✓
Melatonin		(✓—Brings forward sleep onset)
Adenosine		✓
Noradrenaline	✓	
Dopamine	✓	
Serotonin	✓	
Histamine	✓	
Acetylcholine	✓	
Orexin	✓	

cell bodies are located in brainstem or midbrain centres, with projections to the thalamus and higher centres. These arousing neurotransmitters are noradrenaline, serotonin, acetylcholine, dopamine and histamine. In addition, the orexin system with cell bodies in the hypothalamus promotes wakefulness through regulating arousal 'pathways' (and inhibiting sedative ones) (Samuels and Szabadi 2008; Saper et al. 2005). Sleep can be promoted by blocking the postsynaptic actions of these arousal neurotransmitters. Sleep is also regulated by a number of arousal-reducing neurotransmitters (see Table 8.1); primary amongst these is gamma-aminobutyric acid (GABA), the most prolific inhibitory neurotransmitter in the brain. Most of the medications we use in insomnia either increase GABA function or inhibit arousal function via these neurotransmitters.

8.3   Drugs Which Increase Function of Sleep-Promoting Neurotransmitters

The majority of brain cells are inhibited by GABA, so increasing its function reduces arousal and produces sleep and eventually anaesthesia. There are many sub-sets of GABA neurons distributed throughout the brain, but a particular cluster in the hypothalamus (ventrolateral preoptic nucleus) can be considered to be the sleep 'switch' (Saper et al. 2005). These neurons switch off brain arousal systems at the level of the cell bodies and therefore promote sleep. GABA receptors in the cortex can also promote sedation and sleep by inhibiting the target neurons of the arousal system.

The inhibitory effects of GABA are mediated through the GABA-A receptor, which is a complex of proteins with a binding site for a number of sleep-promoting drugs, in particular the *benzodiazepine receptor agonists* (which include benzodiazepines themselves and the so-called 'Z' drugs like zolpidem and zopiclone) which enhance the effects of GABA's actions at the GABA-A receptor, by an action called positive allosteric modulation. This is why they are known as GABA-PAMs.

8.3.1 Benzodiazepine-Receptor Agonists (GABA-A-Positive Allosteric Modulators)

These drugs are licensed for use in insomnia as they have been proven to improve sleep in clinical trials. They all work in the same way but differ in their speed of onset and duration of action. The faster the drug enters the brain, the sooner sleep is induced. As well as inducing sleep, these drugs are anticonvulsant and antianxiety and produce muscle relaxation, ataxia and memory impairment, while they are in the brain. The latter three are not usually a problem, while people are asleep in bed, but if the effects outlast sleep, then these side effects are undesirable. Therefore, it is important to consider both speed of onset and duration of action when choosing a drug.

The ease of waking and the propensity to daytime carry-over ('hangover') effects are determined by the duration of action—most typically defined by the elimination half-life of the drugs (see Tables 8.2 and 8.3) and the dose taken. Drugs with half-lives of more than 6h tend to leave sufficient residual drug in the brain to cause hangover in the morning. This was particularly the case with the first benzodiazepine agonists such as nitrazepam which was associated with daytime sedation and falls (Trewin et al. 1992). The rationale for developing the Z-drugs was in part to make shorter half-life benzodiazepine agonists with minimal carry-over effects (Nutt 2005). This was largely achieved although there is some hangover seen with zopiclone (Staner et al. 2005). The very short half-life of zaleplon means that it could be taken as little as 5h before the desired time of arising, without the risk of hangover impairment (Walsh et al. 2000). However, at the time of writing, this drug is no longer on the market.

A very short half-life limits a drug's duration of action on sleep, and zaleplon and, to some extent, zolpidem are not particularly effective at maintaining sleep throughout the night. A controlled release formulation of zolpidem (currently only available in the USA) prolongs its nocturnal actions and enhances sleep continuity, though only by tens of minutes (Greenblatt et al. 2006). Individual factors seem

Table 8.2 Sleep-promoting neurotransmitters

Endogenous sleep-promoting neurotransmitter	Examples of drugs increasing function and promoting sleep	Examples of drugs decreasing function and promoting wakefulness
GABA	Benzodiezepine receptor agonists (positive allosteric modulators) e.g. temazepam, zopidone	None
Melatonin	Melatonin M1 and M2 receptor agonists (e.g. melatonin, ramelteon) (bring sleep onset forward)	None
Adenosine	None	Adenosine receptor antagonist (caffeine)

Table 8.3 Wake-promoting neurotransmitters

Endogenous wakefulness-promoting neurotransmitter	Examples of drugs increasing function and promoting wakefulness	Examples of drugs decreasing function and promoting sleep and/or daytime sedation
Noradrenaline	Uptake blocker (e.g. atomoxetine); uptake blocker and neurotransmitter releaser (e.g. amphetamines)	Alpha-1 receptor antagonists (e.g. prazosin, but also e.g. chlorpromazine, clozapine)
Dopamine	Uptake blocker (e.g. modafinil); uptake blocker and neurotransmitter releaser (e.g. amphetamines)	None
Serotonin	Uptake blocker (SRI) but mild effect and often just early in treatment	$5HT_2$ antagonists (e.g. trazodone). 5HTP
Histamine	H3 receptor antagonist (e.g. pitolisant) (H3 is an autoreceptor and therefore antagonizing it increases histamine cell firing)	H1 antagonists (e.g. low-dose doxepin)
Acetylcholine	None	Muscarinic receptor antagonist (e.g. amitriptyline, olanzapine)
Orexin	None	Orexin receptor antagonist (e.g. suvorexant)

important, and some people are more susceptible to carry-over than others, probably due to individual differences either in the rate of drug clearance, which can vary by as much a twofold between subjects, or sensitivity to drug actions; there are also gender differences with women being more susceptible to the hangover effects, particularly relating to driving (Booth et al. 2016).

8.3.2   Tolerance, Dependence and Withdrawal Considerations with GABA-Acting Drugs

Dose escalation above recommended doses in patients with insomnia alone is uncommon, and tolerance to drug effects is not a frequent problem in clinical experience; many patients use the same dose of sleep medication for months or years and still feel it works.

Animal and human research demonstrates that brain receptor function changes in response to chronic treatment with benzodiazepine receptor agonists, and this takes time to return to premedication levels after cessation of medication. There is evidence from animal studies that chronic administration of benzodiazepines produces adaptive changes in the receptor which attenuate the effects of the endogenous neurotransmitter GABA and so produce symptoms on withdrawal (Bateson 2002).

Considerations of dependence are very much contingent on what happens when treatment is stopped. A psychological dependence is seen in many patients, and some are unwilling to stop treatment. If they do stop, there can be relapse, where the patient's original symptoms return, or rebound of symptoms, where for one or two nights there is a worsening of sleep disturbance, with longer sleep onset latency and increased waking during sleep. This is commonly reported by patients and has been documented in some research studies (Soldatos et al. 1999; Hajak et al. 2009). It is also seen in healthy volunteers who have been taking zopiclone or zolpidem for 3 weeks and then stop (Voderholzer et al. 2001). More rarely, there is a longer withdrawal syndrome. All of these can be ameliorated by resuming medication. The withdrawal syndrome is characterized by the emergence of symptoms not previously experienced, such as agitation, headache, dizziness, dysphoria, irritability, fatigue, depersonalization and hypersensitivity to noise and visual stimuli. This syndrome typically resolves within a few weeks, but in some patients it persists, and this may be related to personality traits and cognitive factors (Murphy and Tyrer 1991).

8.3.3   Melatonin

Melatonin is a natural hormone that is produced in the pineal gland and which has an important role in regulating circadian rhythms (Dijk and von Schantz 2005; Cajochen et al. 2003). The circadian pacemaker in the suprachiasmatic nucleus (SCN) of the hypothalamus drives melatonin synthesis and secretion from the pineal gland. Once melatonin appears in the plasma, it enters the brain and binds to melatonin receptors in the hypothalamus, forming a feedback loop. The SCN contains melatonin 1 and melatonin 2 receptors, and much research is ongoing about their role in sleep-wake regulation and circadian rhythms. Giving melatonin tablets has both phase-shifting effects, thus changing the timing of the biological clock, and direct effects to promote sleep onset. A slow-release formulation of melatonin has been licensed on the basis of improved sleep continuity and daytime well-being in people aged over 55 years with insomnia. Numerous melatonin preparations are available off the shelf in many countries. Ramelteon, a synthetic melatonin agonist, is available in the USA. There are very few side effects of melatonin; in particular there are no effects on movement or memory.

8.3.4   Adenosine

Another sleep-promoting neurotransmitter is adenosine. Brain levels of this rise during the day and are thought to lead to sleepiness, which increases the longer the time since the last sleep. The arousing and sleep-impairing effects of caffeine (Landolt et al. 2004) are thought to be due to antagonism of adenosine-A2 receptors, so attenuating this natural process (Porkka-Heiskanen et al. 2002). Caffeine is a useful translational model for insomnia as its effects in rodents are very similar to those in humans and could be used to screen potential new treatments (Paterson et al. 2007). However, there is no adenosine agonist drug available for use in humans, though this may be a target for future drugs.

8.4   Drugs Which Decrease Function of Wakefulness-Promoting Neurotransmitters

8.4.1   Histamine (H1 Receptor Antagonists)

Histamine is a wakefulness-promoting neurotransmitter; antihistamines block histamine H1 receptors in the brain and peripherally. These have been used for many years as over-the-counter sleep remedies. There is sparse evidence that the older drugs improve sleep, and the drugs used (mainly promethazine, diphenhydramine, alimemazine) have effects on many other neurotransmitter systems as well as histamine. Thus, they can have unpleasant side effects; promethazine is a dopamine D2 antagonist, like other phenothiazines such as chlorpromazine, and so there is a risk of movement disorder and tardive dyskinesia. It and the other over-the-counter antihistamines also have effects on noradrenergic and cholinergic receptors in the brain and body, thus giving rise to cardiovascular effects in those at risk, particularly if taken in overdose.

One of the most potent H1 antagonists is doxepin, an old drug of tricyclic structure used in depression. It has been used over the past few years as a PET tracer, because in tiny doses labelled with radioactivity, it will occupy nearly all of the H1 receptors in the brain (Nakamura et al. 1998). In 2010 a preparation of this drug containing approximately 1/40th of the dose for depression was licensed in the USA for insomnia after positive clinical trials. At this dose, all the other neurotransmitter actions of the depression drug (neurotransmitter uptake inhibition and actions at noradrenergic and cholinergic receptors) would be minimal, whereas those on histamine would prevail. It has shown good effects on sleep onset and also on waking in the early morning, which are explained by the action of blocking histamine receptors to enhance sleep at the borders of sleep, but not generally during the main part of the night when histamine neurons are quiescent.

8.4.2   Orexin

Orexin (sometimes called hypocretin) neurons in the hypothalamus have an important role in maintaining wakefulness, and they are not active during sleep. In narcolepsy, particularly narcolepsy with cataplexy, these neurons are dramatically reduced or absent. Antagonists of the orexin receptors (OR1 and OR2) have been studied for many years because of this proven role in sleep (Brisbare-Roch et al. 2007), and one such (suvorexant) has been licensed for use in insomnia after positive clinical trials. This is a unique mechanism, in that it targets a known population of neurons involved in sleep, unlike the GABA drugs, for instance, which affect the whole brain. This drug has some effects on morning wakefulness however because of its half-life (see Fig. 8.1). Other drugs with similar action are in development.

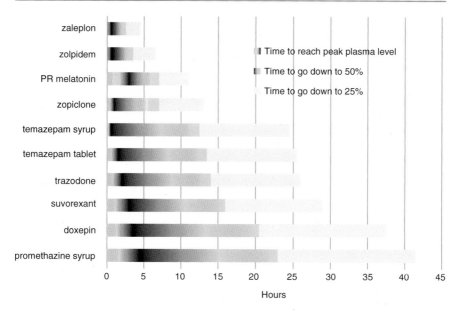

Fig. 8.1 Speed of onset and duration of action of some drugs used in insomnia

8.4.3   Drugs for Depression Used in Insomnia

Drugs for depression which are antagonists of the 5-HT2 receptor (and thus reduce serotonin function) seem to improve sleep in depression, but the evidence base is small, and none is licensed for this indication.

Low doses (subtherapeutic for depression) of sedating drugs, particularly amitriptyline, dosulepin and doxepin, have been used for decades to treat insomnia. This is particularly common practice in primary care in the UK, where amitriptyline 10 or 25 mg is also used for long periods in many patients with chronic illness, particularly those with pain syndromes. At this dose, amitriptyline is probably acting mostly as a histamine H1 receptor antagonist although a degree of 5-HT2 and cholinergic muscarinic antagonism may also contribute. There are no controlled studies of efficacy of low-dose amitriptyline in insomnia, and drugs with tricyclic structures are more likely to be lethal than licensed insomnia drugs in overdose (Nutt 2005).

Trazodone is an antagonist at 5-HT1A, 5-HT2 and alpha-1 adrenergic receptors as well as a weak 5-HT reuptake inhibitor and is the second most prescribed medication for insomnia in the USA. It has a perceived absence of risk and is cheap, and there are no restrictions on use duration, but 25–30% patients experience difficulty tolerating trazodone, and dropout rates tend to be higher than for benzodiazepine or Z-drugs. Several studies have found beneficial effects on sleep; these have mainly been in insomnia comorbid with depression, with one in primary insomnia (Walsh et al. 1998). Some clinicians use a small dose of trazodone to counteract sleep-disturbing effects of serotonin reuptake inhibitors.

Trimipramine is a drug with tricyclic structure which blocks alpha-1 adrenergic, histamine H1, dopamine D2, serotonin 5-HT2 and cholinergic receptors. One controlled trial (Riemann et al. 2002) in insomnia at doses of 50–200 mg for 4 weeks found a significant improvement in sleep efficiency as measured by polysomnography, paralleled by subjective improvements. Side effects were described as marginal.

Paroxetine, a serotonin reuptake inhibitor, was studied in patients with insomnia aged over 55 years, at a median dose of 20 mg for 6 weeks (Reynolds et al. 2006), with subjective sleep quality and daytime well-being improved. This seeming paradoxical action of paroxetine to improve sleep is probably related to its good efficacy in many anxiety disorders where it seems to reduce recurrent thinking and ruminations.

8.5   When to Prescribe Drugs for Insomnia

In order to address the issue of when it is appropriate to prescribe a sleep-promoting drug, it is necessary to differentiate between acute prescribing and chronic prescribing. The risks and side effects that may be unacceptable in the long term may be tolerable and manageable if the medication is only used for a short period of time. Short-term prescribing may be appropriate where there is a clear, time-limited stressor that is driving the insomnia, and therefore the insomnia is likely to resolve when that stressor is removed. Similarly, some patients may benefit from occasional doses when their insomnia is sporadic.

It may also be appropriate to use a short course of sleep medication in chronic insomnia if the patient is awaiting a more definitive intervention such as cognitive behaviour therapy for insomnia. However, the value of short-term prescribing in chronic insomnia is questionable. Sleeping tablets can be effective as long as they are being taken, but there is rarely any sustained improvement once the medication is stopped (Riemann and Perlis 2009). Therefore, the common practice of giving someone with chronic insomnia a 'two week course of hypnotics to reset their sleep cycle' seldom works.

What this means is that when prescribing for chronic insomnia, one either needs an exit strategy, such as CBT for insomnia, or one needs to be comfortable with the idea of prescribing the medication in the long term. Many clinicians baulk at the idea of prescribing benzodiazepine agonists for the long term, and in many countries these are not licensed for long-term use. However, when one considers that insomnia is often a chronic and debilitating condition, one should not automatically dismiss the idea of chronic prescribing. Severe insomnia's impact on quality of life is on a par with major depression (Katz and McHorney 2002), and many patients are willing to accept the risks of chronic medication use if it improves their overall quality of life. Indeed, clinicians are rarely uncomfortable with chronic prescriptions of antidepressants, mood stabilizers and antipsychotics; when insomnia is viewed as a serious psychiatric illness in its own right, the idea of chronic medical treatment seems less troubling.

There is also the question of whether the proactive treatment of insomnia with hypnotics may reduce the risks of other psychiatric symptoms. The evidence that insomnia is a risk factor for other psychiatric conditions is mounting, particularly in relation to depression (Baglioni et al. 2011; Neckelmann et al. 2007). Comorbid insomnia worsens depression outcomes (Pigeon et al. 2008), and treating insomnia comorbid with depression improves the depressive symptoms and prognosis (Manber and Chambers 2009). However, it has not yet been definitively shown that treating insomnia in patients without comorbid psychiatric illnesses is preventative. In practice, however, this should not change one's management of insomnia. Given its significant negative impact on quality of life, insomnia should be treated aggressively regardless of whether it leads to other psychiatric (or physical) illnesses.

The other scenario to consider is the use of hypnotics in the acutely unwell psychiatric patient. These are often prescribed as short-term or as-needed doses in the acute treatment of patients with severe depression, mania or psychosis. From a patient's perspective, this can be very helpful; while many psychiatric drugs can take days or weeks before they start to noticeably improve the patient's symptoms, hypnotics can provide relief from one of their symptoms immediately. However, there are two factors that should be borne in mind. Firstly, acutely unwell patients are likely to be taking a number of medications, and therefore the risk of dangerous interactions is significantly increased, particularly if they are on other sedative drugs such as benzodiazepines. Secondly, hypnotics should only be prescribed if they improve the patient's symptoms and should not be used as a form of behavioural management or as emergency sedation. Staffing levels on psychiatric wards are generally lower at night, and while it is tempting to give patients hypnotics to help the staff manage the ward at night, this is clearly inappropriate.

There is also the risk of overdose to be considered in suicidal patients, and therefore only limited supplies of hypnotics should be given to this population. Ideally, these should be monitored and controlled by another person to minimize the risk of stockpiling the medication. There is mounting evidence that insomnia may be an independent risk factor for suicide (Woznica et al. 2015), but there is a lack of data on whether the treatment of insomnia with hypnotics reduces this risk.

Whether or not a hypnotic is effective, one should always assume that it renders the patient incapable of making clear decisions or taking responsibility. Therefore, one should check that the patient will not be responsible for the care of a child or have similar responsibilities during the night. Even if they are rousable on the hypnotic, they may not be sufficiently compos mentis to be able to look after that child. Similarly, patients should be told very clearly that they should not drive, cook or do any other potentially dangerous activity after taking the medication until they are absolutely certain that the sedative effects of the medication have worn off.

8.5.1   Does the Patient Need a Hypnotic?

A good guiding principle in prescribing is to avoid polypharmacy wherever possible. Therefore, if one is also selecting an antipsychotic, antidepressant or mood stabilizer in a patient with comorbid insomnia, one should consider whether it may be appropriate to select a psychiatric drug with sedative side effects. While the evidence for the use of these drugs in insomnia is somewhat limited, if all else is equal, a sedative drug may be a wise choice. It is the experience of one of the authors (HS) that trazodone and mirtazapine can be effective in many patients for treating both the mood disorder and the sleep disorder in patients with depression and comorbid insomnia. These two drugs have been shown to cause less sleep disturbance than the more activating antidepressants (Manber and Chambers 2009).

Insomnia is a not uncommon side effect of selective serotonin reuptake inhibitors (SSRIs), serotonin and noradrenaline reuptake inhibitors (SNRIs) and noradrenaline reuptake inhibitors (Manber and Chambers 2009). If prescribing one of these drugs, it may be worth considering a short course of sleep-promoting medication during the early stages of treatment when the insomnia tends to be worse.

There is also some evidence that combining benzodiazepine receptor agonists with antidepressants may improve or accelerate the response to the antidepressant in depressed patients. Combining eszopiclone with fluoxetine leads to a more rapid response and a greater magnitude of response to the fluoxetine (Fava et al. 2006). Similarly, the combination of eszopiclone and fluoxetine leads to a greater improvement in generalized anxiety disorder than placebo and fluoxetine (Pollack et al. 2008). The improvements in depression and anxiety were maintained even when the sleep questions were removed from the rating scales. Interestingly, a study looking at the impact of zolpidem controlled release in combination with escitalopram in depression showed improvements in insomnia but not in the depression (Fava et al. 2011) raising the possibility that the effects seen with eszopiclone may be mediated by some other properties of the medication and not its impact on sleep.

8.5.2   Selecting a Medication for Insomnia

The choice of medication is largely dictated by when you want it to work and how important it is to avoid residual sedation the next day. Amongst the commonly used benzodiazepine receptor agonists, there is very little difference in the time taken to reach maximum plasma concentration (Tmax), and therefore the time to onset of action will be much the same. In practice this means that the majority of these drugs will be most effective in the first couple of hours after taking the pill. They are therefore likely to be equally effective for sleep onset insomnia, and, in those patients with pure sleep onset insomnia, it makes sense to try a short-acting hypnotic first. However, when looking to treat middle-of-the-night insomnia or early-morning waking, the half-life becomes important, and here there are significant differences between drugs. A longer half-life drug is likely to be more effective for maintaining sleep in the middle and end of the night. However, the trade-off is that the longer half-life drugs are more likely to lead to daytime sedation the next day. One needs to balance the need for sedation in the latter part of the night with the desirability of avoiding daytime sedation.

It is vital to ask patients about their routines and responsibilities in the mornings. In particular, one should enquire about driving. Clearly the impact of a sleep medication on driving performance will depend on the nature of the drug, the dose, the half-life and the time between taking the drug and driving (Roth et al. 2014). The benzodiazepines, as a rule, impair next-morning driving, particularly if they have half-lives greater than 6h. Zopiclone 7.5 mg has been consistently shown to impair driving performance the morning after taking a dose, and this impairment lasts for 11h after taking the medication (Leufkens and Vermeeren 2014), though driving in the afternoon appears to carry less risk than in the morning (Verster and van de Loo 2017). Interestingly, this impairment in driving can occur even if subjects report that they did not feel any drowsier than usual, and so subjective reports of daytime effects need to be treated with caution (Leufkens and Vermeeren 2014). The situation with zolpidem is more complicated as the US Food and Drug Administration has cautioned that it may affect driving in the morning, but objective studies of driving the day after taking zolpidem have not found this, as long as the drug is taken at bedtime. If it is taken in the middle of the night, driving is adversely affected (Verster and van de Loo 2017). Therefore, a good rule of thumb is that driving should always be avoided if a sleeping tablet is taken in the middle of the night. The melatonin agonist, ramelteon, also affects driving in the morning (Verster and van de Loo 2017).

Hence, it is important to warn patients of the potential for sleep medications to affect driving performance. We should always advise our patients never to drive if sleepy, but as mentioned above, their driving may be affected even if they do not feel sleepy. Therefore, if they are taking a hypnotic, they need to exercise extra caution even in the absence of subjective sleepiness.

8.5.3 Hypnotics and Sleep Apnoea

Any comorbid sleep disorder will add a layer of complexity to the prescribing process, but obstructive sleep apnoea (OSA) deserves particular attention. In OSA, patients will choke in their sleep which will lead to an arousal where they reopen their airway. Some patients will have their arousal before they experience an oxygen desaturation, while others may experience quite profound desaturations before an arousal is triggered. Hypnotics are liable to increase the arousal threshold, and therefore they may prolong the duration of the desaturations. Furthermore, benzodiazepines have muscle-relaxing properties, and this can exacerbate the sleep apnoea; this has been shown in some, though not all, studies. It is thought that zolpidem, which is more specific to the α-1 subunit, causes less muscle relaxation and may therefore be safer in untreated sleep apnoea. Hence, it is essential to screen patients for potential sleep apnoea if one is considering using hypnotics. However, once the patient is established on an effective treatment for their sleep apnoea, such as continuous positive airway pressure (CPAP), the use of these drugs does not appear to worsen the sleep apnoea; indeed there is some evidence that using them in the early stages of CPAP treatment may increase long-term compliance with the CPAP (Luyster et al. 2010).

8.5.4 How to Initiate, Titrate and Monitor Hypnotics

Unless the situation is urgent, it is sensible to start with the lowest dose of any medication. However, it is important to explain to the patient that if the medication does not work at the lower dose, it may yet become effective at the higher end of the dose range. If it doesn't work when they first start the medication, they may develop anxiety that all medication is ineffective for them which will negate much of the effect of the medication even when given at an adequate dose.

If the patient is living in the community, and they do not need to start the medication immediately, it is sensible to suggest that they start the medication on a night when they have few responsibilities the next day and in particular when they don't have to drive the next day. This will allow them to gauge how the medication affects their daytime function.

Ideally one should review the patient within a few days of starting the medication to screen for side effects and check that it is effective. This involves not only asking about the medication's impact on sleep but also its effect on daytime symptoms. In suicidal patients a limited supply of medication should be issued at any one time, and having an early review is essential.

There is rarely a case to be made for exceeding the licensed dose of a hypnotic and if a patient develops tolerance to a drug, it is probably better to switch to a different class of drug than to escalate the dose beyond the recommended maximum (Wilson et al. 2010). It is also advisable for the patient to take occasional drug holidays if there is concern about dependence developing, though the patient should be warned about the possibility of rebound insomnia (see below) during these periods.

8.5.5 When and How to Discontinue Hypnotics

Before stopping the medication, it is essential to be certain that one is stopping for the right reasons. Appropriate triggers for stopping medication include:

- Unacceptable side effects
- Signs of dependence
- Loss of efficacy
- Resolution of the insomnia (difficult to ascertain if hypnotics are taken nightly)
- Initiation of alternative therapy, e.g. cognitive behaviour therapy for insomnia and sedative antidepressant
- Patient's request

Therefore, the medication should be stopped if the risks or side effects outweigh the benefits, if the insomnia resolves or if an alternative effective treatment is put in place.

If the patient is using the medication on an as-needed basis, then they will have very little difficulty coming off the medication. In patients who have been using the medication on a nightly basis, the situation is more complex due to the risk of rebound insomnia. This is a temporary worsening of the insomnia with symptoms more severe than one would expect based on the patient's underlying insomnia. Not all patients will experience rebound insomnia, and it has not been described in all drugs; however, it is wise to warn patients about the potential for rebound insomnia. When patients understand that this exacerbation of symptoms is temporary (typically lasting no more than a few days), they are generally able to tolerate it and persist with the plan.

There are relatively few studies comparing discontinuation methods, and, to a large extent, one needs to be guided by the patient. Some patients are motivated and able to stop medication immediately, but many prefer a gradual reduction. A 25% reduction in dose, or frequency of use, every 1–2 weeks is a sensible guideline, but some patients may need to reduce more slowly than this. In order to do a gradual reduction, one should prescribe the medication in the smallest possible denomination. For example, if reducing zopiclone 7.5 mg, it is difficult to do a 25% reduction if one has to cut one 7.5 mg tablet into quarters. Therefore, one should prescribe two 3.75 mg tablets which would allow the patient to reduce the dose by taking one and a half tablets, then one tablet and then a half tablet.

During the reduction, one should monitor the patient's sleep and mental state closely. If sleep deteriorates significantly, the pace of the reduction should be decreased to minimize distress to the patient. This is particularly important in patients with comorbid psychiatric disorders as there may be a risk of adversely affecting their mental state if their insomnia is not well managed. A practice that one of the authors (HS) uses is to reduce the dose of medication by 25% when, and only when, the sleep efficiency as measured by a sleep diary reaches 90%. This means the medication is only reduced when the patient's sleep is relatively solid and therefore able to tolerate a reduction in medication. It also makes it very clear when one should reduce. One of the difficulties patients experience is indecision about whether it is the right or wrong time to reduce medication, and they will often get very anxious about this. Having a clear numerical trigger for dose reduction relieves them of the burden of having to make this decision. An alternative approach is to set target dates for each reduction at the start of the treatment. However, the clinician should be prepared to adjust these targets based on the patient's response and life circumstances.

Hypnotics are quite unusual drugs in that patients often report that they work even when they don't take them! Just having a supply of them in the cupboard gives them the reassurance that, if they are really struggling, they are available; this safety net then allows them to sleep well. There may therefore be a case for having a supply of tablets for emergencies once the patient has stopped regular use. However, it does mean there is still an element of psychological dependence on the medication and if the patient is keen to overcome this, they will need to discard the medication at some point. They will therefore need to learn to be comfortable with the idea that they will not sleep perfectly every single night and acceptance of this is an important part of the psychological treatment of insomnia. Patients need to learn that nobody sleeps well every night and that they can cope with the occasional bad night. Once they appreciate this, they will be less tempted to use medication on the nights when they are sleeping badly.

There is some evidence to suggest that melatonin can be a useful 'step-down' drug when reducing benzodiazepine receptor agonist hypnotics, particularly in the elderly using hypnotic doses of these drugs (Cardinali et al. 2002), but not all studies have confirmed this (Wright et al. 2015). In a placebo-controlled, randomized and blinded trial of melatonin in schizophrenic and bipolar patients with long-term benzodiazepine use, melatonin did not increase the rate of benzodiazepine discontinuation (Baandrup et al. 2015).

The concomitant use of cognitive behaviour therapy for insomnia may increase the likelihood of successful hypnotic discontinuation (Belanger 2009; Morgan et al. 2003). This may be due to the frequent contact between the patient and the therapist or the fact that patients are simply less likely to need the medication if their insomnia is effectively treated. However, the generalizability of these studies to patients with comorbid psychiatric conditions is yet to be adequately studied.

8.6   Managing Dependence

There is enormous concern amongst doctors and patients about the risk of dependence on benzodiazepine receptor agonists. This anxiety is not without foundation, but the common perception that dependence is inevitable on these medications is not borne out by the literature or clinical experience. The first issue to be addressed is the confusion between chronic, appropriate use of hypnotics and dependence. Hypnotics can effectively treat insomnia but rarely cure it. This is analogous to many other psychiatric drugs such as antipsychotics in schizophrenia or mood stabilizers in bipolar disorder. Insomnia is often a chronic condition that requires a chronic treatment. Therefore, when a patient seeks hypnotics, or when they come asking for a repeat prescription, this should not necessarily be seen as a sign of addiction but may simply be a patient seeking an effective treatment for a distressing disorder.

However, one should always be alert for warning signs that might indicate the patient is engaging in harmful use of the drug. Using doses above the recommended maximum dose for any one drug, using multiple medications, combining hypnotics with alcohol or other sedatives and chaotic use are all causes for concern. When a patient reports using more than the recommended dose, one would expect that they would run out of medication before their next repeat prescription is due, and one should ask what the patient does to manage the nights when they have run out of prescription medications. Some patients choose to have some medication-free nights where they get little or no sleep so that they can have nights where they can take higher doses of the drug and get better sleep; naturally this is still a significant concern as there is a risk of death from overdose. However, other patients fill the gap by using alternative sedatives, illegally bought hypnotics, hypnotics prescribed for a friend or family member or hypnotics obtained from multiple doctors. This should be explored carefully as all of these practices carry significant risks and rationalizing medication requires a clear understanding of where the medication is coming from.

Managing harmful use and addiction may require a combined approach with input from addiction services and sleep services. While most hypnotics can be safely stopped without tapering the dose, many patients won't tolerate this, and those on high doses of benzodiazepines may need to do a very gradual taper to minimize the risk of seizures. Some clinics switch the hypnotic to an equivalent dose of diazepam, a longer-acting benzodiazepine, which allows for a very gradual taper. However, as most patients who abuse hypnotics are self-medicating for insomnia, it is important to address the insomnia as well. Patients need to learn to tolerate a degree of sleep loss in order to come off the medication, and using cognitive behaviour therapy for insomnia may lead to more successful hypnotic discontinuation by treating the main driver of their hypnotic use (Morin et al. 1995).

8.6.1   Prescribing Medication for Insomnia in Psychiatric Disorders

Despite the fact that insomnia is a common comorbid disorder in patients with psychiatric illness, the study of effective treatment in this population is still in its very early stages. To some extent, this may be due to the common perception by psychiatrists that insomnia is a symptom of the psychiatric disorder and should therefore respond to the standard treatment for that disorder. Another obstacle is the difficulty disentangling the effects of insomnia and comorbid psychiatric disorders. In addition, patients with comorbid psychiatric disorders are highly likely to be on at least one other drug which may interact with any hypnotic they are given. It is therefore very difficult to make definite statements about the efficacy and safety of these drugs in specific psychiatric disorders, and it is not clear whether the treatment of insomnia in the presence of comorbid psychiatric disorders is particularly different from prescribing in insomnia alone. Nevertheless, what follows is a brief survey of the prescribing strategies that have been studied in some of the more common psychiatric disorders.

8.6.2   Schizophrenia

Sleep disturbance in schizophrenia is often complicated by adverse life circumstances such as unemployment and social isolation which lead to a lack of structure in the day. Poor sleep quality is a significant predictor of poor quality of life and function (Xiang et al. 2009).

It is always preferable to avoid polypharmacy, and so, in patients with schizophrenia and insomnia, it is worth considering whether one could select an antipsychotic that will treat the insomnia as well as the schizophrenia. The majority of antipsychotics have been shown to improve sleep parameters, and this is true of the typical antipsychotics as well as the atypical antipsychotics. Improvements in sleep parameters have been found, for example, in haloperidol, chlorpromazine, fluphenazine, clozapine, olanzapine, risperidone, paliperidone (Benson 2008) and quetiapine (Anderson and Vande Griend 2014). It should be noted that not all the studies were performed in patients with schizophrenia or insomnia.

There is a marked absence of evidence on the best way to manage insomnia in acutely unwell schizophrenic patients. One study on inpatients with schizophrenia examined the impact of switching from typical to atypical antipsychotics. It showed improvements in the Pittsburgh Sleep Quality Index (PSQI) for patients on quetiapine, risperidone and olanzapine, with the effect being greater in older patients (Yamashita et al. 2005). It should be noted that these patients were on antipsychotic doses of these medications, and so it is unclear if the improvement in their sleep was due to the direct effects of the medications on their sleep or the improvement in their psychiatric symptoms.

In patients with stable schizophrenia, it is not uncommon for there to be residual insomnia. Two studies have looked at the effect of switching these patients from typical (D2 antagonists) to atypical (dopamine serotonin antagonists) antipsychotics, in particular to risperidone (Haffmans et al. 2001), paliperidone (Luthringer et al. 2007) and olanzapine (Salin-Pascual et al. 1999). All these drugs improved sleep architecture and sleep continuity. Once again these were used at antipsychotic doses.

There have been a few studies on the efficacy of hypnotics in stable schizophrenic patients. A small study on six chronic schizophrenic men showed that switching from benzodiazepines to zopiclone reduced stage 1 and increased stage 2 sleep, improved total scores on the Brief Psychiatric Rating Scale and reduced negative symptom scores (Naofumi et al. 1994). However, this study used 15 mg of zopiclone which is higher than the current recommended maximum dose. A larger study of 39 stable patients with schizophrenia or schizoaffective disorder who were randomized to either eszopiclone 3 mg or placebo showed greater improvements in the Insomnia Severity Index in the eszopiclone group, though there was no significant difference in their sleep diary data. The eszopiclone group also demonstrated improvements in cognitive function. Once the active drug was stopped, the improvement in sleep was maintained, but the cognitive improvements receded (Tek et al. 2014).

Evidence pointing to reduced levels of melatonin in schizophrenics has led to interest in melatonin to improve sleep in this population. In a randomized, double-blind, crossover trial of 19 patients with schizophrenia, 2 mg of slow-release melatonin for 3 weeks was shown to improve actigraphically measured sleep efficiency. The improvement was only seen in those patients who had poor sleep efficiency at baseline (Shamir et al. 2000). A placebo-controlled trial of 40 stable schizophrenic patients using 3–12 mg melatonin over 15 nights showed subjective improvements in sleep quality and continuity as well as increased total sleep time without any daytime hangover (Suresh Kumar et al. 2007). Given the favourable side effect profile of melatonin, and the relative paucity of interactions with other drugs, it may be sensible to consider this as a first-line treatment for insomnia in stable schizophrenic patients.

8.6.3   Bipolar Disorder

Prescribing for insomnia in bipolar disorder is complicated by the fact that what may be effective, for example, in the depressive phase, may not be effective in the manic or euthymic phases. In addition, as poor sleep may precipitate a manic episode (Wehr et al. 1987), it makes the management of insomnia more urgent than it might otherwise be. Once again, the principle of using as few medications as possible applies, particularly as it is not uncommon for bipolar patients to be on multiple medications to manage their underlying condition. As many mood stabilizers have sedation as a side effect, it makes sense, where possible, to load these medications at night.

A small placebo-controlled study of ramelteon 8 mg in patients with mild to moderate mania and sleep disturbance did not find any improvement in sleep though the study may have been underpowered (McElroy et al. 2011). Disappointing results for ramelteon were also found in a retrospective study (Schaffer et al. 2011) though this study did not differentiate between the different phases of the bipolar disorder. The same study found that zolpidem, zolpidem controlled release (CR) and eszopiclone were generally safe and effective. However, a more recent placebo-controlled trial of ramelteon in euthymic bipolar patients experiencing sleep difficulties (but not primary insomnia) showed that subjects on ramelteon were half as likely to relapse during the 24-week study period as those on placebo. Interestingly, there was not a significant difference between the groups on the Pittsburgh Sleep Quality Index (PSQI), though the authors postulate that this may have been due to the patients being on other sedative psychotropic drugs (Norris et al. 2013). It is also possible that the ramelteon acted not as a sleep inducer but as a circadian rhythm stabilizer.

There has been more work done on the treatment of insomnia in bipolar depression. A retrospective study of bipolar patients attending a lithium clinic showed that, despite being on a mood stabilizer, patients prescribed sedative antidepressants for their insomnia had a greater risk of manic relapse. Those patients prescribed anxiolytic or benzodiazepine agonist medication for their insomnia had a lower risk of relapse and longer periods of mood stability (Saiz-Ruiz et al. 1994).

Quetiapine has a small evidence base for improving sleep in bipolar depression. A post hoc analysis of the BOLDER (BipOLar DEpRession) I and II trials which examined quetiapine monotherapy at fixed doses of 300 or 600 mg showed significant improvements in the PSQI at days 29 and 57 in patients on quetiapine relative to those on placebo (Endicott et al. 2008). As the PSQI changes correlated with improvements in depressive and anxiety symptoms, it is not possible to determine if the improvements in sleep were due to a hypnotic effect of the drug or due to a general improvement in well-being (Anderson and Vande Griend 2014). Data from the EMBOLDEN (Efficacy of Monotherapy Seroquel in BipOLar DEpressioN) II also showed an improvement in sleep on quetiapine 300 and 600 mg vs. paroxetine or placebo (McElroy et al. 2010). Once again, the nature of the study makes it difficult to determine the mechanism and exact nature of this improvement.

8.6.4 Anxiety Disorders and Post-traumatic Stress Disorder

Despite the fact that panic attacks commonly arise from sleep and can lead to insomnia, there have been no studies looking specifically at treating insomnia in this population, though the nocturnal symptoms do appear to respond to the psychotropic drugs prescribed for panic disorder (Krystal et al. 2017).

Sleep in generalized anxiety disorder (GAD) has been better studied. A placebo-controlled trial of quetiapine XR in GAD demonstrated significant improvements in the PSQI in the quetiapine XR group relative to the placebo group. As there was no active comparator in this study, it is difficult to know if this was due to global improvements in the GAD (Sheehan et al. 2013). A trial in GAD patients comparing quazepam 15–30 mg with triazolam 0.25–0.5 mg over 4 weeks demonstrated reduced sleep onset latency for quazepam but not triazolam. Sleep efficiency was initially improved with both drugs; this improvement was maintained for quazepam, but tolerance developed to the triazolam, and thus this effect was lost with time. Rebound insomnia was only observed in the first night after stopping triazolam. Both drugs improved anxiety which remained improved during a 2-week posttreatment placebo period (Saletu et al. 1994). In contrast to this, a study comparing zopiclone and triazolam with placebo in GAD did find that triazolam was superior to placebo for sleep onset latency. However, the triazolam group experienced increased inter-dose anxiety, and other sleep improvements did not reach significance. Zopiclone was significantly better than placebo on most sleep parameters, and, while there was inter-dose anxiety, it was not as severe as with triazolam (Fontaine et al. 1990).

A large multicentre double-blind, placebo-controlled study of zolpidem extended release in combination with open-label escitalopram in patients with GAD and insomnia found significant improvements in total sleep time over an 8-week study period in the zolpidem group. It did not, however, have any effect on anxiety levels (Fava et al. 2009). Conversely, in a previous study of similar design with eszopiclone and escitalopram in GAD, the eszopiclone group not only experienced significantly better sleep and daytime function but also experienced a greater reduction in anxiety and a more rapid response to the escitalopram. After 8 weeks the eszopiclone was withdrawn, and sleep, though still improved, was no longer significantly different from the placebo group. However, the differences in anxiety measures were maintained even after eszopiclone discontinuation (Pollack et al. 2008). This raises the question as to whether eszopiclone has specific antianxiety action that is lacking in zolpidem. In both the above studies, the hypnotics were generally well tolerated, efficacy was maintained across the 8 weeks of the study, and rebound insomnia was not a significant problem on withdrawing the drug.

Post-traumatic stress disorder (PTSD) commonly presents with both insomnia and nightmares. Indeed, sleep disturbance can predict the onset of PTSD following trauma, and treating these sleep symptoms may have beneficial effects on daytime symptoms. While some sleep symptoms may respond to antidepressants alone, insomnia can be exacerbated by some antidepressants, and more targeted therapy for the insomnia is often warranted (Lipinska et al. 2016).

There is some evidence for the use of trazodone to reduce both nightmares and insomnia in PTSD (James and Mendelson 2004), and our clinical experience with this medication is that it can be useful in these patients. As priapism is a potential side effect of this medication, one should warn patients about it and discontinue the drug if it occurs. As improvement in insomnia symptoms can correlate with the reduction in nightmares (Warner et al. 2001), it is possible that specifically targeting nightmares, for example, with prazosin (Singh et al. 2016), may improve insomnia. Similarly, there is low-level evidence that clonidine can reduce nightmares and sleep complaints (Lipinska et al. 2016).

Olanzapine and risperidone have been shown to reduce sleep-related symptoms of PTSD when taken in combination with SSRIs but seem to be less effective when taken as monotherapy. There is also some evidence for the use of quetiapine (Lipinska et al. 2016).

Perhaps surprisingly, evidence for the efficacy of benzodiazepines in improving sleep in PTSD is lacking. In fact, alprazolam and clonazepam were not shown to be superior to placebo (Lipinska et al. 2016). However, a brief trial of eszopiclone demonstrated improvements in sleep latency and PSQI scores relative to placebo (Pollack et al. 2011).

8.6.5 Major Depressive Disorder

Patients with depression have high rates of insomnia (Benca 2008) which can persist once the depression has resolved (Buysse 2008). There is an increased awareness of the need to treat insomnia as a disorder comorbid with, rather than secondary to depression. The situation is complicated by the fact that many commonly used antidepressants exacerbate insomnia, and therefore one either needs to choose antidepressants with sedation as a side effect to minimize the risk of insomnia or have a strategy to manage this insomnia.

It is common in clinical practice to prescribe benzodiazepine receptor agonist hypnotics in combination with antidepressants, particularly in the early stages of treatment. Multiple studies have found this approach to be effective at improving patients' sleep without interfering with the effect of the antidepressant (Howland 2011). In fact, eszopiclone led to improvements in sleep and an improved response to fluoxetine in depressed patients, an effect that has not been found with other non-benzodiazepine hypnotics (Fava et al. 2006). Although studies have found benefit in combining antidepressants with benzodiazepine hypnotics, both in terms of sleep and antidepressant response (Jindal 2009), it is unclear to what extent the anxiolytic action of the benzodiazepines is responsible for this effect.

Monotherapy of both depression and insomnia is often a desirable treatment strategy as it reduces the risk of drug interactions, as well as the cost and complexity of the treatment regime. Amitriptyline and trimipramine have been shown to improve mood and sleep in patients with depression and insomnia (Jindal 2009). However, this must be balanced against the relatively high burden of side effects with these tricyclic antidepressants.

Agomelatine, which has melatonin agonist properties, has some data to support its use in depression with disrupted sleep. It appears to improve subjective and objective measures of sleep and does so very early on in the treatment (Quera-Salva et al. 2010). However, it is important to note that these improvements were demonstrated primarily in studies comparing agomelatine to SSRIs and SNRIs, which are known to be disruptive to sleep, particularly in the early stages of treatment. Nevertheless it may be a useful option if further sleep disruption in the early stages of treatment is undesirable.

Mirtazapine leads to early improvements in sleep continuity and increases in slow-wave sleep in depressed patients. There is some debate about whether these improvements are maintained relative to other antidepressants in the long term; however, the rapid improvement in sleep is clearly an advantage (Jindal 2009). It can also be prescribed in combination with other antidepressants such as SSRIs and so is sometimes used to manage the insomnia associated with these drugs as well as providing additional antidepressant action. While mirtazapine is sedative and can therefore improve insomnia, its antihistaminergic activity can exacerbate restless legs. Therefore, before prescribing mirtazapine in depressed patients with insomnia, one should exclude restless legs as the cause of their insomnia.

Trazodone is widely prescribed off label for the management of insomnia in some countries. It has very little abuse potential and a relatively short half-life (Stahl 2009), and it may be combined with other antidepressants to reduce the burden of insomnia. It is less liable to produce weight gain than mirtazapine and is generally well tolerated (Stahl 2014). Although it does have some histamine antagonist properties, our clinical experience is that exacerbation of restless legs is rarely a problem. It appears to be a good choice of antidepressant in patients with depression and sleep disturbances (Fagiolini 2012).

8.6.6 Dementia

Sleep disturbance in patients with dementia presents a unique and complex challenge. In addition to the impact of the dementia itself, one also needs to bear in mind the complexities of prescribing in adults who are likely to have multiple comorbidities and are on multiple medications. Furthermore, sleep disturbance in home-dwelling patients with dementia leads to sleep disruption for their families and is a source of great distress; it can lead to depression in carers and is a frequent trigger for the decision to move the patient out of the community into a care home (Cipriani et al. 2015). It is therefore tempting to consider hypnotics in this group to allow them to stay at home longer and delay the necessity for nursing home admission. On the other hand, it is questionable whether hypnotics should be used to manage behavioural symptoms if the patient is not distressed by their night-time wakefulness.

There are also a number of issues which relate to hypnotic prescribing in elderly patients in general which apply to elderly patients with dementia. The first is that their clearance of most drugs is likely to be reduced leading to prolonged half-lives and higher risk of overdose or unwanted daytime sedation. It should be noted that this is not unique to benzodiazepine receptor agonists but is just as true of sedative antidepressants. Therefore, starting at the lowest possible dose is always wise, as is having frequent breaks from the medication.

One of the biggest concerns in this population is the risk of falls, and there is a significant body of evidence that sedative medication use is associated with increased falls, presumably due to sedation, hypotension and impairments in concentration, coordination and reaction time (Kozono et al. 2016). One criticism of the data linking hypnotics with falls is that studies have generally not examined the temporal relationship between administration of the drug and the falls. There is also evidence that insomnia itself is a risk factor for falls (Avidan et al. 2005; Walsh 2017). It is therefore possible that, in some patients, the risk of falls when wandering unsupervised at night may outweigh the risk from the medication, though the relative risks are difficult to quantify.

Unfortunately the available evidence with regard to medical management of insomnia in this population has failed to generate any consistent results. To some extent this is to be expected as the causes of insomnia in these patients are likely to be as varied as in non-demented patients but with the added burden of the neurodegenerative process, the loss of daytime activities and time cues and the increased burden of comorbid medical and psychiatric disorders. It can be difficult, for example, in more advanced cases to differentiate between insomnia and restless legs, and it is possible that some of the negative studies included patients with restless legs who were less likely to respond to insomnia medication.

Given the relatively benign side effect profile of melatonin and the fact that melatonin levels decline with age, there has been a great deal of interest in the use of melatonin for sleep disturbance in patients with dementia (Cipriani et al. 2015). Certainly, 2 mg of prolonged release melatonin has been shown to improve sleep onset latency, sleep quality and daytime symptoms in older adults without dementia (Wade et al. 2007) and does not impair postural stability within the first 4h of dosing (Otmani et al. 2012). However, findings in dementia have been contradictory. For example, in patients with Alzheimer's disease, 3 mg of melatonin increased sleep time and reduced night-time activity, but this did not translate into noticeable daytime improvements in activity levels, napping or cognition (Asayama et al. 2003). However, given the risk of wandering and of falls in this population, the reduced night-time activity may be a desirable outcome in itself. But another study showed no benefit of 6 mg slow-release melatonin in dementia patients; however, it should be noted that this study included patients with vascular and Lewy body dementia as well as Alzheimer's (Serfaty et al. 2002).

A common practice is to treat insomnia in dementia patients with sedative antidepressants as they are perceived to be safer. However, this is not necessarily the case. Antidepressants tend to have longer half-lives and can lead to significant daytime sedation, they may have anticholinergic effects which impair cognition further, and many have considerable cardiovascular side effects such as hypotension which can raise the risk of falls. There is also scant evidence that they work in this population.

Overall, it is recommended that behavioural interventions such as limiting daytime naps, exposure to bright light during the day and avoidance of bright light at night should be the first line in treating insomnia in dementia (Neikrug and Ancoli-Israel 2010); however, there may be times when medication is warranted. Despite the contradictory evidence, it is probably wise to use melatonin as a first line given its relatively mild side effect profile. If stronger drugs are required, one should aim to use shorter-acting drugs to minimize daytime side effects. However, it is vital to monitor the response to the medication early in the treatment and review it frequently. If the medication is ineffective, one runs the risk of having a patient who is sedated by the medication but still ambulant at night, and this is likely to raise the risk of falls even more.

8.6.7 Substance Misuse Disorders

Insomnia can be a symptom of both active substance misuse and withdrawal. For example, in alcohol misuse, the prevalence of insomnia is high in both active and abstinent drinkers (Zhabenko et al. 2012; Cohn et al. 2003). Many alcohol misusers may be using that substance to self-medicate their insomnia, and insomnia is a risk factor for relapse following abstinence (Brower et al. 2001). The impact of sedative or stimulant substances on sleep is complex and variable, and this makes it difficult to draw generalized conclusions about the optimum strategy for medicating insomnia in substance misusers. However, there are a few issues which are common to most patients with substance misuse disorders.

The first issue that often arises is whether the use of hypnotic medication is contraindicated due to the risk of addiction to that medication. In patients who have a history of addiction, one wants to avoid adding to the burden of addictions. There is a perception that hypnotic drugs are highly addictive, though this is not borne out by the evidence (Wilson et al. 2010); however, the risks may be higher in substance misusers.

In some cases one may choose to take a harm minimization approach. For example, if a patient is drinking to try to sleep, then it may be safer for them to be prescribed a sleep medication as it is less likely to have adverse physical and psychosocial effects than excessive alcohol. If this approach is taken, one must ensure that the patient stops using the alcohol when they start the medication as the combination of alcohol or drugs with hypnotics carries significant risk. Selecting the patients who will benefit from this strategy can be difficult, but a helpful indicator may be the pattern of their substance use. If they are taking a sedative substance at night only, then it is more likely that they are self-medicating for insomnia and may significantly reduce their substance use if prescribed a sleep-promoting medication. However, patients that use a sedative substance throughout the day are less likely to be using it purely for sleep and may therefore be less likely to stop that substance if given a hypnotic.

The other approach is to utilize other sleep-promoting drugs, such as sedative antidepressants, which may be less likely to lead to dependence. Trazodone is widely used to treat insomnia in substance misuse clinics. However, a study of trazodone 50–150 mg in patients with sleep disturbance undergoing alcohol detoxification showed that, while it did improve sleep, it was also associated with fewer days' abstinence and more alcohol consumed on non-abstinent days than placebo (Friedmann 2008).

8.6.8 Learning Disability

Given the very wide range of conditions within the category of learning disability, it is difficult to make general statements about the management of insomnia in this group. There are very few controlled trials in the field; however, melatonin has the strongest evidence base (Wilson et al. 2010). Indeed, melatonin has been shown to be effective at improving not only insomnia symptoms but, at 5 mg in adults and 2.5 mg in children, can reduce daytime challenging behaviour, presumably as a result of the improved sleep (Braam et al. 2010).

Special mention should be made of Smith-Magenis syndrome, a syndrome caused by interstitial deletions of chromosome 17p11.2. These patients have a reversal of their melatonin rhythm with melatonin being secreted during the day and very disrupted sleep at night. These patients can be successfully treated with an evening dose of slow-release melatonin and a morning dose of acebutolol, as β-blockers inhibit melatonin secretion (De Leersnyder et al. 2003).

Choosing a medication in adults with learning disabilities need not necessarily be much different from the process in other adults. The particular cause of the learning disability is only one factor in that patient's insomnia. The choice may therefore be dictated as much by the type of insomnia, the side effects acceptable to the patient and the desired half-life of the drug as by the learning disability.

References

Anderson SL, Vande Griend JP. Quetiapine for insomnia: a review of the literature. Am J Health Syst Pharm. 2014;71(5):394–402.

Asayama K, et al. Double blind study of melatonin effects on the sleep-wake rhythm, cognitive and non-cognitive functions in Alzheimer type dementia. J Nippon Med Sch. 2003;70(4):334–41.

Avidan AY, et al. Insomnia and hypnotic use, recorded in the minimum data set, as predictors of falls and hip fractures in Michigan nursing homes. J Am Geriatr Soc. 2005;53(6):955–62.

Baandrup L, et al. Prolonged-release melatonin versus placebo for benzodiazepine discontinuation in patients with schizophrenia or bipolar disorder: a randomised, placebo-controlled, blinded trial. World J Biol Psychiatry. 2015;17:1–11.

Baglioni C, et al. Insomnia as a predictor of depression: a meta-analytic evaluation of longitudinal epidemiological studies. J Affect Disord. 2011;135(1–3):10–9.

Bateson AN. Basic pharmacologic mechanisms involved in benzodiazepine tolerance and withdrawal. Curr Pharm Des. 2002;8:5–21.

Benca RM, Peterson MJ. Insomnia and depression. Sleep Med. 2008;9(1):3–9. https://doi.org/10.1016/S1389-9457(08)70010-8.

Benson KL. Sleep in schizophrenia. Sleep Med Clin. 2008;3(2):251–60.

Bélanger L, Belleville G, Morin C. Management of hypnotic discontinuation in chronic insomnia. Sleep Med Clin. 2009;4(4):583–92. https://doi.org/10.1016/j.jsmc.2009.07.011.

Booth JN III, Behring M, Cantor RS, et al. Zolpidem use and motor vehicle collisions in older drivers. Sleep Med. 2016;20:98–102.

Braam W, et al. Melatonin decreases daytime challenging behaviour in persons with intellectual disability and chronic insomnia. J Intellect Disabil Res. 2010;54(1):52–9. https://doi.org/10.1111/j.1365-2788.2009.01223.x.

Brisbare-Roch C, Dingemanse J, Koberstein R, et al. Promotion of sleep by targeting the orexin system in rats, dogs and humans. Nat Med. 2007;13:150–5.

Brower KJ, et al. Insomnia, self-medication, and relapse to alcoholism. Am J Psychiatr. 2001;158(3):399–404.

Buysse DJ, et al. Prevalence, course, and comorbidity of insomnia and depression in young adults. Sleep. 2008;31(4):473–80. https://doi.org/10.5167/uzh-10110.

Cajochen C, Krauchi K, Wirz-Justice A. Role of melatonin in the regulation of human circadian rhythms and sleep. J Neuroendocrinol. 2003;15:432–7.

Cardinali DP, et al. A double blind-placebo controlled study on melatonin efficacy to reduce anxiolytic benzodiazepine use in the elderly. Neuroendocrinol Lett. 2002;23(1):55–60.

Cipriani G, et al. Sleep disturbances and dementia. Psychogeriatrics. 2015;15(1):65–74.

Cohn T, Foster J, Peters T. Sequential studies of sleep disturbance and quality of life in abstaining alcoholics. Addict Biol. 2003;8(4):455–62.

De Leersnyder H, et al. Beta 1-adrenergic antagonists and melatonin reset the clock and restore sleep in a circadian disorder, Smith-Magenis syndrome. J Med Genet. 2003;40(1):74–8. Available at: http://www.pubmedcentral.nih.gov/articlerender.fcgi?artid=1735264&tool=pmcentrez&rendertype=abstract

Dijk DJ, von Schantz M. Timing and consolidation of human sleep, wakefulness, and performance by a symphony of oscillators. J Biol Rhythm. 2005;20:279–90.

Endicott J, et al. Quetiapine monotherapy in the treatment of depressive episodes of bipolar I and II disorder: improvements in quality of life and quality of sleep. J Affect Disord. 2008;111(2–3):306–19.

Fagiolini A, et al. Rediscovering trazodone for the treatment of major depressive disorder. CNS Drugs. 2012;26(12):1033–49.

Fava M, McCall WV, Krystal A, et al. Eszopiclone co-administered with fluoxetine in patients with insomnia coexisting with major depressive disorder. Biol Psychiatry. 2006;59(11):1052e60.

Fava M, et al. Zolpidem extended-release improves sleep and next-day symptoms in comorbid insomnia and generalized anxiety disorder. J Clin Psychopharmacol. 2009;29(3):222–30.

Fava M, Asnis GM, Shrivastava RK, et al. Improved insomnia symptoms and sleep-related next-day functioning in patients with comorbid major depressive disorder and insomnia following concomitant zolpidem extended-release 12.5 mg and escitalopram treatment: a randomized controlled trial. J Clin Psychiatry. 2011;72(7):914–28.

Fontaine R, et al. Zopiclone and triazolam in insomnia associated with generalized anxiety disorder: a placebo-controlled evaluation of efficacy and daytime anxiety. Int Clin Psychopharmacol. 1990;5(3):173–83.

Friedmann PD. Trazodone for sleep disturbance after alcohol detoxification: a double blind, placebo-controlled trial. Alcohol Clin Exp Res. 2008;32:1652.

Greenblatt DJ, Legangneux E, Harmatz JS, et al. Dynamics and kinetics of a modified-release formulation of zolpidem: comparison with immediate-release standard zolpidem and placebo. J Clin Pharmacol. 2006;46:1469–80.

Haffmans PMJ, et al. The effect of risperidone versus haloperidol on sleep patterns of schizophrenic patients — results of a double-blind, randomised pilot trial. Eur Neuropsychopharmacol. 2001;11:S260.

Hajak G, Hedner J, Eglin M, et al. A 2-week efficacy and safety study of gaboxadol and zolpidem using electronic diaries in primary insomnia outpatients. Sleep Med. 2009;10:705–12.

Howland RH. Sleep interventions for the treatment of depression. J Psychosoc Nurs Ment Health Serv. 2011;49:17–20. https://doi.org/10.3928/02793695-20101208–01.

James SP, Mendelson WB. The use of trazodone as a hypnotic: a critical review. J Clin Psychiatry. 2004;65(6):752–5.

Jindal RD. Insomnia in patients with depression: some pathophysiological and treatment considerations. CNS Drugs. 2009;23(4):309–29.

Katz D, McHorney C. The relationship between insomnia and health-related quality of life in patients with chronic illness. J Fam Pract. 2002;51(3):229–35.

Kozono A, et al. Relationship of prescribed drugs with the risk of fall in inpatients. Yakugaku Zasshi. 2016;136(5):769–76. Available at: http://www.ncbi.nlm.nih.gov/pubmed/27150933. Accessed 5 June 2017

Krystal AD, Stein MB, Szabo ST. Chapter 136 – Anxiety disorders and posttraumatic stress disorder. In: Kryger M, Roth T, Dement W, editors. Principles and practice of sleep medicine. Philadelphia: Saunders; 2017. p. 1341–51.

Landolt HP, Retey JV, Tonz K, et al. Caffeine attenuates waking and sleep electroencephalographic markers of sleep homeostasis in humans. Neuropsychopharmacology. 2004;29:1933–9.

Leufkens TRM, Vermeeren A. Zopiclone's residual effects on actual driving performance in a standardized test: a pooled analysis of age and sex effects in 4 placebo-controlled studies. Clin Ther. 2014;36(1):141–50.

Lipinska G, Baldwin DS, Thomas KGF. Pharmacology for sleep disturbance in PTSD. Hum Psychopharmacol Clin Exp. 2016;31(2):156–63.

Luthringer R, et al. A double-blind, placebo-controlled, randomized study evaluating the effect of paliperidone extended-release tablets on sleep architecture in patients with schizophrenia. Int Clin Psychopharmacol. 2007;22(5):299–308.

Luyster FS, et al. Comorbid insomnia and obstructive sleep apnea: challenges for clinical practice and research. J Clin Sleep Med. 2010;6(2):196–204.

Manber R, Chambers AS. Insomnia and depression: a multifaceted interplay. Curr Psychiatry Rep. 2009;11(6):437–42.

McElroy SL, et al. A double-blind, placebo-controlled study of quetiapine and paroxetine as monotherapy in adults with bipolar depression (EMBOLDEN II). J Clin Psychiatry. 2010;71(2):163–74.

McElroy SL, et al. A randomized, placebo-controlled study of adjunctive ramelteon in ambulatory bipolar I disorder with manic symptoms and sleep disturbance. Int Clin Psychopharmacol. 2011;26(1):48–53.

Morgan K, et al. Psychological treatment for insomnia in the management of long-term hypnotic drug use: a pragmatic randomised controlled trial. Br J Gen Pract. 2003;53(497):923–8.

Morin CM, et al. Cognitive behavior therapy to facilitate benzodiazepine discontinuation among hypnotic-dependent patients with insomnia. Behav Ther. 1995;26(4):733–45.

Murphy SM, Tyrer P. A double-blind comparison of the effects of gradual withdrawal of lorazepam, diazepam and bromazepam in benzodiazepine dependence. Br J Psychiatry. 1991;158:511–6.

Nakamura T, Hayashi Y, Watabe H, et al. Estimation of organ cumulated activities and absorbed doses on intakes of several 11C labelled radiopharmaceuticals from external measurement with thermoluminescent dosimeters. Phys Med Biol. 1998;43:389–405.

Naofumi K, et al. Effects of zopiclone on sleep and symptoms in schizophrenia: comparison with benzodiazepine hypnotics. Prog Neuro-Psychopharmacol Biol Psychiatry. 1994;18(3):477–90.

Neckelmann D, Mykletun A, Dahl AA. Chronic insomnia as a risk factor for developing anxiety and depression. Sleep. 2007;30(7):873–80.

Neikrug AB, Ancoli-Israel S. Sleep disorders in the older adult - a mini-review. Gerontology. 2010;56(2):181–9.

Norris ER, et al. A double-blind, randomized, placebo-controlled trial of adjunctive ramelteon for the treatment of insomnia and mood stability in patients with euthymic bipolar disorder. J Affect Disord. 2013;144(1–2):141–7.

Nutt DJ. Death by tricyclic: the real antidepressant scandal? J Psychopharmacol. 2005;19:123–4.

Otmani S, et al. Effects of prolonged-release melatonin and zolpidem on postural stability in older adults. Hum Psychopharmacol Clin Exp. 2012;27(3):270–6.

Paterson LM, Wilson SJ, Nutt DJ, et al. A translational, caffeine-induced model of onset insomnia in rats and healthy volunteers. Psychopharmacology. 2007;191:943–50.

Pigeon WR, Hegel M, Unützer J, et al. Is insomnia a perpetuating factor for late-life depression in the IMPACT cohort? Sleep. 2008;31:481–8.

Pollack M, Kinrys G, Krystal A, et al. Eszopiclone co-administered with escitalopram in patients with insomnia and comorbid generalized anxiety disorder. Arch Gen Psychiatry. 2008;65(5):551–62.

Pollack MH, et al. Eszopiclone for the treatment of posttraumatic stress disorder and associated insomnia: a randomized, double-blind, placebo-controlled trial. J Clin Psychiatry. 2011;72(7):892–7.

Porkka-Heiskanen T, Alanko L, Kalinchuk A, et al. Adenosine and sleep. Sleep Med Rev. 2002;6:321–32.

Quera-Salva M-A, Lemoine P, Guilleminault C. Impact of the novel antidepressant agomelatine on disturbed sleep-wake cycles in depressed patients. Hum Psychopharmacol Clin Exp. 2010;25(3):222–9. Available at: http://www.ncbi.nlm.nih.gov/pubmed/20373473. Accessed 9 Mar 2017

Reynolds CF III, Buysse DJ, Miller MD, et al. Paroxetine treatment of primary insomnia in older adults. Am J Geriatr Psychiatry. 2006;14:803–7.

Riemann D, Perlis ML. The treatments of chronic insomnia: a review of benzodiazepine receptor agonists and psychological and behavioral therapies. Sleep Med Rev. 2009;13(3):205–14.

Riemann D, Voderholzer U, Cohrs S, et al. Trimipramine in primary insomnia: results of a polysomnographic double-blind controlled study. Pharmacopsychiatry. 2002;35:165–74.

Roth T, Eklov SD, Drake CL, Verster JC. Meta-analysis of on the road experimental studies of hypnotics: effects of time after intake, dose, and half-life. Traffic Inj Prev. 2014;15(5):439–45.

Saiz-Ruiz J, Cebollada A, Ibañez A. Sleep disorders in bipolar depression: hypnotics vs sedative antidepressants. J Psychosom Res. 1994;38:55–60.

Saletu B, et al. Insomnia in generalized anxiety disorder: polysomnographic, psychometric and clinical investigations before, during and after therapy with a long- versus a short-half-life benzodiazepine (quazepam versus triazolam). Neuropsychobiology. 1994;29(2):69–90.

Salin-Pascual RJ, Herrera-Estrella M, Galicia-Polo L, et al. Olanzapine acute administration in schizophrenic patients increases delta sleep and sleep efficiency. Biol Psychiatry. 1999;46:141–3.

Samuels ER, Szabadi E. Functional neuroanatomy of the noradrenergic locus coeruleus: its roles in the regulation of arousal and autonomic function. Part II: Physiological and pharmacological manipulations and pathological alterations of locus coeruleus activity in humans. Curr Neuropharmacol. 2008;6:254–85.

Saper CB, Scammell TE, Lu J. Hypothalamic regulation of sleep and circadian rhythms. Nature. 2005;437:1257–63.

Schaffer CB, et al. Efficacy and safety of nonbenzodiazepine hypnotics for chronic insomnia in patients with bipolar disorder. J Affect Disord. 2011;128(3):305–8.

Serfaty M, et al. Double blind randomised placebo controlled trial of low dose melatonin for sleep disorders in dementia. Int J Geriatr Psychiatry. 2002;17(12):1120–7. Available at: http://doi.wiley.com/10.1002/gps.760. Accessed 27 Apr 2017

Shamir E, et al. Melatonin improves sleep quality of patients with chronic schizophrenia. J Clin Psychiatry. 2000;61(5):373–7.

Sheehan DV, et al. Effects of extended-release quetiapine fumarate on long-term functioning and sleep quality in patients with Generalized Anxiety Disorder (GAD): data from a randomized-withdrawal, placebo-controlled maintenance study. J Affect Disord. 2013;151(3):906–13.

Singh B, Hughes AJ, Mehta G, et al. Efficacy of prazosin in posttraumatic stress disorder: a systematic review and meta-analysis. Prim Care Companion CNS Disord. 2016. https://doi.org/10.4088/PCC.16r01943.

Soldatos CR, Dikeos DG, Whitehead A. Tolerance and rebound insomnia with rapidly eliminated hypnotics: a meta-analysis of sleep laboratory studies. Int Clin Psychopharmacol. 1999;14:287–303.

Stahl SM. Mechanism of action of trazodone: a multifunctional drug. CNS Spectr. 2009;14(10):536–46.

Stahl SM. Stahl's essential psychopharmacology: prescriber's guide. 2014. Available at: http://www.cambridge.org/ro/titles/prescribers-guide-stahls-essential-psychopharmacology-5th-edition/. Accessed 9 Mar 2017.

Staner L, Ertle S, Boeijinga P, et al. Next-day residual effects of hypnotics in DSM-IV primary insomnia: a driving simulator study with simultaneous electroencephalogram monitoring. Psychopharmacology. 2005;181:790–8.

Suresh Kumar PN, et al. Melatonin in schizophrenic outpatients with insomnia: a double-blind, placebo-controlled study. J Clin Psychiatry. 2007;68(2):237–41.

Tek C, et al. The impact of eszopiclone on sleep and cognition in patients with schizophrenia and insomnia: a double-blind, randomized, placebo-controlled trial. Schizophr Res. 2014;160(1):180–5.

Trewin VF, Lawrence CJ, Veitch GB. An investigation of the association of benzodiazepines and other hypnotics with the incidence of falls in the elderly. J Clin Pharm Ther. 1992;17:129–33.

Verster JC, van de Loo AJAE. Chapter 46 – Effects of hypnotic drugs on driving performance. In: Kryger M, Roth T, Dement W, editors. Principles and practice of sleep medicine. Philadelphia: Saunders; 2017. p. 499–505.e3.

Voderholzer U, Riemann D, Hornyak M, et al. A double-blind, randomized and placebo-controlled study on the polysomnographic withdrawal effects of zopiclone, zolpidem and triazolam in healthy subjects. Eur Arch Psychiatry Clin Neurosci. 2001;251:117–23.

Wade AG, et al. Efficacy of prolonged release melatonin in insomnia patients aged 55–80 years: quality of sleep and next-day alertness outcomes. Curr Med Res Opin. 2007;23(10):2597–605. Available at: http://www.tandfonline.com/doi/full/10.1185/030079907X233098. Accessed 5 June 2017

Walsh JK. Chapter 87 – Pharmacologic treatment of insomnia: benzodiazepine receptor agonists. In: Kryger M, Roth T, Dement W, editors. Principles and practice of sleep medicine. Philadelphia: Saunders; 2017. p. 832–841.e4.

Walsh JK, Erman M, Erwin CW, et al. Subjective hypnotic efficacy of trazodone and zolpidem in DSM-III-R primary insomnia. Human Psychopharmacol Clin Exp. 1998;13:191–8.

Walsh JK, Pollak CP, Scharf MB, et al. Lack of residual sedation following middle-of-the-night zaleplon administration in sleep maintenance insomnia. Clin Neuropharmacol. 2000;23:17–21.

Warner MD, Dorn MR, Peabody CA. Survey on the usefulness of trazodone in patients with PTSD with insomnia or nightmares. Pharmacopsychiatry. 2001;34(4):128–31.

Wehr TA, Sack DA, Rosenthal NE. Sleep reduction as a final common pathway in the genesis of mania. Am J Psychiatry. 1987;144(2):201–4.

Wilson SJ, et al. British Association for Psychopharmacology consensus statement on evidence-based treatment of insomnia, parasomnias and circadian rhythm disorders. J Psychopharmacol (Oxford, England). 2010;24(11):1577–601.

Woznica AA, et al. The insomnia and suicide link: toward an enhanced understanding of this relationship. Sleep Med Rev. 2015;22:37–46.

Wright A, et al. The effect of melatonin on benzodiazepine discontinuation and sleep quality in adults attempting to discontinue benzodiazepines: a systematic review and meta-analysis. Drugs Aging. 2015;32(12):1009–18.

Xiang Y-T, et al. Prevalence and correlates of insomnia and its impact on quality of life in Chinese schizophrenia patients. Sleep. 2009;32(1):105–9.

Yamashita H, et al. Influence of aging on the improvement of subjective sleep quality by atypical antipsychotic drugs in patients with schizophrenia: comparison of middle-aged and older adults. Am J Geriatr Psychiatry. 2005;13(5):377–84.

Zhabenko N, Wojnar M, Brower KJ. Prevalence and correlates of insomnia in a polish sample of alcohol-dependent patients. Alcohol Clin Exp Res. 2012;36(9):1600–7. Available at: http://www.ncbi.nlm.nih.gov/pubmed/22471339. Accessed 27 Apr 2017

Cognitive Behaviour Therapy for Insomnia in Co-morbid Psychiatric Disorders

9

David O'Regan

9.1 Introduction

Whilst the link between insomnia and psychopathology has long been observed, our understanding of their dynamic relationship is continually evolving. The vast majority of insomnia—the most prevalent sleep disorder in the general population—exists as co-morbid insomnia (Roth and Roehrs 2003). Up to 45% of individuals with insomnia have a co-morbid psychiatric disorder (Sarsour et al. 2010), and up to 86% have a co-morbid medical illness (Taylor et al. 2007a, b). Co-morbid insomnia is therefore the rule rather than the exception. Compared to chronic medical illnesses, psychiatric disorders are more significantly associated with insomnia severity (Sarsour et al. 2010).

Insomnia may increase the risk of developing a psychiatric illness (Baglioni et al. 2011; Ruhrmann et al. 2010), exacerbate its severity and reduce the efficacy of its treatment (e.g. Dew et al. 1997; Thase et al. 1997; Pigeon et al. 2008). Moreover, insomnia can persist long after the co-morbid condition has resolved, only to later precipitate its relapse (Brower et al. 2001; Perlis et al. 1997). Conversely, cognitive and behavioural treatment of the co-morbid insomnia may not only improve the sleep disorder but also the co-morbid psychiatric condition (e.g. Manber et al. 2008; Ulmer et al. 2011; Myers et al. 2011).

The current evidence argues that insomnia should be conceptualized and addressed as a diagnostic entity in its own right, rather than as a symptom of a psychiatric disorder. This chapter reviews the reciprocal interactions between insomnia and psychiatric disorders, particularly depression, post-traumatic stress disorder (PTSD), alcohol dependence and psychosis. We focus on the evidence to support the use of cognitive behavioural therapy for insomnia (CBT-I) in treating co-morbid insomnia, as well as its benefits for co-morbid psychiatric disorders. Finally, we discuss some practical considerations for the implementation of CBT-I in treating co-morbid insomnia.

D. O'Regan
Insomnia Clinic, Royal London Hospital for Integrated Medicine and Sleep Disorders Centre, Guy's and St Thomas' NHS Foundation Trust, London, UK
e-mail: DavidO'Regan@nhs.net

© Springer-Verlag GmbH Germany, part of Springer Nature 2018
H. Selsick (ed.), *Sleep Disorders in Psychiatric Patients*,
https://doi.org/10.1007/978-3-642-54836-9_9

9.1.1 Insomnia as a Co-morbid, Rather Than 'Secondary', Condition

As clinicians, we commonly encounter insomnia symptoms in the context of 'primary' presenting psychiatric disorders. In the UK, our principal diagnostic manual (i.e. the International Classification of Diseases-10) encourages us to conceptualize insomnia as being 'secondary' to, or encapsulated within, the main presenting psychiatric condition. Yet, this tenet of insomnia as always being 'secondary to' or arising from the co-occurring psychiatric disorder is a simplistic one, which remains unvalidated (see Lichstein 2006; Lichstein et al. 2000 for further discussion). Consequently, in the new Diagnostic and Statistical Manual of Mental Disorders-V, primary insomnia has been renamed insomnia disorder in an attempt to avoid this differentiation of 'primary' and 'secondary' insomnia.

In truth, we know surprisingly little about the ways in which insomnia and co-occurring psychiatric conditions interact and affect one another. However, retaining our view of insomnia as a *purely* secondary condition implies that it is therapeutically untouchable until we first resolve the primary condition. Such reasoning is potentially flawed and further runs the risk of doing a disservice to our patients. For example, in the case of depression, it has been shown that insomnia is a common residual symptom amongst patients who have otherwise achieved remission from depression-focused therapy (Carney et al. 2007; Nierenberg et al. 1999). Moreover, we know that insomnia not only adversely affects quality of life but is also an important independent risk factor in developing a further depressive episode (Perlis et al. 1997).

The evolution of insomnia from a 'secondary' condition to a co-morbid one is therefore clinically important. By targeting insomnia in its own right, we may not only resolve the sleep disturbance and its consequences but also promote resolution and prevent relapse of the co-occurring condition. For example, an exciting pilot trial using CBT-I in patients with persistent persecutory delusions and insomnia showed that CBT-I not only reduced the sleep disturbance but also reduced the psychotic symptom load (Myers et al. 2011). Furthermore, the daytime symptoms of insomnia (e.g. fatigue and irritability) may not only act to exacerbate co-morbid mental illness but also adversely interfere with engagement in therapeutic strategies.

9.1.2 Evidence for CBT in the Management of Insomnia with Co-morbid Psychiatric Disorders

Since the 1980s, compelling evidence has gathered strength for the efficacy of CBT-I in the treatment of uncomplicated insomnia, i.e. when it presents as a stand-alone condition. Moreover, CBT-I shows longer-term benefits than pharmacotherapy (Jacobs et al. 2004), has few physical side effects (though fatigue can be troublesome in the initial stages of CBT-I) and is preferred by patients (Vincent and Lionberg 2001). The American Academy of Sleep Medicine's (AASM) task force report summarized that CBT-I in uncomplicated cases is associated with an improvement in 70% of patients and is maintained for at least 6 months post-treatment (Riemann and Perlis 2009; Chesson et al. 1999). Importantly, these improvements are not only seen in sleep parameters but also in daytime functioning.

By contrast, the evidence for CBT-I in treating co-morbid insomnia is in its relative infancy. It was first officially recognized in the 2006 AASM report, which included 11 studies, four of which were randomized controlled trials (Chesson et al. 1999). Notably, these studies demonstrated efficacy for CBT-I when insomnia presented with both psychiatric and medical co-morbidities.

Since 2006, there has been a steady strengthening of the evidence for the efficacy of CBT for the treatment of insomnia occurring with a variety of co-morbid psychiatric disorders. Included in this group are studies focused on specific psychiatric illnesses (e.g. depression, PTSD, alcohol dependence and psychosis), as well as for mixed mental disorders. These are individually discussed later in the chapter.

9.1.3   An Outline of CBT for the Treatment of Chronic Insomnia

A plethora of behavioural and cognitive techniques have been validated for the treatment of chronic insomnia. These include stimulus control, sleep rescheduling, relaxation-based therapy, cognitive therapy and general sleep hygiene and education (Morin et al. 2006a, b).

The techniques are aligned to Spielman's conceptual model of chronic insomnia, i.e. the '3P' model (Spielman et al. 1987). According to this model, several *predisposing* (e.g. anxious personality traits), *precipitating* (e.g. adverse life events, psychiatric illness) and *perpetuating* (e.g. daytime napping, spending excessive time in bed, erratic sleep schedules) factors are involved in the development of insomnia (see Fig. 9.1). Central to the model is the theory that, irrespective of the precipitating

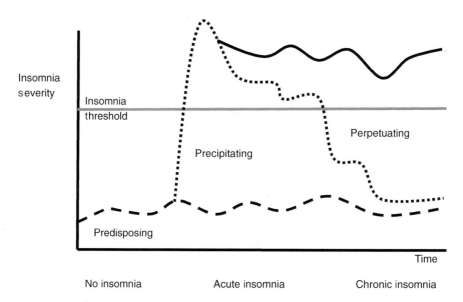

Fig. 9.1 The '3P' model of insomnia. A dynamic version of the conceptual model of insomnia demonstrating how predisposing, precipitating and perpetuating factors combine to initiate and maintain insomnia over time. Adapted from Spielman et al. (1987)

event(s), behavioural and psychological factors develop and act to maintain the insomnia over time. In the specific case of co-morbid insomnia, these maintaining factors may operate independent of the co-morbid psychiatric illness to drive the insomnia. So, even if the co-morbid condition was the original precipitant, insomnia can develop partial or total independence from it.

The different CBT-I techniques mentioned are designed to target the maintaining factors which perpetuate insomnia. In this way, CBT-I does not focus or dwell on the precipitant(s), which some patients find surprising. Figure 9.2 shows how the various behavioural and cognitive techniques strive to tackle the perpetuating factors. These varying techniques are readily integrated into one multimodal treatment package, for example, CBT-I, and have become the mainstay of psychological treatment for insomnia (Edinger and Means 2005). By having so many different techniques within the one treatment package, we stand a greater chance of addressing a wide range of maintaining factors.

In our clinic, we monitor patient progression via the validated Insomnia Severity Index (ISI; Bastien et al. 2001), which is brief and easy to complete. The ISI indicates sleep difficulties involving both day and night functioning and covers the Diagnostic and Statistical Manual of Mental Disorders-IV insomnia criteria. It consists of seven self-rated items evaluating the perceived severity of insomnia on a five-point scale (ranging from 0, i.e. *not at all*, to 4, i.e. *very much*). Total scores range from 0 to 28 and are categorized into 'no clinically significant insomnia' (0–7),

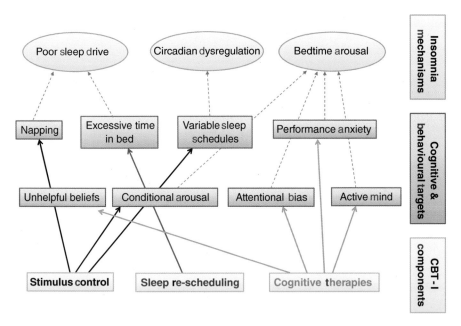

Fig. 9.2 A diagram of how the various components of CBT-I target the perpetuating cognitive and behavioural factors which drive insomnia. Chronic insomnia is postulated to be the result of one or more of poor sleep drive, circadian dysfunction and excessive bedtime arousal

'subthreshold insomnia' (8–14), 'moderate clinical insomnia' (15–21) and 'severe clinical insomnia' (22–28).

Our patients also keep sleep diaries to principally calculate their average sleep efficiency (i.e. time asleep/time in bed × 100) over the course of 1 week (Kales and Kales 1984). This also allows us (and the patient) to monitor their total sleep time, sleep onset latency and wakefulness after sleep onset.

9.1.4   CBT for Insomnia Associated with Depressive Disorders

It is very common for patients presenting with depression to also report difficulty initiating and/or maintaining sleep. In fact, epidemiological evidence suggests that up to 90% of patients presenting with depression also suffer from insomnia (Tsuno et al. 2005; Riemann and Voderholzer 2003). This finding is perhaps to be expected, given that both depression and insomnia share the same neurotransmitter pathophysiology (principally involving serotonergic and dopaminergic systems; Harvey et al. 2011). Moreover, insomnia has been clearly shown to be a risk factor for the development of depression, with an overall odds ratio of 2.1 (95 percent confidence intervals of 1.9–2.4; Baglioni et al. 2011). The association is so common that some primary care physicians base their diagnosis of depression solely on the presence of insomnia (Krupinski and Tiller 2001).

Depressed patients with insomnia have significantly poorer clinical outcomes with respect to symptom ratings, attrition and remission rates and the stability of response to treatment when compared to depressed patients without insomnia (Dew et al. 1997; Thase et al. 1997). Furthermore, there is a growing evidence to demonstrate that insomnia is not just a correlate or symptom of depression. Rather, it affects the course of the depressive illness and the response to treatment, and when insomnia is unresolved, it poses an important risk factor for relapse (de Wild-Hartmann et al. 2013; Pigeon et al. 2008; Perlis et al. 1997). Insomnia is further associated with both suicidal thinking (McCall et al. 2010) and completed suicide (Bjørngaard et al. 2011; Fawcett et al. 1990). Understandably, therefore, there has been much interest in the usefulness of CBT-I in patients with depression.

As noted previously, the AASM in 2006 first suggested the potential benefits of CBT for insomnia on improving the mood of patients with depression. This work has been subsequently built upon by an encouraging, albeit small, case series study (Taylor et al. 2007a, b; see Table 9.1 for further details).

The strongest evidence, however, comes from two recent randomized controlled trials. In the first, a pilot study of 30 patients with major depression was randomly assigned to a combined treatment of CBT-I and anti-depressant medication *or* a combination of sham psychotherapy for insomnia and anti-depressant medication (Manber et al. 2008). Both the CBT-I and sham psychological treatments were administered for the same length of time and at the same frequency. As expected, CBT-I was effective in reducing insomnia symptoms, so much so, that remission (as measured by normal ISI scores) was significantly higher in patients receiving CBT-I (50% vs 8%). Therefore, the addition of CBT-I provided enhanced sleep outcomes, as compared to those who just received anti-depressant medication alone

Table 9.1 Characteristics of studies supporting CBT-I for patients with co-morbid psychiatric disorders

Co-morbid psychiatric diagnosis	Author et al., year	Randomization	Control group	CBT components	Treatment sessions	Treatment format	Outcome measures
Depression	Morawetz (2003)	No	–	Sleep education, sleep hygiene, sleep scheduling, stimulus control, cognitive therapy, relaxation	6	Self-help (book and audio cassette)	Sleep diary
Depression	Taylor et al. (2007a, b)	No	–	Sleep hygiene, stimulus control, relaxation	6	Individual	Sleep diary, Beck Depression Inventory
Depression	Manber et al. (2008)	Yes	Sleep education, sleep hygiene	Sleep education, sleep hygiene, sleep scheduling, stimulus control, genitive therapy, relaxation, relapse prevention	7	Individual	Sleep diary, ISI, actigraphy, HRSD$_{17}$
Depression	Watanabe et al. (2011)	Yes	TAU	Sleep education, sleep hygiene, sleep rescheduling, stimulus control, relapse prevention	4	Individual	Sleep diary, ISI, PSQI, HDRS, GRID-HAMD, medication (anti-depressant and hypnotic) use
PTSD	DeViva et al. (2005)	No	–	Stimulus control, sleep rescheduling, cognitive restructuring, sleep hygiene	5	Individual	Sleep diary
PTSD	Ulmer et al. (2011)	Yes	TAU	Sleep hygiene, sleep rescheduling, stimulus control, imagery rehearsal therapy	6 over 12 weeks	Individual	Electronic sleep diary, ISI, PSQI, PCL-M, PHQ-2
Alcohol dependence	Greeff and Conradie (1998)	Yes	No treatment	Relaxation	10	Group	Questionnaire
Alcohol dependence	Currie et al. (2004)	Yes	Wait list	Sleep education, sleep hygiene, stimulus control, sleep restriction, cognitive therapy, relaxation	5	Individual or self-help (book) with telephone support	Sleep diary, actigraph, PSQI

Alcohol dependence	Arnedt et al. (2007)	No	No	Sleep education (including effects of alcohol on sleep), sleep hygiene, stimulus control, sleep restriction, cognitive therapy, relapse prevention	8	Individual (four face-to-face and four via telephone)	Sleep diary, ISI, DBAS-SF, questionnaires on fatigue, anxiety, depression, interviews regarding alcohol intake
Alcohol dependence	Arnedt et al. (2011)	Yes	Behavioural placebo treatment	Sleep education (including effects of alcohol on sleep), sleep hygiene, stimulus control, sleep restriction, cognitive therapy, relapse prevention	8	Individual	Sleep diary, ISI, questionnaires on daytime functioning, drinking and treatment fidelity
Psychosis	Myers et al. (2011)	No	–	Sleep education, sleep hygiene, stimulus control, relaxation, relapse prevention	4	Individual	ISI, PSQI, G-PTS, PSYRATS, CAPS, DASS
BPAD	Harvey et al. (2015)	Yes	Psycho-education	Sleep education, case formulation, stimulus control, sleep restriction (limited to 6.5h in bed), relaxation therapy, cognitive therapy, improving daytime functioning, relapse prevention	8	Individual	SCID, YMRS, IDS-C, ISI. Sleep Diary, PSQI, PROMIS-D, SDS, Q-LES-Q-SF, CEQ

Abbreviations: *ISI* Insomnia Severity Index, *HRSD₁₇* - 17 item Hamilton Rating Scale for Depression, *PSQI* Pittsburgh Sleep Questionnaire Index, *GRID-HAMD* GRID-Hamilton Depression Rating Scale, *TAU* Treatment as Usual, *PTSD* post-traumatic stress disorder, *PCL-M* PTSD Checklist Military Version, *PHQ-2* Patient Health Questionnaire Version 2, *DBAS-SF* dysfunctional beliefs and attitudes about sleep—short form, *G-PTS* Green Paranoid Thought Scales, *PSYRATS* Psychotic Symptom Rating Scale: Delusions Subscale, *CAPS* Cardiff Anomalous Perception Scale, *DASS* Depression Anxiety Stress Scale, *BPAD* Bipolar Affective Disorder, *SCID* Structured Clinical Interview for the Diagnostic and Statistical Manual Version V, *YMRS* Young Mania Rating Scale, *IDS-C* Inventory of Depressive Symptomatology—Clinician, *PROMIS-SD* Patient-Reported Outcomes Measurement Information System—Sleep Disturbance, *SDS* Sheehan Disability Scale, *Q-LES-Q-SF* Quality of Life Enjoyment and Satisfaction Questionnaire, *CEQ* Credibility/Expectancy Questionnaire (i.e. two active treatments are better than one). Moreover, depression remission (as measured by the Hamilton Rating Scale for Depression [HRSD]) was approximately twice as high for those receiving CBT-I (61.5% vs 33.3%). Even when items relating to sleep in the HRSD were removed, the effect size was equivalent (i.e. the improvement in HRSD scores did not just occur because sleep parameters had improved). Hence, CBT-I markedly enhanced the depression treatment response (Table 9.1).

The second larger trial, undertaken by Watanabe et al. (2011), echoed this conclusion. In their trial, 73 outpatients with depression and co-morbid insomnia, which was refractory to adequate pharmacotherapy, were randomized to treatment as usual *or* treatment as usual plus four weekly 1-h individual sessions of CBT-I. After treatment, the CBT-I group had significantly lower insomnia and depression scores (even after sleep items were removed), as well as higher remission rates for both insomnia and depression.

These studies clearly suggest that independent targeting of both conditions provides the optimal outcome for patients suffering from co-morbid insomnia and depression. Moreover, they tally with previous pharmacotherapy studies, which also demonstrated that independent treatment of insomnia in patients with depression is possible and results in better depression outcomes (Fava et al. 2006).

9.1.4.1 CBT for Insomnia Associated with Bipolar Affective Disorder

Sleep difficulties go hand-in-hand with bipolar affective disorder (BPAD) and can be challenging to manage, as they do not always respond to pharmacotherapy (Gruber et al. 2011). Reduced need for sleep is a symptom of mania, which worsens as the episode unfolds (Jackson et al. 2003); and both insomnia and hypersomnia are seen during episodes of depression (American Psychiatric Association 2012). Even between episodes, up to 70% of patients with BPAD report significant sleep difficulties (Harvey et al. 2005), which are associated with mood symptoms, impaired daytime functioning, relapse, and suicide attempts (Sylvia et al. 2012).

In their pilot randomised control trial, Harvey and colleagues are the first to compare two psychosocial treatments (i.e. modified CBT-I vs. psycho-education) for patients with inter-episode BPAD and co-morbid insomnia (Harvey et al. 2015). During the 6-month follow-up, patients assigned to CBT-I (n = 30) had fewer days in a bipolar episode (3.3 days vs. 25.5 days) compared to those in the psycho-education group (n = 28). Furthermore, patients who underwent CBT-I showed enhanced mood stability, improved daytime functioning, and had a significantly lower hypomania/mania relapse rate (4.6% vs. 31.6%). Immediately post-treatment, the CBT-I group had higher rates of insomnia remission (72.7% vs. 14.3%), which remained higher at 6 months follow-up (63.6% vs. 21.1%).

Although the study size was small (which is emphasised by the authors), it clearly demonstrates the value of developing treatments aimed to improve sleep in patients with BPAD. By treating the co-morbid insomnia, BPAD symptoms and daytime functioning were improved.

9.1.5   CBT for Insomnia Associated with PTSD

PTSD is another psychiatric condition that is associated with a marked sleep disturbance. As in the case for depression, there is evidence that debilitating insomnia
persists in a substantial number of patients who have otherwise achieved remission
from PTSD (Zayfert and DeViva 2004). Moreover, there is a growing evidence to
suggest that independently targeting the co-morbid insomnia in PTSD helps to not
only improve the specific sleep disturbance but also the PTSD itself (Germain et al.
2007; Swanson et al. 2009).

In interpreting these studies, it is important to note that CBT-I was combined
with imagery rehearsal therapy,[1] a treatment designed to reduce sleep-disruptive
nightmares. It is therefore difficult to precisely tease out which improvements in
sleep can be specifically attributed to the insomnia-targeting part of the treatment.
Nonetheless, the emerging consensus again suggests that two active treatments (i.e.
targeting insomnia and PTSD) are better than one (i.e. targeting PTSD alone).

Building on earlier studies (see Table 9.1 for details), Ulmer et al. (2011) examined the effects of CBT-I and imagery rehearsal therapy on a large sample of veterans. In their control group, veterans received treatment as usual, i.e. pharmacotherapy
such as hypnotics and/or anxiolytics, etc. The treatment group also received these
pharmacological interventions as well as a comprehensive intervention for sleep
disturbance. The latter consisted of six biweekly 1-h individual sessions of CBT-I
(the first three sessions) and imagery rehearsal therapy (the subsequent three sessions). Unlike the control group, improvements in both clinically validated sleep-
related outcomes *and* PTSD symptoms were observed in patients receiving the
sleep-targeted therapy. Once again, therefore, by independently targeting insomnia,
a concurrent improvement in the co-morbid psychiatric condition was also achieved.

9.1.6   CBT for Insomnia Associated with Alcohol Dependence

Recovery from alcohol dependence is also frequently associated with prominent
insomnia. In fact, between 36% and 72% of all abstinent patients in this group experience a clinically significant insomnia (Ford and Kamerow 1989). Moreover, just as
in the case of depression and PTSD, sleep disturbances may exist for a substantial
period of time, long after alcohol-dependent patients have achieved abstinence
(Drummond et al. 1998). Unsurprisingly, such difficult and persistent sleep difficulties may unfortunately result in a return to alcohol consumption (Brower et al. 2001).

Studies examining the efficacy of CBT-I in recovering alcohol-dependent
patients are limited in number (see Table 9.1 for details). Currie et al. investigated
60 recovering patients with alcohol dependence using individual CBT-I, a self-help
manual and a wait-list control condition ($n = 20$ each; Currie et al. 2004). The active
treatment conditions improved sleep efficiency, sleep onset latency and sleep quality; however, no effect on the relapse prevention was observed.

---

[1] Imagery or dream rehearsal therapy is a cognitive approach that encourages the patient to recall
the nightmare, 'change the nightmare any way you wish' and then rehearse the 'new dream' whilst
awake.

More recently, Arnedt et al. (2007) performed an uncontrolled pilot study in which they found that individual CBT-I was effective in improving sleep efficiency and sleep onset latency in a small group of seven abstinent patients. Furthermore, there were no alcohol relapses observed during treatment. A second study of this research group used a randomized controlled design in a larger group of patients ($n = 17$, $n = 9$ in the CBT-I group and $n = 8$ in the behavioural placebo group; Arnedt et al. 2011). They reported that CBT-I improved objective and subjective sleep parameters in the treatment group, with an additional improvement in daytime ratings of general fatigue. However, as in the investigation of Currie et al., CBT-I had little impact on alcohol consumption.

These early studies question whether CBT-I aids in relapse prevention in individuals with alcohol dependence. However, the small sample sizes need to be borne in mind, and further research is clearly required before any firm conclusions can be drawn.

9.1.7   CBT for Insomnia Associated with Psychosis

Sleep disturbance is common in individuals with psychosis (Benca et al. 1991; Chouinard et al. 2004). One study showed that 44% of outpatients with schizophreniform disorders had a co-morbid insomnia (Palmese et al. 2011), which was, in turn, independently associated with a lower quality of life. Sleep disturbances also importantly appear to be a risk factor for the development of schizophrenia (Ruhrmann et al. 2010) and are further likely to exacerbate psychotic experiences (Freeman et al. 2010). Moreover, insomnia predicts a worsening of positive symptoms following antipsychotic withdrawal (Chemerinski et al. 2002).

Despite the clinical importance of insomnia, there is currently a paucity of evidence for the efficacy of CBT-I in psychotic disorders. As touched on previously, one promising pilot trial has shown that CBT-I (encompassing psycho-education, sleep hygiene and stimulus control) resulted in a clinically significant reduction in insomnia *and* psychotic symptoms (Myers et al. 2011). Furthermore, these improvements were maintained for at least 1 month post-therapy. As in the other psychiatric disorders we have discussed, here again, CBT-I resulted in positive benefits for the co-morbid psychiatric condition.

9.2   Practical Considerations for the Implementation of CBT for Insomnia

9.2.1   Accessing Therapy

Despite the overwhelming clinical evidence for CBT-I (e.g. Morin et al. 1994, 1999, 2006a), its acceptance by patients (Vincent and Lionberg 2001) and proven cost-effectiveness (Daley et al. 2009), the majority of individuals with insomnia still remain untreated (Morin et al. 2006b). Barriers to seeking and offering appropriate treatment arise from a combination of patient, clinician and policymaker factors. For example, only about a third of individuals with insomnia seek professional help

(Ancoli-Israel and Roth 1999; Morin et al. 2006b). Reasons for this include a tendency for patients to belittle their sleep problems, as well as a perceived lack of effective treatment options (Stinson et al. 2006).

Even when individuals do present for help, assessment and treatment of chronic insomnia are frequently inadequate in primary care (Sateia and Nowell 2004). This in part may reflect the state of our current clinical guidelines. In the UK, it is recommended that non-medical treatments are considered before hypnotics; however, there is little further information regarding these (National Institute for Clinical Excellence 2004). Even when professionals are aware of CBT-I, there are few available services (Lamberg 2008). Perhaps more pertinent to this chapter, the commonly held view of insomnia being a secondary condition to other psychiatric disorders has seen funding and development of services focused on the latter (National Institute for Health 2005).

Given these obstacles, the challenges become ones of maximizing the use of available resources, increasing patient access to appropriate therapy and disseminating practical and useful information to other healthcare professionals.

9.2.2 Anatomy of CBT-I

CBT-I is typically delivered in the context of five to six once-weekly therapy sessions (see Fig. 9.3 and Table 9.2; for more in-depth guides, see Perlis et al. 2008;

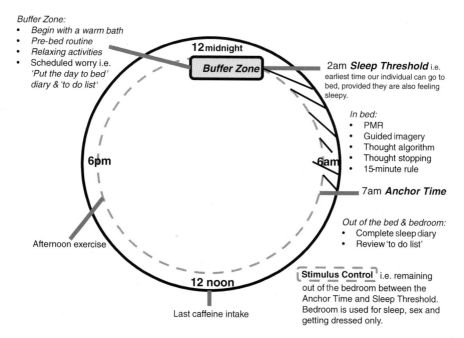

Fig. 9.3 Diagram illustrating how the various components of CBT-I fit into a 24-h period for an individual with a sleep threshold time of 2 a.m. and an anchor time of 7 a.m. *CBT-I* cognitive behavioural therapy, *PMR* progressive muscular relaxation

Table 9.2 Components of a typical group CBT-I treatment package

Session 1: Sleep and CBT-I education
Education about the nature and science of sleep, and explanation of the CBT-I model, including:

- Why we treat insomnia with CBT-I
- How insomnia originates and is maintained (explanation of the '3P' model)
- An explanation of the normal age-related sleep changes
- The stages of sleep and REM sleep (i.e. explanation of the normal hypnogram)
- The daytime consequences of inadequate sleep
- How insomnia differs from sleep deprivation—this can be strikingly potent in alleviating anxieties about the long-term effects of insomnia on one's physical health
- How to assess how much sleep is enough
- Exploration of popular sleep myths (e.g. 'everyone needs 8 h per night'; 'insomnia damages your brain')
- How common sleep problems are
- Introduction to maintaining a sleep diary (see Appendix C)

Session 2: Sleep hygiene education, stimulus control, anchoring the day and the 15-min rule[a]
Exploring habits/behaviours associated with sleep interference and ways of reducing/eliminating them. These include dietary factors (e.g. caffeine and alcohol intake), other lifestyle factors (e.g. nicotine use before bed, lack of a bedtime routine) and bedroom factors (e.g. noise, temperature, clock watching)
Stimulus control helps people to reduce the association of the bedroom as being a place of wakeful, purposeful activity. It limits bed and bedroom activities to sleep, sex and getting dressed only. It further emphasizes the importance of only going to bed when sleepy
'Anchoring the day' teaches the importance of rising at (or before) a set time each morning, 7 days a week, regardless of how well an individual has slept the previous night
The 15-min rule encourages individuals to leave the bedroom and to engage in a relaxing activity if they have not fallen asleep after 15 min (a time period they guess, rather than calculate via an alarm or via clock watching, etc.). Individuals return to bed when they feel sleepy again. This rule is maintained throughout the night

Session 3: Sleep rescheduling and progressive muscular relaxation
In sleep rescheduling, the initial requirement is to limit the time in bed to the average estimated time spent asleep each night (calculated from each individual's sleep diary; a minimum lower limit is set to 5 h). This generally increases the individual's sleep threshold, i.e. the earliest time they can go to bed *provided* they are also feeling sleepy. The aim here is to bring the total sleep time as close as possible to the time spent in bed. As the sleep efficiency improves, the time spent in bed can be increased
Progressive muscular relaxation is introduced and supported by a CD guide which is given to individuals

Session 4: Sleep cognitions
Encouraging individuals to include a 'buffer zone' (usually lasting 1.5–2 h) before their sleep threshold. During this buffer zone, they implement a pre-bed routine (e.g. commencing with a warm bath) and 'put the day to bed' by dealing constructively with worries or anxieties arising from the day, e.g. via use of a reflective diary of what has gone well and not so well during the day. This 'buffer zone' is used solely for relaxation, and as a 'wind-down' period, during which all work-related and stimulating activities are stopped
We also teach individuals how to cope with unwanted thoughts or worries that arise during the night, e.g. via use of a thought algorithm and via thought-stopping techniques, e.g. the 'The' technique

Table 9.2 (continued)

Session 5: Further relaxation techniques, bringing it all together and forward planning
Further relaxation techniques are taught, e.g. guided imagery
We review all of the techniques discussed by drawing a map of a typical day, indicating where each technique and strategy can be used (see Fig. 9.3)
We remind patients how to use their sleep efficiencies to alter their sleep threshold times[b], provide time for individual queries, give guidance on realistic expectations over the coming weeks and give encouragement
Some patients may be anxious that therapy is ending at this point and that they will be on their own until their 3-month follow-up review. Advising bibliotherapy (e.g. Colin Espie's 'Overcoming insomnia and sleep problems; a self-help guide using Cognitive Behavioral Techniques') can be useful to address these anxieties

CBT-I cognitive behavioural therapy for insomnia, *REM* rapid eye movement
[a]Sleep efficiency (SE, time asleep/time in bed × 100) is usually ≥90% in individuals without insomnia. For individuals undergoing CBT-I with an SE of ≥90%, we advise a reduction of their sleep threshold time by 15 min. When the SE is between 85% and 89.9%, we advise maintaining the same sleep threshold time. Finally, when the SE is ≤84.9%, we advise bringing the sleep threshold time forward by 15 min. Eventually, adjusting the sleep threshold time by 15 min in either direction will not affect the SE; maintenance of a weekly sleep diary can be stopped at this point
[b]For patients taking hypnotic medication, Sessions 1 and 2 may be completed over three sessions to allow for discussion and support of how and when to withdraw hypnotics

Espie 2010). Thereafter, the number of follow-up visits depends on the insomnia severity, co-morbidity and patient motivation. Whilst acute uncomplicated insomnia might require less time and can typically be managed in a non-specialist setting (Espie et al. 2007, 2008), more complex cases probably require the input of behavioural sleep medicine specialists.

Since individual face-to-face therapy with a sleep specialist is not always feasible, research has focused on the viability of alternative treatment delivery models. There is now evidence to support self-help approaches, using printed materials (Belleville et al. 2007; Mimeault and Morin 1999), videos (Savard et al. 2011) or Internet-based programmes (Ritterband et al. 2009). These are helpful either on their own or when supplemented by professional administered therapy. Other efficacious and cost-effective treatment modalities include telephone conversations (Bastien et al. 2004) and group therapy (Currie et al. 2004). Finally, there is also a growing evidence to support the use of a brief two-session CBT-I intervention (Edinger and Sampson 2003) as well as a single day-long intensive CBT-I workshop (Swift et al. 2012).

Each treatment modality has its own specific characteristics and unique advantages (e.g. increased social support in group therapy). These need to be considered during the initial assessment of the patient's needs so that a successful therapeutic outcome can be achieved. Some patients might require little guidance, whereas others might need a more intensive and structured approach. Regardless of the therapy entry level, there should be scope to move between modalities as required, i.e. the provision of a stepped-care approach (Espie 2009).

Ultimately, the success of CBT-I depends on the patient's ability to adhere to treatment recommendations. To optimize outcomes, follow-up consultations are often necessary to monitor progress, to address concordance difficulties and to provide guidance and support.

9.2.3   Who Is Appropriate for CBT-I in Co-morbid Insomnia?

Following an accurate diagnosis of insomnia (i.e. never assume that all persons referred for CBT-I have insomnia!), the next step is to determine if an individual is appropriate for CBT-I. This involves consideration of general selection criteria (applicable to most psychological and behavioural therapies), as well as specific conditions relating to both insomnia and the co-morbid condition.

In terms of general selection criteria, individuals presenting with the following are *usually* excluded: terminal illness, suicidality, current alcohol and substance misuse, cognitive impairment (usually with a Mini-Mental State Examination score of ≤25) as well as those undergoing another form of active psychological therapy. However, one could take a more creative viewpoint and consider the utility of groups specifically targeted for patients with addiction problems, the involvement of carers in those with cognitive impairment or learning disability and the joint working with mainstream psychiatric services in the acutely ill and suicidal. Moreover, there is plenty of scope to incorporate aspects of CBT-I into the patient's current psychological therapy, e.g. a patient undergoing depression-focused psychotherapy could readily incorporate CBT-I strategies.

Insomnia may also present as a part of *another* unstable or undiagnosed intrinsic sleep disorder, e.g. sleep apnoea, restless legs syndrome or periodic limb movement disorder. Whilst individuals presenting with these conditions require further assessment (e.g. via a polysomnogram) and specific treatment, they may also benefit from the addition of CBT-I (Pigeon and Yurcheshen 2009; Sanchez et al. 2009). Therefore, regardless of the sleep disorder diagnosis, *most* therapists would probably agree that appropriate individuals for CBT-I are those who present with the following:

- Difficulty in falling and/or staying asleep
- A report of one or more of the following:
  Regularly extending their sleep opportunity to compensate for sleep loss and/or
  Staying in bed for protracted periods of time whilst awake and/or
  Engaging in behaviours other than sleep and sex in the bed and bedroom
- Evidence of conditioned arousal, e.g. individuals suddenly feeling awake on entering their bedroom and/or sleeping much better when away from home
- Evidence of poor sleep hygiene, i.e. those behaviours which reduce sleep propensity, e.g. use of stimulants at night time, using alcohol as a hypnotic, giving bed space/dominance to pets, etc.

In terms of the co-morbid disorder, psychiatric and/or medical conditions that are relatively stable or treated are appropriate for consideration. Unstable psychiatric conditions are generally those that require imminent hospitalization or necessitated recent inpatient treatment, i.e. within the last 3 months. CBT-I in this early recovery period may play a role, but it is likely that the patient will require additional support and close supervision.

Whilst CBT-I is relatively free from side effects, it is not entirely without risk. For example, sleep rescheduling may trigger manic episodes in vulnerable individuals (e.g. Colombo et al. 1990) and needs to be carefully administered with enhanced monitoring, as discussed in more detail in the next section. Also, patients with nocturnal panic are particularly susceptible to the paradoxical phenomenon of relaxation-induced anxiety (Heide and Borkovec 1983). This can occur in about 15% of individuals attempting relaxation therapies and needs to be managed clinically.

9.2.4 Special Considerations for Conducting CBT-I in Co-morbid Psychiatric Disorders

9.2.4.1 Depression

A patient with depression may experience low energy levels and reduced motivation as part of their illness. These symptoms may readily interfere with concordance to some of the behavioural changes as prescribed in CBT-I, e.g. sleep rescheduling, maintaining a consistent anchor time and adhering to the 15-minute rule. Sleep, and/or resting in bed, may also be viewed as the only periods of respite from the distress of the depressive illness. Here, increased longing for sleep can lead to increased effort in trying to sleep, which can lead to hyperarousal in bed and sleep interference. Overcoming these challenges requires open acknowledgement of the concordance difficulties, a clear explanation of the intended purpose of the behavioural strategies and flexibility in the mode of CBT-I delivery. With regard to the latter, it may be necessary to separately address some of the depressed cognitions which are impacting on CBT-I concordance. Additionally, a gentler implementation of the behavioural strategies may also be helpful. For example, in the case of sleep rescheduling, increasing bedtimes in weekly increments of 15 min may be more tolerable than immediately setting a sleep threshold which is hours later than the patient's current bedtime.

9.2.4.2 Bipolar-Affective Disorder

It is worth considering the potential impact of sleep re-scheduling in patients prone to hypomania or mania. Partial disruptions to sleep continuity (e.g. following the birth of a new born infant) and sleep deprivation are both well-described precipitators of hypomania/mania (Berger et al. 1997; Wehr 1990). For example, the risk of triggering a manic episode posed by sleep deprivation is similar to that posed by switching anti-depressants (about 5%; Colombo et al. 1990). It is therefore probably prudent to advise gentler sleep re-scheduling regimes as outlined earlier. For patients with a rapid cycling bipolar illness, there is evidence to suggest that scheduling regular nightly extended periods of bed rest in the dark may be helpful in achieving mood stabilisation (Wehr et al. 1998).

9.2.4.3 Anxiety

Some very anxious patients may struggle to cope with sleep rescheduling. This technique aims to consolidate sleep by increasing sleep debt, which in turn 'fuels' sleep. Initially, the person is therefore advised to reduce their time in bed by matching it to their current average sleep time (as calculated from their sleep diaries). Such limitations to the time spent in bed can be *very* anxiety provoking, to the point where it counteracts the effects of sleep debt, and may even worsen the insomnia. To circumnavigate this potential, we set a minimum lower limit of 5 h in bed; so even if a person calculates his/her current sleep time as being 2 h, we would recommend that his/her sleep threshold be set to 5 h (and not 2 h) before their chosen anchor time. However, a highly anxious person might find this intolerable, and we would then encourage them to increase their current bedtime in weekly 15-min increments.

For the severely anxious individual, focusing on stimulus control as the main CBT-I intervention may be less anxiogenic than sleep rescheduling. Stimulus control shifts the location of anxiety from the bedroom to another room and may therefore lessen the association of the bedroom as a place of worry and heightened anxiety. Remembering to schedule 'worry time' in the 'buffer zone' may also reduce presleep intrusive thoughts and worries. Finally, it will be important to highlight the relevance of relaxation and cognitive restructuring techniques to this patient group.

9.2.4.4 PTSD

Co-morbid insomnia with PTSD may additionally be complicated by a fear of going to sleep as it may involve re-experiencing traumatic nightmares. This fear may lead to prolonged sleep onset latency and irregular bedtimes. It may be particularly pronounced in those patients who experienced trauma in a sleep-related context, e.g. in some cases of sexual abuse. Combining imagery rehearsal therapy (to desensitize and diminish the arousal associated with nightmares) with CBT-I has been shown to overcome this difficulty and to result in favourable outcomes for patients with co-morbid insomnia and PTSD (e.g. Ulmer et al. 2011).

9.2.4.5 Alcohol Dependence

Specific psycho-education may be valuable in helping to set realistic expectations in patients who are recovering from alcohol dependence. Initially, alcohol cessation can result in a significant and severe sleep fragmentation, whilst a milder sleep fragmentation can be experienced for up to 2 years afterwards (Gillin and Drummond 2000; Adamson and Burdick 1973). Warning patients in advance about this potential sleep loss can be beneficial. It can further help to stimulate an open discussion about what is tolerable in terms of sleep changes, which may in turn lead to consideration of combined pharmacotherapy. CBT-I should not initially be expected to produce the same immediate hypnotic effect as alcohol, and combined pharmacotherapy may help to avert an alcoholic relapse. Longer-term, sleep rescheduling is likely to be advantageous in helping to reduce fragmented sleep patterns in patients recovering from alcohol dependence.

9.2.4.6 Psychosis

Finally, for patients suffering from co-morbid insomnia and psychotic disorders, clarity and flexibility in CBT-I delivery are probably key. In their pilot study, Myers et al. (2011) report using a simplified model of CBT-I centred on stimulus control as the main therapeutic intervention. This was supplemented by more general sleep hygiene and education advice. In a patient cohort that may have particular difficulty in initiating, making and adapting to cognitive and behavioural changes, it is probably advisable to adhere to a single main message, e.g. 'only use your bedroom for sleep and sex'. Such straight-forward and clear take-home messages are also easier to disseminate to allied mental health professionals (e.g. key workers, care coordinators and accommodation staff), who may play a valuable role in helping to encourage concordance.

9.2.5 CBT for Insomnia with Older Adults

Insomnia is more prevalent in older adults and, perhaps unsurprisingly, is more likely to be co-morbid with other medical and/or psychiatric disorders. Studies demonstrate that older adults treated with CBT-I show similar treatment size effects when compared to their younger middle-aged counterparts (Irwin et al. 2006). Moreover, there is also evidence to support insomnia treatment as being beneficial to later life co-morbid conditions and to increasing quality of life measures (Lichstein et al. 2000).

Some evidence suggests that CBT-I should be adapted in order to optimize outcomes in older adults. In a systematic review, McCurry and colleagues concluded that multimodal CBT and sleep rescheduling alone met criteria for empirically validated therapies, whereas evidence was insufficient to support cognitive therapy, relaxation or sleep hygiene education as stand-alone therapies for insomnia in older adults (McCurry et al. 2007). These findings mirror studies for the treatment of other psychological conditions in older age, where outcomes appear to favour more behaviourally orientated strategies (Oude Voshaar 2013).

Finally, many older adults with insomnia are long-term users of hypnotics, especially benzodiazepines. The use of CBT-I in this group has been shown to significantly reduce the quantity and frequency of benzodiazepine use, promote sustained abstinence as well as minimize the risk of rebound insomnia (Soeffing et al. 2008).

9.2.6 Combined CBT-I and Pharmacotherapy

CBT-I and pharmacotherapy can have complementary roles in the management of both uncomplicated and co-morbid insomnia. Combined approaches should optimize outcomes by taking advantage of the more immediate and potent effects of hypnotic agents and the more sustained effects of behavioural interventions.

Findings from studies that directly contrast the effects of CBT and medication for insomnia (e.g. Morin et al. 1999) show that these two therapies are effective in the short term, with medication producing faster results in the acute (first week) phase of treatment, whereas they are equally effective in the medium term (weeks four to eight of treatment). Individuals given CBT-I maintain their improvements with time, whereas those given hypnotics alone tend to relapse after discontinuation. Combined interventions have a slight advantage compared with single modalities during initial treatment, but this advantage does not always persist with time.

Whilst a discussion of suitable pharmacotherapeutic agents falls outside the remit of this chapter (see Morin and Benca 2012, for further discussion), polypharmacy can be avoided by selecting (where possible) dual-function medications, i.e. those which target the co-morbid disorder, and also act as hypnotics, e.g. in the case of co-morbid depression and insomnia, use of a sedating anti-depressant such as trazodone or mirtazapine may be beneficial.

Of course, there may be times when sedating psychotropic medication is not suitable for the co-morbid disorder, and an additional hypnotic medication will be required. Judging when to stop hypnotics in this scenario can be difficult, and the best option appears to be to discontinue them whilst patients are still receiving CBT-I. In our clinic, we add an extra therapy session to the course of group CBT-I in order to facilitate this (see Table 9.2).

9.2.7 Is There a Role for CBT-I in Co-morbid Paradoxical Insomnia?

Paradoxical insomnia (previously termed 'sleep state misperception') is a complaint of *severe* insomnia, which is disproportionate to the presence of objective sleep disturbance or daytime impairment (AASM 2005). Hypervigilance occurs as the patient is trying to sleep, and subsequent physiological and/or perceptual deficits result in impaired sleep/wake discrimination, leading to an underestimation of the time spent asleep (Bonne and Arand 1997).

Despite being a prevalent (up to 43%) subtype of chronic insomnia, it is a notoriously difficult condition to assess (owing in part to a lack of standardized diagnostic criteria) and to treat (Dorsey and Bootzin 1997; Edinger and Sampson 2003). To our knowledge, there are no published data in regard to its co-occurrence with other psychiatric disorders. There are also no standard treatments for paradoxical insomnia, and it typically responds poorly to usual CBT-I approaches.

Recent therapeutic efforts have focused on enhancing the patient's ability to discriminate between sleep/wake periods (Geyer et al. 2008). In their case series study, Geyer et al. (2011) followed a course of CBT-I with a novel sleep education technique, where they utilized a polysomnogram with video, to help patients explore the discrepancy between their reported and observed sleep experiences. For two of the four patients, this resulted in a meaningful improvement in their ISI scores and in their self-reported sleep onset latency and total sleep times. Although this was a small case series study, it provides therapeutic hope for patients with paradoxical insomnia, as well as for the clinicians treating them. A randomized controlled trial comparing CBT-I, this novel sleep education technique and a combination of both therapies would shed much-needed light on how best to approach this challenging condition.

Conclusion

Insomnia and psychiatric disorders are commonly intertwined. CBT-I is a well-established treatment for insomnia and, increasingly, appears to also benefit co-morbid psychiatric conditions. The basic challenges for us as clinicians remain ones of recognizing co-morbid insomnia and providing access to therapy for our patients.

Other treatment modalities, such as Acceptance and Commitment Therapy and Mindfulness and Intensive Sleep Retraining, have yet to demonstrate their equivalence to CBT-I in resolving insomnia, including co-morbid psychiatric conditions.

Future research, via large-scale randomized controlled trials, is required to expand our knowledge of the clinical effectiveness of CBT-I in the treatment of co-morbid insomnia and psychiatric disorders.

References

Adamson J, Burdick JA. Sleep of dry alcoholics. Arch Gen Psychiatry. 1973;28:146–9.

American Academy of Sleep Medicine. International classification of sleep disorders, 2nd ed.: Diagnostic and coding manual. Westchester, IL: Author; 2005.

American Psychiatric Association. Diagnostic and statistical manual of mental disorders. 5th ed; 2012. Author

Ancoli-Israel S, Roth T. Characteristics of insomnia in the United States: results of the 1991 National Sleep Foundation survey. Sleep. 1999;22:347–53.

Arnedt JT, Conroy D, Rutt J, et al. An open trial of cognitive-behavioral treatment for insomnia co-morbid with alcohol dependence. Sleep Med. 2007;8(2):176–80.

Arnedt JT, Conroy DA, Armitage R, Brower KJ. Cognitive-behavioral therapy for insomnia in alcohol dependent patients: a randomized controlled pilot trial. Behav Res Ther. 2011;49(4):227–33.

Baglioni C, Battagliese G, Feige B, et al. Insomnia as a predictor of depression: a meta-analytic evaluation of longitudinal epidemiological studies. J Affect Disord. 2011;135:10–9.

Bastien CH, Vallières A, Morin CM. Validation of the Insomnia Severity Index as an outcome measure for insomnia research. Sleep Med. 2001;2(4):297–307.

Bastien CH, Morin CM, Ouellet MC, et al. Cognitive-behavioral therapy for insomnia: comparison of individual therapy, group therapy, and telephone consultations. J Consult Clin Psychol. 2004;72:653–9.

Belleville G, Guay C, Guay B, et al. Hypnotic taper with or without self-help treatment: a randomized clinical trial. J Consult Clin Psychol. 2007;75:325–35.

Benca RM, Obermeyer WH, Thisted RA, Gillin JC. Sleep and psychiatric disorders. Arch Gen Psychiatry. 1991;49:651–68.

Berger M, Vollmann J, Hohagen F, et al. Sleep deprivation combined with consecutive sleep phase advance as a fast-acting therapy in depression: an open pilot trial in medicated and unmedicated patients. Am J Psychiatry. 1997;154(6):870–2.

Bjørngaard JH, Bjerkeset O, Romundstad P, Gunnell D. Sleeping problems and suicide in 75,000 Norwegian adults: a 20 year follow-up of the HUNT I study. Sleep. 2011;34(9):1155.

Bonne MH, Arand DL. Physiological activation in patients with sleep state misperception. Psychosom Med. 1997;59:533–40.

Brower KJ, Aldrich MS, Robinson EA, et al. Insomnia, self-medication, and relapse to alcoholism. Am J Psychiatry. 2001;158(3):399–404.

Carney CE, Segal ZV, Edinger JD, Kyrstal AD. A comparison of rates of residual insomnia symptoms following pharmacotherapy or cognitive-behavioural-therapy for major depressive disorder. J Clin Psychiatry. 2007;68(2):254–60.

Chemerinski E, Ho BC, Flaum M, et al. Insomnia as a predictor for symptom worsening following antipsychotic withdrawal in schizophrenia. Compr Psychiatry. 2002;43:393–6.

Chesson AL, Anderson WM, Littner M, et al. Practice parameters for the nonpharmacologic treatment of chronic insomnia. An American Academy of Sleep Medicine report. Standards of Practice Committee of the American Academy of Sleep Medicine. Sleep. 1999;22(8):1128–33.

Chouinard S, Poulin J, Stip E, Godbout R. Sleep in untreated patients with schizophrenia: a meta-analysis. Schizophr Bull. 2004;30:957–67.

Colombo C, Benedetti F, Barbini B, et al. Rate of switch from depression into mania after therapeutic sleep deprivation in bipolar depression. Psychiatry Res. 1990;86(3):267–70.

Currie SR, Clark S, Hodgins DC, El-Guebaly N. Randomized controlled trial of brief cognitive-behavioural interventions for insomnia in recovering alcoholics. Addiction. 2004;99:1121–32.

Daley M, Morin CM, Leblanc M, et al. The economic burden of insomnia: direct and indirect costs for individuals with insomnia syndrome, insomnia symptoms, and good sleepers. Sleep. 2009;32:55–64.

DeViva JC, Zayfert C, Pigeon WR, Mellman TA. Treatment of residual insomnia after CBT for PTSD: case studies. J Trauma Stress. 2005;18(2):155–9.

Dew MA, Reynolds CF, Houck PR, et al. Temporal profiles of the course of depression during treatment. Predictors of pathways toward recovery in the elderly. Arch Gen Psychiatry. 1997;54:1016–24.

Dorsey CM, Bootzin RR. Subjective and psychophysiologic insomnia: an examination of sleep tendency and personality. Biol Psychiatry. 1997;41:209–16.

Drummond SP, Gillin JC, Smith TL, DeModena A. The sleep of abstinent pure primary alcoholic patients: natural course and relationship to relapse. Alcohol Clin Exp Res. 1998;22(8):1796–802.

Edinger JD, Means MK. Cognitive-behavioural therapy for primary insomnia. Clin Psychol Rev. 2005;25(5):539–58.

Edinger JD, Sampson WS. A primary care "friendly" cognitive behaviour insomnia therapy. Sleep. 2003;26:177–82.

Espie CA. "Stepped care": a health technology solution for delivering cognitive behavioral therapy as a first line insomnia treatment. Sleep. 2009;32:1549–58.

Espie CA. Overcoming insomnia and sleep problems; a self-help guide using cognitive behavioural techniques. London: Constable and Robinson LTD; 2010.

Espie CA, MacMahon KM, Kelly HL, et al. Randomized clinical effectiveness trial of nurse-administered small-group cognitive behavior therapy for persistent insomnia in general practice. Sleep. 2007;30:574–84.

Espie CA, Fleming L, Cassidy J, et al. Randomized controlled clinical effectiveness trial of cognitive behavior therapy compared with treatment as usual for persistent insomnia in patients with cancer. J Clin Oncol. 2008;26:4651–8.

Fava M, McCall WV, Krystal A, et al. Eszopiclone co-administered with fluoxetine in patients with insomnia coexisting with major depressive disorder. Biol Psychiatry. 2006;59:1052–60.

Fawcett J, Scheftner WA, Fogg L, et al. Time-related predictors of suicide in major affective disorder. Am J Psychiatry. 1990;147:1189–94.

Ford DE, Kamerow DB. Epidemiologic study of sleep disturbances and psychiatric disorders. An opportunity for prevention? JAMA. 1989;262(11):1479–84.

Freeman D, Brugha T, Meltzer H, et al. Persecutory ideation and insomnia: findings from the second British National Survey of Psychiatric Morbidity. J Psychiatr Res. 2010;44(15): 1021–6.

Germain A, Shear MK, Hall M, Buysse DJ. Effects of a brief behavioural treatment for PTSD-related sleep disturbances: a pilot study. Behav Res Ther. 2007;45(3):627–32.

Geyer JD, Lichstein KL, Carney PR, et al. Paradoxical insomnia. Casebook of sleep medicine—a learning companion to the international classification of sleep disorders, diagnostic and coding manual. 2nd ed. Westchester, IL: American Academy of Sleep Medicine; 2008. p. 25–8.

Geyer JD, Lichstein KL, Ruiter ME, et al. Sleep education for paradoxical insomnia. Behav Sleep Med. 2011;9(4):266–72.

Gillin JC, Drummond SPA. Medication and substance abuse. In: Kryger M, Roth T, Dement W, editors. Principles and practices of sleep medicine. 2nd ed. Philadelphia, PA: W.B. Saunders Company; 2000.

Greeff AP, Conradie WS. Use of progressive relaxation training for chronic alcoholics with insomnia. Psychol Rep. 1998;82(2):407–12.

Gruber J, Miklowitz DJ, Harvey AG, et al. Sleep matters: sleep functioning and course of illness in bipolar disorder. J Affect Disord. 2011;134:416–20.

Harvey AG, Schmidt DA, Scarnà A, et al. Sleep-related functioning in euthymic patients with bipolar disorder, patients with insomnia, and subjects without sleep problems. Am J Psychiatry. 2005;162:50–7.

Harvey AG, Murray G, Chandler RA, Soehner A. Sleep disturbance as transdiagnostic: consideration of neurobiological mechanisms. Clin Psychol Rev. 2011;31:225–35.

Harvey AG, Soehner AM, Kaplan KA, et al. Treating insomnia improves mood state, sleep, and functioning in bipolar disorder: a pilot randomized controlled trial. J Consult Clin Psychol. 2015;83(3):564–77.

Heide FJ, Borkovec TD. Relaxation-induced anxiety: paradoxical anxiety enhancement due to relaxation training. J Consult Clin Psychol. 1983;51(2):171–82.

Irwin MR, Cole JC, Nicassio PM, et al. Comparative meta-analysis of behavioral interventions for insomnia and their efficacy in middle-aged adults and in older adults 55+ years of age. Health Psychol. 2006;25:3–14.

Jackson A, Cavanagh J, Scott J. A systematic review of manic and depressive prodromes. J Affect Disord. 2003;74:209–17.

Jacobs GD, Pace-Schott EF, Stickgold R, et al. Cognitive behavior therapy and pharmacotherapy for insomnia; a randomized controlled trial and direct comparison. Arch Intern Med. 2004;164:1888–96.

Kales A, Kales JD. Evaluation and treatment of insomnia. New York, NY: Oxford University Press; 1984.

Krupinski J, Tiller JW. The identification and treatment of depression by general practitioners. Aust N Z J Psychiatry. 2001;35(6):827–32.

Lamberg L. Despite effectiveness, behavioural therapy for chronic insomnia still under used. JAMA. 2008;300:2474–5.

Lichstein KL. Secondary insomnia: a myth dismissed. Sleep Med Rev. 2006;10(1):3–5.

Lichstein KL, Wislon NM, Johnson CT. Psychological treatment of secondary insomnia. Psychol Aging. 2000;15(2):232–40.

Manber R, Edinger JD, Gress JL, et al. Cognitive behavioral therapy for insomnia enhances depression outcome in patients with comorbid major depressive disorder and insomnia. Sleep. 2008;31(4):489–95.

McCall WV, Blocker JN, D'Agostino R Jr, et al. Insomnia severity is an indicator of suicidal ideation during a depression clinical trial. Sleep Med. 2010;11:822–7.

McCurry SM, Logsdon RG, Teri L, et al. Evidence-based psychological treatments for insomnia in older adults. Psychol Aging. 2007;22:18–27.

Mimeault V, Morin CM. Self-help treatment for insomnia: bibliotherapy with and without professional guidance. J Consult Clin Psychol. 1999;67:511–9.

Morawetz D. Insomnia and depression: which comes first? Sleep Res Online. 2003;5:77–81.

Morin CM, Benca R. Chronic insomnia. Lancet. 2012;379:1129–41.

Morin CM, Culbert PJ, Schwartz SM. Nonpharmacological interventions for insomnia: a meta-analysis of treatment efficacy. Am J Psychiatry. 1994;151:1172–80.

Morin CM, Hauri PJ, Espie CA, et al. Nonpharmacologic treatment of chronic insomnia. Sleep. 1999;22:1134–56.

Morin CM, Bootzin RR, Buysse DJ, et al. Psychological and behavioural treatment of insomnia: update of the recent evidence (1998–2004). Sleep. 2006a;29(11):1398–414.

Morin CM, Leblanc M, Daley M, et al. Epidemiology of insomnia: prevalence, self-help treatments, consultations, and determinants of help-seeking behaviors. Sleep Med. 2006b;7:123–30.

Myers E, Startup H, Freeman D. Cognitive behavioural treatment of insomnia in individuals with persistent persecutory delusions: a pilot trial. J Behav Ther Exp Psychiatry. 2011;42(3):330–6.

National Institute for Clinical Excellence (NICE). TA77: guidance on the use of zaleplon, zolpidem and zopiclone for the short-term management of insomnia. London: NICE; 2004.

National Institute of Health (NIH). Manifestations and management of chronic insomnia in adults. State Sci Statements. 2005;22:1–36.

Nierenberg AA, Keefe BR, Leslie VC, et al. Residual symptoms in depressed patients who respond acutely to fluoxetine. J Clin Psychiatry. 1999;60(4):221–5.

Oude Voshaar RC. Lack of interventions for anxiety in older people. Br J Psychiatry. 2013;203:8–9.

Palmese LB, DeGeorge PC, Ratliff JC, et al. Insomnia is frequent in schizophrenia and associated with night eating and obesity. Schizophr Res. 2011;133:238–43.

Perlis ML, Giles DE, Buysee DJ, Tu X, Kupfer DJ. Self-reported sleep disturbance as a prodormal symptom in recurrent depression. J Affect Disord. 1997;42:209–12.

Perlis ML, Jungquist C, Smith MT, et al. Cognitive behavioural treatment of insomnia: a session-by-session guide. New York, NY: Springer; 2008.

Pigeon WR, Yurcheshen M. Behavioral sleep medicine interventions for restless legs syndrome and periodic limb movement disorder. Sleep Med Clin. 2009;1(4):487–94.

Pigeon WR, Hegel M, Unützer J, et al. Is insomnia a perpetuating factor for late-life depression in the IMPACT cohort? Sleep. 2008;31:481–8.

Riemann D, Perlis ML. The treatments of chronic insomnia: a review of benzodiazepine receptor agonists and psychological and behavioural therapies. Sleep Med Rev. 2009;13(3):205–14.

Riemann D, Voderholzer U. Primary insomnia: a risk factor to develop depression? J Affect Disord. 2003;76:255–9.

Ritterband LM, Thorndike FP, Gonder-Frederick LA, et al. Efficacy of an internet-based behavioral intervention for adults with insomnia. Arch Gen Psychiatry. 2009;66:692–8.

Roth T, Roehrs T. Insomnia: epidemiology, characteristics, and consequences. Clin Cornerstone. 2003;5(3):5–15.

Ruhrmann S, Schultze-Lutter F, Salokangas RK, et al. Prediction of psychosis in adolescents and young adults at high risk. Arch Gen Psychiatry. 2010;67:241–51.

Sanchez AI, Martinez P, Miro E, et al. CPAP and behavioral therapies in patients with obstructive sleep apnea: effects on daytime sleepiness, mood, and cognitive function. Sleep Med Rev. 2009;13:223–33.

Sarsour K, Morin CM, Foley K, et al. Association of insomnia severity and co-morbid medical and psychiatric disorders in a health plan-based sample: Insomnia severity and co-morbidities. Sleep Med. 2010;11(1):69–74.

Sateia MJ, Nowell PD. Insomnia. Lancet. 2004;364:1959–73.

Savard J, Villa J, Simard S, et al. Feasibility of a self-help treatment for insomnia co-morbid with cancer. Psychooncology. 2011;20(9):1013–9.

Soeffing JP, Lichstein KL, Nau SD, et al. Psychological treatment of insomnia in hypnotic-dependant older adults. Sleep Med. 2008;9:165–71.

Spielman AJ, Caruso LS, Glovinsky PB. A behavioural perspective on insomnia treatment. Psychiatr Clin North Am. 1987;10(4):541–53.

Stinson K, Tang NKY, Harvey AG. Barriers to treatment seeking in primary insomnia in the United Kingdom: a cross-sectional perspective. Sleep. 2006;29:1643–6.

Swanson LM, Favoutire TK, Horin E, Arnedt JT. A combined group treatment for nightmares and insomnia in combat veterans: a pilot study. J Trauma Stress. 2009;22(6):639–42.

Swift N, Stewart R, Andiappan M, et al. The effectiveness of community day-long CBT-I workshops for participants with insomnia symptoms: a randomized controlled trial. J Sleep Res. 2012;21:270–80.

Sylvia LG, Dupuy JM, Ostacher MJ, et al. Sleep disturbance in euthymic bipolar patients. J Psychopharmacol. 2012;26:1108–12.

Taylor DJ, Lichstein KL, Weinstock J, et al. A pilot study of cognitive-behavioural therapy of insomnia in people with mild depression. Behav Ther. 2007a;38(1):49–57.

Taylor DJ, Mallory LJ, Lichstein KL, et al. Co-morbidity of chronic insomnia with medical problems. Sleep. 2007b;30(2):213–8.

Thase ME, Buysse DJ, Frank E, et al. Which depressed patients will respond to interpersonal psychotherapy? The role of abnormal EEG sleep profiles. Am J Psychiatry. 1997;154:502–9.

Tsuno N, Besset A, Ritchie K. Sleep and depression. J Clin Psychiatry. 2005;66:1254–69.

Ulmer CS, Edinger JD, Calhoun PS. A multi-component cognitive-behavioural intervention for sleep disturbance in veterans with PTSD: a pilot stud. J Clin Sleep Med. 2011;7(1):57–68.

Vincent N, Lionberg C. Treatment preference and patient satisfaction in chronic insomnia. Sleep. 2001;11:488–96.

Watanabe N, Furukawa TA, Shimodera S, et al. Brief behavioral therapy for refractory insomnia in residual depression: an assessor-blind, randomized controlled trial. J Clin Psychiatry. 2011;72:1651–8.

Wehr T. Effects of wakefulness and sleep on depression and mania. In: Montplaisir J, Godbout R, editors. Sleep and biological rhythms: basic mechanisms and application to psychiatry. New York, NY: Oxford University Press; 1990. p. 42–86.

Wehr TA, Turner EH, Shimada JM, et al. Treatment of rapidly cycling bipolar patient by using extended bed rest and darkness to stabilize the timing and duration of sleep. Biol Psychiatry. 1998;43(11):822–8.

de Wild-Hartmann JA, Wichers M, van Bemmel AL, et al. Day-to-day associations between subjective sleep and affect in regard to future depression in a female population-based sample. Br J Psychiatry. 2013;202(6):407–12.

Zayfert C, DeViva JC. Residual insomnia following cognitive behavioural therapy for PTSD. J Trauma Stress. 2004;17(1):69–73.

Restless Legs Syndrome

10

Guy D. Leschziner

10.1 Introduction

Restless legs syndrome (RLS) is a common neurological disorder characterized by the urge to move the legs, or indeed other body parts, usually accompanied by a range of unpleasant sensations (Leschziner and Gringras 2012). These clinical features are typically under a circadian influence and worsen in the evening or night; they are transiently or partially relieved by movement and are worsened by immobility. RLS is a common cause of insomnia—both sleep initiation and sleep maintenance problems—unrefreshing sleep and excessive daytime sleepiness.

Despite its frequency, it is often unrecognized or misdiagnosed, in part due to lack of awareness of the condition, but also as a result of a wide spectrum of symptoms and signs. However, prompt diagnosis and management has a large impact on morbidity and quality of life.

10.2 Clinical Features

RLS, first identified by Ekbom (1945), is essentially a clinical diagnosis without specific biological markers. Diagnosis is based upon four essential criteria, as defined by the International Restless Legs Syndrome Study Group (Allen et al. 2003):

- The urge to move legs, accompanied by uncomfortable or unpleasant sensations. Other body parts can be affected in addition to the lower limbs.
- The urge to move or unpleasant sensations during periods of immobility or sleep.

G. D. Leschziner, M.A., Ph.D., F.R.C.P.
Department of Neurology and Sleep Disorders Centre, Guy's and St Thomas'
NHS Foundation Trust, London, UK
e-mail: Guy.Leschziner@gstt.nhs.uk

© Springer-Verlag GmbH Germany, part of Springer Nature 2018
H. Selsick (ed.), *Sleep Disorders in Psychiatric Patients*,
https://doi.org/10.1007/978-3-642-54836-9_10

175

- Movement of the affected limbs results in a partial or transient relief of symptoms.
- The symptoms worsen in the evening or night—this feature may not persist but should have been present initially.

The nature of the sensory symptoms varies greatly. In some individuals, it presents with a non-specific discomfort, although patients may use a variety of terms to describe their sensations: a sensation of pulling, jittering, worms or insects, moving, tingling, itching, aching, bubbling, fidgeting, electric current sensations, tightness and throbbing (Garcia-Borreguero et al. 2011). In others, the symptoms can be extremely painful. Although the legs are the commonest anatomical site of involvement, the upper limbs, abdomen or even face can be involved (Michaud et al. 2000; Perez-Diaz et al. 2011).

In fact, in secondary care, insomnia is the most frequent presentation of RLS, affecting 79% of patients (Holmes et al. 2007). Excessive daytime sleepiness is a feature of up to a third of individuals (Hening et al. 2007). As a result, patients may sometimes present with features secondary to poor sleep, such as fatigue, poor concentration or even depression.

The symptoms of RLS may present at any age. The disorder is probably underdiagnosed in children, given that 38% of affected adults have reported the onset of symptoms before the age of 20 and 10% before the age of 10 (Montplaisir et al. 1997). Some children who have been diagnosed as having 'growing pains' meet the diagnostic criteria for RLS (Walters 2002). The sleep disturbance associated with this disorder in childhood can manifest as difficulty falling asleep, bedtime resistance or night-time awakenings, and symptoms are often associated with attention-deficit/hyperactivity disorder (Chervin et al. 2002). Diagnosis in children can be problematic, since describing their sensations in their own words can prove difficult for the very young, and other supporting information often needs to be taken into account. However, the prevalence of RLS increases with age, and the typical course is of a paroxysmal disorder that gradually becomes chronic and progressive. Periodic remission is more common in the young (Allen et al. 2003), and many patients do not experience daily symptoms until 40–60 years of age. One major issue in the elderly, in the context of dementia, is that patients often cannot self-report RLS symptoms, and differentiating RLS-related sleep disturbance from sundowning is problematic (Hadjigeorgiou and Scarmeas 2015).

In addition to the motor restlessness that patients describe, 80–90% of RLS sufferers also experience frank leg movements, which usually arise in sleep but can also occur in wakefulness (Montplaisir et al. 1997). These leg movements are involuntary and typically involve periodic flexion of the hip and knee, dorsiflexion of the foot and extension of the hallux, although these movements are frequently more subtle, and may simply manifest as minimal extension of the hallux. These movements, if arising in sleep, may result in frequent arousals from sleep causing unrefreshing sleep or complete awakenings resulting in fragmented sleep and sleep maintenance issues. They may also impact on the sleep of the bed partner. They are defined as periodic limb movements of sleep (PLMS) if the movements meet certain criteria: lasting between 0.5 and 5 s and with at least four movements in a 90-s period (Iber et al. 2007). A periodic limb movement index of 5–25/h is considered mild, and over 50/h is considered severe.

However, PLMS may occur in isolation, in the absence of symptoms of RLS. The prevalence of periodic limb movement disorder (PLMD)—the clinical consequences of PLMS—is unknown, as it requires polysomnography to diagnose, but PLMS is relatively common, occurring in approximately one third of patients over 60 years of age (Ohayon and Roth 2002). In the context of the sleep clinic setting, frequent PLMS is a common cause of sleep maintenance insomnia and unrefreshing sleep, and the majority of patients with PLMD will not have RLS symptoms.

10.3   Differential Diagnosis

A variety of conditions may mimic RLS. Potential mimics include peripheral neuropathy, cramps, varicose veins, akathisia (a feeling of motor restlessness associated with neuroleptic drugs), fibromyalgia, anxiety and vascular or neurogenic claudication secondary to spinal stenosis (Table 10.1). Therefore, it is imperative that a proper history is elucidated, that the symptoms meet all four diagnostic criteria and that a general and neurological examination is undertaken to exclude these possibilities. On the basis of the diagnostic criteria alone, the specificity is estimated at 85 % (Hening et al. 2009), and so mimics are not necessarily excluded.

10.4   Impact of RLS on Health

RLS has a large impact on quality of life, similar to that of type 2 diabetes and osteoarthritis (Happe et al. 2009; Allen et al. 2005). Increased symptom severity is associated with serious psychological impairment in multiple psychological domains (Scholz et al. 2011). Patients with the disorder have longer adjusted sleep latencies and a higher arousal index than controls (Winkelman et al. 2009), and they report difficulty initiating sleep, difficulty maintaining sleep and unrefreshing sleep two to three times more often than controls (Ohayon et al. 2012).

Emerging evidence also suggests that RLS is associated with metabolic dysregulation, autonomic dysfunction and risk of cardiovascular disease. The syndrome is strongly and positively related to cardiovascular disease, is probably associated with diabetes and impaired glucose tolerance and may be modestly associated with body mass index and dyslipidaemia (Innes et al. 2012). However, the direction of the association is unclear. The syndrome may lead to increased risk for these disorders, perhaps via chronic activation of the sympathetic nervous system and the hypothalamic-pituitary-adrenal axis; these conditions may increase the risk for the syndrome; or RLS may be linked to these conditions through shared risk factors.

Table 10.1 Differential diagnosis

Meeting criteria	Comment		Disorder
Urge to move and unpleasant sensations in the legs Symptoms begin/worsen during periods of rest or inactivity Symptoms relieved with movement Symptoms worse in the evening/night	Definite RLS	Awake symptom diagnosis made by clinical history; uncomfortable urge to move with or without deep creepy-crawling sensation brought on at time of inactivity or rest (sitting or lying); immediate relief either complete or partial with movement; symptomatic relief is persistent as long as movement continues; presence of circadian pattern with peak around midnight and nadir in the morning	RLS
Urge to move Symptoms begin/worsen during periods of rest or inactivity Symptoms relieved with movement Orthostatic hypotension	Neurological disorder with 'urge to move'	Feeling of restlessness which may be localized in legs, brought on by sitting still; should not occur while lying down but might be relieved by movement; occurs in patients with orthostatic hypotension	Hypotensive akathisia
Unpleasant sensations in the legs Symptoms relieved with movement Symptoms worse in the evening/night No positive response to dopaminergic drugs	Pain disorder	Dysesthesias and pain in the legs, frequently one sided, often radicular arrangement of sensory symptoms, atrophic changes of musculature, no urge to move the legs, symptoms can be initiated by sitting and lying and improve by movement, usually neurological and neurophysiological deficits, does not respond to dopaminergic therapy	Radiculopathy
Unpleasant sensations in the legs Symptoms relieved with movement Symptoms worse in the evening/night	Vascular disorder	Dysesthesias and pain in the legs. May appear to occur with or after rest but is associated with or occurs after periods of standing/walking; intensity increased by movement and usually relieved by prolonging rest often best in a lying position, no urge to move, no circadian pattern, usually no sleep disturbances, frequently associated with skin alterations and oedemas. Often associated with vascular disease, circadian pattern if any relates more to activity levels	Vascular claudication, neurogenic claudication

Table 10.1 (continued)

Meeting criteria	Comment		Disorder
Urge to move Symptoms begin/worsen during periods of rest or inactivity Periodic limb movements History of neuroleptics	Neurological disorder with 'urge to move'	Looks like very severe RLS affecting the whole body, but usually without any sensations of pain reported by RLS patients often no relief with movement, should have a history of specific medication exposure	Neuroleptic-induced akathisia
Unpleasant sensations in the legs Symptoms begin/worsen during periods of rest or inactivity No positive response to dopaminergic drugs	Pain disorder	Sensory symptoms commonly reported as numbness, burning and pain; not as common in RLS; numbness is rare in RLS, no urge to move; sensory symptoms usually present throughout the day, less frequent at night; complete and persistent relief is not obtained while walking or during sustained movement	Neuropathy
No periodic limb movements			
Unpleasant sensations in the legs Symptoms begin/worsen during periods of rest or inactivity	Pain disorder	Patients after surgeries frequently do not remember the origin of their complaints. They almost always report symptoms in the legs or in the back, when lying or sitting or during movement	Chronic pain syndrome (lumbar, cervical)
Unpleasant sensations in the legs Symptoms relieved with movement	Disorders without 'urge to move'	Often comes on with prolonged sitting or lying in the same position but usually relieved by a simple change in position, unlike RLS, which often returns when change of position, movement, or walking is not continued, no circadian pattern	Positional discomfort
Symptoms relieved with movement Symptoms worse in the evening/night	Neurological disorder with 'urge to move'	Leg cramps or charley horse cramps can come on at night and are relieved with stretching or walking; no urge to move; experienced as a usually painful muscular contraction, often involving the calf muscles, unlike RLS sensations; sudden onset, occurs not regularly, short duration, usually palpable contractions	Nocturnal leg cramps

(continued)

Table 10.1 (continued)

Meeting criteria	Comment		Disorder
Unpleasant sensations in the legs Symptoms worse in the evening/night Sleep disturbance	Sleep-related disorders	Involuntary muscle (myoclonic) twitch which occurs during falling asleep, described as an electric shock or falling sensation which can cause movements of legs and arms. Occurring once or twice per night, frequent in the population	Hypnic jerks
Unpleasant sensations in the legs Symptoms worse in the evening/night Sleep disturbance	Psychiatric disorders	Depressive disorder with somatic symptoms like psychomotor agitation and diverse somatic complaints, circadian pattern with early awakening in the morning, daytime sleepiness	Depression, various forms with somatic syndrome
Urge to move No positive response to dopaminergic drugs No sleep disturbance	Neurological disorder with 'urge to move'	Occurs in subjects who fidget, especially when bored or anxious, but usually do not experience associated sensory symptoms, discomfort or conscious urge to move; symptoms do not bother the subject, usually lacks a circadian pattern, more of a type of psychic restlessness, less sleep disturbances, no response to dopaminergic medication	Volitional movements, foot tapping, leg rocking
Urge to move No positive response to dopaminergic drugs No periodic limb movements	Disorders without 'urge to move'	Discomfort centred more in joints, may not have prominent circadian pattern as seen in RLS, increase of symptoms during movement, does not respond to dopaminergics, usually no PLMs	Arthritis, lower limb
Urge to move Sleep disturbance	Disorders without 'urge to move'	Multiple, alternating, multiform complaints in muscle groups and joints; sometimes leg maximally involved but mostly whole body affected; frequent sleep disorders, no circadian pattern, no relief by movement, no dopaminergic response	Fibromyalgia
Urge to move	Vascular disorder	Discomfort in legs, some relief with massage or inactivity	Varicose veins

10.5 Epidemiology

The prevalence of RLS remains uncertain, but is clearly high. Studies have used a variety of methods to ascertain cases, ranging from a single question such as 'Do you have restless legs or troublesome twitches of the legs?' to more stringent diagnostic criteria and subsequent case review to rule out differential diagnoses. On the basis of a single question, prevalence has been estimated at 9–15%, whereas studies that tried to rule out alternative diagnoses estimated the prevalence as 1.9–4.6% (Ohayon et al. 2012; Earley and Silber 2010). The prevalence is approximately twice as high in women as in men, and RLS is the most common movement disorder in pregnancy, affecting between 13.5 and 26.6% of pregnant women (Ohayon et al. 2012). To some extent, this is assumed to be related to hormonal fluctuations, since RLS symptoms frequently abate a few days after delivery. However, transient RLS in pregnancy increases the risk of developing RLS later in life by fourfold (Cesnik et al. 2010). The estimated prevalence in school-age children is 2% (Picchietti et al. 2007). Most studies point to a higher prevalence in Northern Europeans and North Americans than in individuals of other ancestries (Yeh et al. 2012).

The majority of RLS cases have an idiopathic basis, and between 20 and 60% of patients report a positive family history of the condition (Rangarajan et al. 2007; Vogl et al. 2006), implying a strong genetic component; this is borne out by more recent studies of RLS genetics (see below). However, a variety of conditions have been associated with higher prevalences of RLS, although the strength of these associations varies. Certainly uraemia secondary to kidney failure is strongly associated, and up to 60% of renal dialysis patients experience symptoms of RLS, despite having a much lower rate of reported family history when compared to the idiopathic RLS population (Kavanagh et al. 2004). Systemic iron deficiency also appears to be associated with RLS and has been identified since Ekbom's original description of RLS—he found that 25% of his original patients were iron deficient (Ekbom 1945). A low serum ferritin, a measure of brain iron stores, albeit imprecise, is associated with patients presenting later in life (Earley et al. 2000a, b). Furthermore, initiation or exacerbation with venesection is well described. As stated above, RLS is also associated with pregnancy, and although the time course of resolution of symptoms suggests a hormonal component, lower haemoglobin levels, lower plasma iron and lower preconception ferritin are associated, suggesting a role for iron deficiency in some pregnant women (Manconi et al. 2004). Peripheral neuropathy, especially small fibre neuropathy, is another robust association with RLS, and myelopathy due to demyelination, spinal trauma, spinal cord tumours and syringomyelia have all been reported to trigger RLS symptoms. Other associations include Parkinson's disease, hereditary ataxias and essential tremor.

10.6   Pathophysiology

The cause of RLS is not fully understood, although clinical observation has informed our understanding of the condition. Dopaminergic agents improve symptoms, and RLS is frequently triggered or exacerbated by dopaminergic antagonists, implying an important role for dopaminergic transmission. Metoclopramide, which crosses the blood-brain barrier, exacerbates RLS symptoms whereas domperidone, which does not, has no influence on RLS, suggesting that the underlying pathophysiological mechanism is located within the central rather than peripheral nervous system. Structural brain imaging, nuclear medicine techniques and post-mortem examination do not demonstrate consistent abnormalities.

However, biochemical studies have largely confirmed evidence of dopaminergic dysregulation in patients with RLS. Studies in animal models and patients have shown increased tyrosine hydroxylase (the rate-limiting enzyme in dopamine synthesis) concentrations in the substantia nigra, decreased numbers of D_2 dopamine receptors in the putamen and increased concentrations of 3-O-methyldopa in the cerebrospinal fluid (Salas et al. 2010), which implies that the syndrome is characterized by upregulation of dopaminergic transmission, with postsynaptic desensitization. Patients with RLS show larger circadian fluctuations in cerebrospinal fluid (CSF) dopamine metabolites (Earley et al. 2006). Additionally, D_2 receptor density in the basal ganglia is inversely correlated with RLS severity (Connor et al. 2009). Despite these biochemical findings, however, PET and SPECT studies of D_2-receptor binding in the basal ganglia do not show consistent changes. It has been proposed that the dopaminergic abnormalities may be localized to the A11 cell group of the subparafascicular nucleus in RLS, which is a modulator of spinal networks (Clemens et al. 2006), and indeed experimental lesioning of this pathway results in an RLS-like picture.

Brain iron is intimately linked to the dopaminergic system, since iron is an essential cofactor in dopamine synthesis (Erikson et al. 2000). Post-mortem examination of the substantia nigra has demonstrated decreased staining for iron and H-ferritin in patients with RLS (Connor et al. 2003), and several studies have shown reduced cerebrospinal fluid levels of ferritin, illustrating low CSF iron stores (Clardy et al. 2006; Earley et al. 2000a, b). Nevertheless, the association between iron and dopaminergic transmission remains uncertain. As detailed above, rat and human studies suggest a hyperdopaminergic state in RLS, with evidence of postsynaptic downregulation (see Khan et al. 2017).

Idiopathic RLS appears to have a strong genetic basis. In addition to frequent reports of a family history, twin studies have shown hereditability estimates of 54–83% (Desai et al. 2004; Ondo et al. 2000). Genome-wide association studies have shown associations with variants in several genes, *MEIS1*, *BTBD9*, *MAP2K5/SKOR1*, *PTPRD* and *TOX3*, but the roles of these genes remain unclear (see Winkelmann et al. 2017). *BTBD9* has also been associated with PLMS (Stefansson et al. 2007).

10.7 Substances and Medications Exacerbating or Triggering RLS

RLS has been associated with a variety of commonly utilized medications, many of which are extremely relevant in the management of patients with psychiatric conditions (Mackie and Winkelman 2015). Anti-depressants in particular are exacerbators of RLS, and although data comparing various drugs is scanty, it appears that high-dose tricyclics venlafaxine and mirtazapine are the most potent aggravating drugs. Unfortunately, these are agents that are commonly prescribed in unrecognized RLS with a predominant picture of sleep initiation or sleep maintenance insomnia. Other drugs used in psychiatric patients that may have an impact on RLS include beta-blockers for anxiety and antipsychotic agents. Antihistamines, often purchased over the counter as sleep-promoting agents, may also exacerbate RLS, resulting in a paradoxical worsening of the insomnia. Further implicated drugs include anti-emetics (with the exception of domperidone, which does not cross the blood-brain barrier) phenytoin and calcium channel antagonists. Caffeine, alcohol and nicotine have all been reported to worsen RLS symptoms.

10.8 Management

After the diagnosis of RLS has been made, efforts should be made to exclude underlying causes such as an iron deficiency state or uraemia. All patients should have renal function and iron studies, including serum ferritin, checked. Any patient with a serum ferritin below 50 µg/L should be commenced on high-dose oral iron supplementation, either in isolation or in conjunction with treatment for RLS (Garcia-Borreguero et al. 2011). Patients should also be screened for any substances or medications that might exacerbate RLS (Mackie and Winkelman 2015), since simple rationalization of medication or a reduction in caffeine, alcohol or nicotine intake may improve symptoms dramatically.

It is important to point out that only 20% of RLS sufferers require specific treatment (Hening et al. 1999). The vast majority of patients can be managed using non-pharmacological techniques. Since tiredness or sleep deprivation in themselves can worsen symptoms, considerable effort should be made to optimize sleep hygiene, and indeed for patients with superimposed psychophysiological insomnia, cognitive behavioural therapy for insomnia may be helpful. As part of sleep hygiene, stimulating substances should be avoided near bedtime. Many patients also experience significant benefit from relaxation therapy, walking or stretching before bedtime, a warm bath in the evening or evening massage of the affected limbs (Mitchell 2011).

The minority of patients require specific treatment, either due to the symptoms of RLS themselves or due to the associated sleep disturbance. Several therapeutic options exist (Winkelman et al. 2016), but in the UK only three agents are licensed for the indication of RLS. These three agents are all dopa agonists: ropinirole, pramipexole and rotigotine, the latter as a topical patch. The dopa agonists have not been directly compared in head-to-head trials but meta-analyses suggest that they are of similar efficacy. The side effect profile is similar for all the agents (common adverse effects include nausea, headache and fatigue), with the exception of rotigotine, which also has a frequent adverse effect of skin reaction to the patch.

The dopa agonists have certain class-specific issues. The impulse control disorders—compulsive gambling, compulsive eating, problem shopping and hypersexuality—are well documented in patients with Parkinson's disease who are treated with these drugs, but more recently these adverse effects have also been described in patients with RLS and indeed have been reported in up to 20% of patients (Cornelius et al. 2010). In Parkinson's disease, risk factors for the development of impulse control disorders include novelty-seeking personality traits, depression and a previous history of substance misuse (Voon et al. 2017).

A further issue for dopa agonists is the phenomenon of augmentation (Garcia-Borreguero et al. 2016; Trenkwalder et al. 2015). Augmentation describes the worsening of RLS symptom severity beyond that expected as part of the natural history of the condition. It is characterized by an earlier time of onset during the day, a worsening of symptom intensity, spreading to other body parts not previously involved such as the arms or face, a shorter latency between rest/immobility and symptom onset, a lessening of the period of relief of symptoms after movement, a shorter duration of treatment effect and a worsening of periodic limb movements of sleep or wakefulness. Rates of augmentation are especially high for levodopa—up to 60% after 6 months—with a median time to augmentation of 71 days, which has led to this treatment modality very much falling out of favour, although it remains licensed for RLS in Germany, Switzerland and Austria. However, even for the dopa agonists, augmentation rates are clinically significant, although once again direct head-to-head trials have not been undertaken. Augmentation rates are of the order of approximately 7% per annum, although perhaps lower for rotigotine if the dose is maintained within the licensed range (Garcia-Borreguero et al. 2016). Augmentation is a dose-related effect and so can be minimized by maintaining as low a dose as possible. It is generally recommended that daily dosages should be kept to a maximum of 2 mg of ropinirole, 500 μg of pramipexole and 3–4 mg of rotigotine. Attention should be paid to the serum ferritin, as the likelihood of augmentation increases with low iron stores (Trenkwalder et al. 2008).

Other classes of drugs do not appear to cause augmentation. However, in the UK, all other therapies are off-label, although in the USA, gabapentin enacarbil has been licensed in the last few years. This is a prodrug of gabapentin, formulated to circumvent issues of poor bioavailability with gabapentin, but is not available in the UK. Gabapentin can however be effective in RLS, particularly when pain is a prominent feature. Pregabalin has recently gained increasing use and has better bioavailability compared to gabapentin. A recent study has suggested that pregabalin is as effective as pramipexole, with low augmentation rates (Allen et al. 2014). It is of course licensed for generalized anxiety disorder and therefore is potentially useful in individuals with prominent anxiety symptoms. Other widely used drugs include the opioids—methadone has been demonstrated to be helpful, with no evidence of significant dosage increase despite a 10-year follow-up (Silver et al. 2011), and more recently oxycodone as a prolonged release formulation with naloxone to prevent gastrointestinal side effects has been shown to be effective (Trenkwalder et al. 2013). The opioids are particularly helpful when there is a prominent pain component and can also be utilized for patients who need occasional treatment only, for example, while on a flight or in a cinema or meeting. They can also be used to cover the withdrawal of dopa agonists when augmentation has occurred. Clonazepam at low dose can be particularly effective for patients with significant insomnia (Garcia-Borreguero et al. 2011), although there remain concerns about dependency, and the long half-life can potentially result in daytime drowsiness.

A variety of other drugs have been tried and certainly anecdotally can be effective, although the evidence base is limited. These include anti-epileptic drugs such as carbamazepine, valproate, topiramate, perampanel, baclofen, clonidine (which is widely used in the paediatric setting) and intravenous iron.

From a psychiatric perspective, treatment of depression coexisting with RLS can be problematic. Bupropion, in contrast to other anti-depressants, has been reported as being helpful in RLS (Lee et al. 2009), presumably due to its dopamine-reuptake inhibitory effects. A single small randomized controlled trial of bupropion has at least suggested that it does not seem to worsen RLS severity (Bayard et al. 2011).

Data for the management of isolated PLMD is much more scanty, but typically the same therapeutic agents are used as for RLS. A recent meta-analysis has demonstrated evidence for the reduction in the periodic limb movement index for the dopa agonists, oxycodone, pregabalin, gabapentin and gabapentin enacarbil (Hornyak et al. 2014). It has been suggested in a small study that the dopa agonists may simply suppress leg movements without significantly impacting on arousals or EEG instability, whereas clonazepam reduces non-REM EEG instability without affecting the limb movements (Manconi et al. 2012). However, in the absence of a significant evidence base, the author's practice is to favour drugs that act to consolidate sleep where there is no coexistent RLS, especially as no drugs are specifically licensed for PLMD. In contrast to RLS, where successful improvement of RLS symptoms is reported by the patient, in isolated PLMD, treatment needs to be guided by improvement in self-reported daytime symptoms, although ankle actigraphy or repeated polysomnography may be required.

Conclusions

The wide spectrum of clinical features of RLS presents a significant diagnostic challenge to medical practitioners. Early recognition and appropriate management can have a significant impact on sleep quality, physical and psychological morbidity and quality of life. The majority of patients with RLS can be managed through non-pharmacological measures and rationalization of medication, but for those requiring specific and targeted pharmacological therapy, there are potential pitfalls in achieving successful symptom control.

References

Allen RP, Picchietti D, Hening WA, Trenkwalder C, Walters AS, Montplaisi J, Restless Legs Syndrome Diagnosis and Epidemiology Workshop at the National Institutes of Health and International Restless Legs Syndrome Study Group. Restless legs syndrome: diagnostic criteria, special considerations, and epidemiology. A report from the restless legs syndrome diagnosis and epidemiology workshop at the National Institutes of Health. Sleep Med. 2003;4(2):101–19.

Allen RP, Walters AS, Montplaisir J, Hening W, Myers A, Bell TJ, Ferini-Strambi L. Restless legs syndrome prevalence and impact: REST general population study. Arch Intern Med. 2005; 165(11):1286–92.

Allen RP, Chen C, Garcia-Borreguero D, Polo O, Dubrava S, Miceli J, Knapp L, Winkelman JW. Comparison of pregabalin with pramipexole for restless legs syndrome. N Engl J Med. 2014;370(7):621–31.

Bayard M, Bailey B, Acharya D, Ambreen F, Duggal S, Kaur T, Rahman ZU, Roller K, Tudiver F. Bupropion and restless legs syndrome: a randomized controlled trial. J Am Board Fam Med. 2011;24(4):422–8.

Cesnik E, Casetta I, Turri M, Govoni V, Granieri E, Strambi LF, Manconi M. Transient RLS during pregnancy is a risk factor for the chronic idiopathic form. Neurology. 2010;75(23):2117–20.

Chervin RD, Archbold KH, Dillon JE, Pituch KJ, Panahi P, Dahl RE, Guilleminault C. Associations between symptoms of inattention, hyperactivity, restless legs, and periodic leg movements. Sleep. 2002;25(2):213–8.

Clardy SL, Earley CJ, Allen RP, Beard JL, Connor JR. Ferritin subunits in CSF are decreased in restless legs syndrome. J Lab Clin Med. 2006;147(2):67–73.

Clemens S, Rye D, Hochman S. Restless legs syndrome: revisiting the dopamine hypothesis from the spinal cord perspective. Neurology. 2006;67(1):125–30.

Connor JR, Boyer PJ, Menzies SL, Dellinger B, Allen RP, Ondo WG, Earley CJ. Neuropathological examination suggests impaired brain iron acquisition in restless legs syndrome. Neurology. 2003;61(3):304–9.

Connor JR, Wang XS, Allen RP, Beard JL, Wiesinger JA, Felt BT, Earley CJ. Altered dopaminergic profile in the putamen and substantia nigra in restless leg syndrome. Brain. 2009;132(Pt 9): 2403–12.

Cornelius JR, Tippmann-Peikert M, Slocumb NL, Frerichs CF, Silber MH. Impulse control disorders with the use of dopaminergic agents in restless legs syndrome: a case-control study. Sleep. 2010;33(1):81–7.

Desai AV, Cherkas LF, Spector TD, Williams AJ. Genetic influences in self-reported symptoms of obstructive sleep apnoea and restless legs: a twin study. Twin Res. 2004;7(6):589–95.

Earley CJ, Hyland K, Allen RP. Circadian changes in CSF dopaminergic measures in restless legs syndrome. Sleep Med. 2006;7(3):263–8.

Earley CJ, Silber MH. Restless legs syndrome: understanding its consequences and the need for better treatment. Sleep Med. 2010;11(9):807–15.

Earley CJ, Allen RP, Beard JL, Connor JR. Insight into the pathophysiology of restless legs syndrome. J Neurosci Res. 2000a;62(5):623–8.

Earley CJ, Connor JR, Beard JL, Malecki EA, Epstein DK, Allen RP. Abnormalities in CSF concentrations of ferritin and transferrin in restless legs syndrome. Neurology. 2000b;54(8): 1698–700.

Ekbom K. Restless legs: a clinical study. Acta Med Scand. 1945;158(Suppl):1–122.

Erikson KM, Jones BC, Beard JL. Iron deficiency alters dopamine transporter functioning in rat striatum. J Nutr. 2000;130(11):2831–7.

Garcia-Borreguero D, Stillman P, Benes H, Buschmann H, Chaudhuri KR, Gonzalez Rodriguez VM, Hogl B, Kohnen R, Monti GC, Stiasny-Kolster K, Trenkwalder C, Williams AM, Zucconi M. Algorithms for the diagnosis and treatment of restless legs syndrome in primary care. BMC Neurol. 2011;11:28.

Garcia-Borreguero D, Silber MH, Winkelman JW, Hogl B, Bainbridge J, Buchfuhrer M, Hadjigeorgiou G, Inoue Y, Manconi M, Oertel W, Ondo W, Winkelmann J, Allen RP. Guidelines for the first-line treatment of restless legs syndrome/Willis-Ekbom disease, prevention and treatment of dopaminergic augmentation: a combined task force of the IRLSSG, EURLSSG, and the RLS-foundation. Sleep Med. 2016;21:1–11.

Hadjigeorgiou GM, Scarmeas N. Restless legs syndrome in the darkness of dementia. Sleep. 2015;38(3):333–4.

Happe S, Reese JP, Stiasny-Kolster K, Peglau I, Mayer G, Klotsche J, Giani G, Geraedts M, Trenkwalder C, Dodel R. Assessing health-related quality of life in patients with restless legs syndrome. Sleep Med. 2009;10(3):295–305.

Hening W, Allen R, Earley C, Kushida C, Picchietti D, Silber M. The treatment of restless legs syndrome and periodic limb movement disorder. An American Academy of Sleep Medicine Review. Sleep. 1999;22(7):970–99.

Hening W, Allen RP, Tenzer P, Winkelman JW. Restless legs syndrome: demographics, presentation, and differential diagnosis. Geriatrics. 2007;62(9):26–9.

Hening WA, Allen RP, Washburn M, Lesage SR, Earley CJ. The four diagnostic criteria for restless legs syndrome are unable to exclude confounding conditions ("mimics"). Sleep Med. 2009;10(9):976–81.

Holmes R, Tluk S, Metta V, Patel P, Rao R, Williams A, Chaudhuri KR. Nature and variants of idiopathic restless legs syndrome: observations from 152 patients referred to secondary care in the UK. J Neural Transm. 2007;114(7):929–34.

Hornyak M, Scholz H, Kohnen R, Bengel J, Kassubek J, Trenkwalder C. What treatment works best for restless legs syndrome? Meta-analyses of dopaminergic and non-dopaminergic medications. Sleep Med Rev. 2014;18(2):153–64.

Iber C, Ancoli-Israel S, Chesson A, Quan SF. The AASM manual for the scoring of sleep and associates events: rules, terminology and technical specifications. Westchester, IL: American Academy of Sleep Medicine; 2007.

Innes KE, Selfe TK, Agarwal P. Restless legs syndrome and conditions associated with metabolic dysregulation, sympathoadrenal dysfunction, and cardiovascular disease risk: a systematic review. Sleep Med Rev. 2012;16(4):309–39.

Kavanagh D, Siddiqui S, Geddes CC. Restless legs syndrome in patients on dialysis. Am J Kidney Dis. 2004;43(5):763–71.

Khan FH, Ahlberg CD, Chow CA, Shah DR, Koo BB. Iron, dopamine, genetics, and hormones in the pathophysiology of restless legs syndrome. J Neurol. 2017;264(8):1634–41.

Lee JJ, Erdos J, Wilkosz MF, Laplante R, Wagoner B. Bupropion as a possible treatment option for restless legs syndrome. Ann Pharmacother. 2009;43(2):370–4.

Leschziner G, Gringras P. Restless legs syndrome. BMJ. 2012;344:E3056.

Mackie S, Winkelman JW. Long-term treatment of restless legs syndrome (RLS): an approach to management of worsening symptoms, loss of efficacy, and augmentation. CNS Drugs. 2015; 29(5):351–7.

Manconi M, Govoni V, De Vito A, Economou NT, Cesnik E, Mollica G, Granieri E. Pregnancy as a risk factor for restless legs syndrome. Sleep Med. 2004;5(3):305–8.

Manconi M, Fulda S, Ferri R, Ferini-Strambi L, Bassetti CL. 7. Dissociation of periodic leg movements from arousals in restless legs syndrome. Clin Neurophysiol. 2012;123(10):E111.

Michaud M, Chabli A, Lavigne G, Montplaisir J. Arm restlessness in patients with restless legs syndrome. Mov Disord. 2000;15(2):289–93.

Mitchell UH. Nondrug-related aspect of treating Ekbom disease, formerly known as restless legs syndrome. Neuropsychiatr Dis Treat. 2011;7:251–7.

Montplaisir J, Boucher S, Poirier G, Lavigne G, Lapierre O, Lesperance P. Clinical, polysomnographic, and genetic characteristics of restless legs syndrome: a study of 133 patients diagnosed with new standard criteria. Mov Disord. 1997;12(1):61–5.

Ohayon MM, Roth T. Prevalence of restless legs syndrome and periodic limb movement disorder in the general population. J Psychosom Res. 2002;53(1):547–54.

Ohayon MM, O'hara R, Vitiello MV. Epidemiology of restless legs syndrome: a synthesis of the literature. Sleep Med Rev. 2012;16(4):283–95.

Ondo WG, Vuong KD, Wang Q. Restless legs syndrome in monozygotic twins: clinical correlates. Neurology. 2000;55(9):1404–6.

Perez-Diaz H, Iranzo A, Rye DB, Santamaria J. Restless abdomen: a phenotypic variant of restless legs syndrome. Neurology. 2011;77(13):1283–6.

Picchietti D, Allen RP, Walters AS, Davidson JE, Myers A, Ferini-Strambi L. Restless legs syndrome: prevalence and impact in children and adolescents—the Peds REST study. Pediatrics. 2007;120(2):253–66.

Rangarajan S, Rangarajan S, D'Souza GA. Restless legs syndrome in an Indian urban population. Sleep Med. 2007;9(1):88–93.

Salas RE, Gamaldo CE, Allen RP. Update in restless legs syndrome. Curr Opin Neurol. 2010;23(4):401–6.

Scholz H, Benes H, Happe S, Bengel J, Kohnen R, Hornyak M. Psychological distress of patients suffering from restless legs syndrome: a cross-sectional study. Health Qual Life Outcomes. 2011;9:73.

Silver N, Allen RP, Senerth J, Earley CJ. A 10-year, longitudinal assessment of dopamine agonists and methadone in the treatment of restless legs syndrome. Sleep Med. 2011;12(5):440–4.

Stefansson H, Rye DB, Hicks A, Petursson H, Ingason A, Thorgeirsson TE, Palsson S, Sigmundsson T, Sigurdsson AP, Eiriksdottir I, Soebech E, Bliwise D, Beck JM, Rosen A, Waddy S, Trotti LM, Iranzo A, Thambisetty M, Hardarson GA, Kristjansson K, Gudmundsson LJ, Thorsteinsdottir U, Kong A, Gulcher JR, Gudbjartsson D, Stefansson K. A genetic risk factor for periodic limb movements in sleep. N Engl J Med. 2007;357(7):639–47.

Trenkwalder C, Högl B, Benes H, Kohnen R. Augmentation in restless legs syndrome is associated with low ferritin. Sleep Med. 2008;9(5):572–4.

Trenkwalder C, Beneš H, Grote L, García-Borreguero D, Högl B, Hopp M, Bosse B, Oksche A, Reimer K, Winkelmann J, Allen RP, Kohnen R. Prolonged release oxycodone-naloxone for treatment of severe restless legs syndrome after failure of previous treatment: a double-blind, randomised, placebo-controlled trial with an open-label extension. Lancet Neurol. 2013;12(12):1141–50.

Trenkwalder C, Winkelmann J, Inoue Y, Paulus W. Restless legs syndrome-current therapies and management of augmentation. Nat Rev Neurol. 2015;11(8):434–45.

Vogl FD, Pichler I, Adel S, Pinggera GK, Bracco S, De Grandi A, Volpato CB, Aridon P, Mayer T, Meitinger T, Klein C, Casari G, Pramstaller PP. Restless legs syndrome: epidemiological and clinicogenetic study in a South Tyrolean population isolate. Mov Disord. 2006;21(8):1189–95.

Voon V, Napier TC, Frank MJ, Sgambato-Faure V, Grace AA, Rodriguez-Oroz M, Obeso J, Bezard E, Fernagut PO. Impulse control disorders and levodopa-induced dyskinesias in Parkinson's disease: an update. LancetNeurol. 2017;16(3):238–50.

Walters AS. Is there a subpopulation of children with growing pains who really have restless legs syndrome? A review of the literature. Sleep Med. 2002;3(2):93–8.

Winkelman JW, Redline S, Baldwin CM, Resnick HE, Newman AB, Gottlieb DJ. Polysomnographic and health-related quality of life correlates of restless legs syndrome in the Sleep Heart Health Study. Sleep. 2009;32(6):772–8.

Winkelman JW, Armstrong MJ, Allen RP, Chaudhuri KR, Ondo W, Trenkwalder C, Zee PC, Gronseth GS, Gloss D, Zesiewicz T. Practice guideline summary: treatment of restless legs syndrome in adults: report of the Guideline Development, Dissemination, and Implementation Subcommittee of the American Academy of Neurology. Neurology. 2016;87(24):2585–93.

Winkelmann J, Schormair B, Xiong L, Dion PA, Rye DB, Rouleau GA. Genetics of restless legs syndrome. Sleep Med. 2017;31:18–22.

Yeh P, Walters AS, Tsuang JW. Restless legs syndrome: a comprehensive overview on its epidemiology, risk factors, and treatment. Sleep Breath. 2012;16(4):987–1007.

Circadian Rhythm Sleep-Wake Disorders

11

Dora Zalai, Bojana Gladanac, and Colin M. Shapiro

11.1 Introduction

The circadian system regulates a range of behavioural, physiological and cellular rhythms that allow organisms to anticipate changes in their physical environment, such as cycles of day and night. These predictive near-24-h oscillations persist in the absence of all environmental cues and are driven by the endogenous master pacemaker located in the suprachiasmatic nucleus (SCN) of the anterior hypothalamus in mammals (Stephan and Zucker 1972; Ralph et al. 1990; Edgar et al. 1993). Within individual SCN neurons, cyclic core clock genes and proteins establish a molecular basis of circadian control through transcriptional, translational and post-translational feedback loops (Reppert and Weaver 2002). This intracellular clock is not only found in the SCN, but in nearly all peripheral tissues of the mammalian body where it establishes tissue-specific gene expression to temporally coordinate physiology. Signals from the central SCN are relayed throughout the brain and body to synchronize these peripheral clocks to appropriate phases through neuronal, hormonal and physiological mechanisms (Buhr and Takahashi 2013). In this manner, the SCN regulates many diverse processes, including daily patterns of sleep, endocrine secretion, glucose homeostasis and core body temperature.

D. Zalai, M.D., Ph.D. (✉)
Department of Psychology, Ryerson University, Toronto, ON, Canada

Sleep and Alertness Clinic, Toronto, ON, Canada
e-mail: dora.zalai@psych.ryerson.ca

B. Gladanac
Melatonin Assessment Testing Laboratory, Toronto, ON, Canada

C. M. Shapiro, M.D., Ph.D.
Youthdale Child and Adolescent Sleep Centre, Toronto, ON, Canada

University of Toronto, Toronto, ON, Canada

© Springer-Verlag GmbH Germany, part of Springer Nature 2018
H. Selsick (ed.), *Sleep Disorders in Psychiatric Patients*,
https://doi.org/10.1007/978-3-642-54836-9_11

In order to properly align these internal rhythms to external 24-h time, the circadian timing system is reset daily by environmental time cues including exercise, food intake and light exposure. Light is the dominant daily entrainment cue that resets the SCN through direct retinal photic pathways via rod, cone and melanopsin-expressing photoreceptors (Gooley et al. 2010). The acute and phase-resetting responses are dependent on the spectral composition, intensity, duration and timing of light exposure (Czeisler and Gooley 2007). Phase-resetting responses to light are often depicted by a phase response curve (PRC), which plots the magnitude of phase shift as a function of the circadian time the light was administered. In humans, light exposure given before the nadir of core body temperature (early in the subjective night) will induce a phase delay of the circadian rhythm, whereas light exposure given after nadir (late in the subjective night or early morning) will induce a phase advance (Czeisler et al. 1986; Khalsa et al. 2003). Given that the endogenous circadian period is, on average, longer than 24 h in humans, we require a daily phase advance of about 10 min in order to entrain to a 24-h solar day (Czeisler et al. 1999; Duffy et al. 2011). By synchronizing the human circadian timing system to external time, optimal performance and alertness can occur during daytime hours, and sleep can occur during the night time.

In humans, the regulation of sleep-wake cycles is dependent on the precise interaction and counterbalance between the circadian system and the homeostatic sleep process (Borbely 1982). Under entrained conditions, as the homeostatic sleep pressure increases with prolonged wakefulness, it is opposed by an increasing circadian wakefulness drive, allowing for a sustained wake episode each day. Conversely, as the homeostatic sleep pressure dissipates with sleep, the circadian propensity to sleep increases, allowing for a consolidated bout of sleep each night (Dijk and Czeisler 1994). Thus, the alignment and opposing interactions of these two independent processes influence waking performance and the timing, quantity and architecture of sleep (Dijk and Czeisler 1994; Dijk and Czeisler 1995; Dijk et al. 1992).

Daily rhythms in sleep and wakefulness are manifestations of the intrinsic biological clock and extrinsic environmental and behavioural rhythms. In circadian rhythm sleep-wake disorders (CRSWD), chronic or recurring changes to daily sleep-wake cycles can result from problems with the intrinsic circadian system or from a misalignment between this intrinsic circadian system and the extrinsic environment with its personal and societal demands. The most common clinical symptoms of CRSWD are insomnia and/or excessive sleepiness that result in considerable impairments in physical, mental, social, occupational and/or other important domains of functioning (International Classification of Sleep Disorders 2014). Excessive sleepiness and difficulties initiating/maintaining sleep are common complaints; therefore, it is important to accurately detect CRSWD using current diagnostic tools. CRSWD can be complex in aetiology and therefore often requires a multifaceted treatment approach that includes both intrinsic and extrinsic factors that can influence the progression and severity of the symptoms. This is highlighted by Clinical Vignette A, which emphasizes the multifaceted aspect of circadian changes and the link to psychiatric presentations.

11.2   Delayed Sleep-Wake Phase Disorder

11.2.1 Description

Delayed sleep-wake phase disorder (DSWPD) is a CRSWD in which there is a habitual delay in the phase of the sleep-wake cycle, such that the major bout of sleep occurs at a later-than-desired clock time. Thus, DSWPD is characterized by recurrent late sleep and correspondingly late rising and an inability to fall asleep and wake up at scheduled times during work or school days (Weitzman et al. 1981). More specifically, when allowed to follow preferred sleep schedules, as on weekends or nonwork days, DSWPD patients demonstrate a significant delay in the major sleep episode, typically falling asleep between 1 and 4 am and awakening in the late morning or afternoon (International Classification of Sleep Disorders 2014). Due to a delayed sleep onset, their sleep is curtailed in the morning (if trying to get up at a socially desirable time) when their circadian sleep propensity and melatonin levels are still elevated. There is sleep inertia (problems of arising at an "appropriate time") and excessive daytime sleepiness.

11.2.2 Risk Factors

As the most common CRSWD, DSWPD represents 5–10% of individuals diagnosed with chronic insomnia disorder in sleep clinics and has an estimated prevalence of 0.13–0.17% in the general population (Schrader et al. 1993; Yazaki et al. 1999). It is more common amongst adolescents and young adults, with studies reporting a prevalence of about 4–16% in these populations (Thorpy et al. 1988; Sivertsen et al. 2013; Saxvig et al. 2012). The shift in diurnal preference, from "morningness" in younger children to "eveningness" in adolescents, appears to be associated with various biological and environmental changes during pubertal development (Crowley et al. 2007).

There are several reports of genetic predispositions to extreme diurnal preference and DSWPD, including polymorphisms and haplotypes in the circadian clock gene *PER3* (Archer et al. 2003; Pereira et al. 2005; Jones et al. 2007; Lazar et al. 2012; Archer et al. 2010; Ebisawa et al. 2001). Moreover, studies have found other genetic variants that appear to be associated with DSWPD, including arylalkylamine N-acetyltransferase which is an important part of the melatonin synthesis pathway (Hohjoh et al. 2003); casein kinase I epsilon, which is a key post-translational modulator of the molecular clock (Takano et al. 2004); and an increased frequency of human leukocyte antigen (HLA-DR1) (Hohjoh et al. 1999).

There is substantial evidence that evening-type individuals are more likely to have affective disorders, including major depression (Drennan et al. 1991; Merikanto et al. 2013), seasonal affective disorder (SAD) (Natale et al. 2005) and bipolar disorder (Wood et al. 2009). Furthermore, "eveningness" may even predict earlier onset and increased severity of these states (Gaspar-Barba et al. 2009; Mansour et al. 2005). A recent report looking at a large cohort of outpatients with a history of mood disorders found that depression severity was significantly associated with delayed sleep-wake and activity rhythms in adolescents and young adults (Robillard et al. 2014). It is therefore not surprising that rates of co-morbidity are high between DSWPD and depression (Thorpy et al. 1988; Takahashi et al. 2000; Regestein and Pavlova 1995), seasonal affective disorder (SAD) (Lee et al. 2011) and bipolar disorder (Dagan et al. 1998). Studies suggest that 40–75% of DSWPD patients are co-diagnosed with depression; however, this can vary based on the sample population (Thorpy et al. 1988; Takahashi et al. 2000; Regestein and Pavlova 1995). Interestingly, individuals with bipolar disorder may display a more pronounced phase delay in the gold standard test of melatonin secretion (dim light melatonin onset, DLMO) and sleep onset than individuals with unipolar depression (Robillard et al. 2013a; Robillard et al. 2013b) (Fig. 11.1). We have recently shown that sleep disturbances (and particularly DSPWD) occur in an adolescent inpatient psychiatric facility in inpatients with a more complex psychopathology. This suggests that DSWPD may be linked with severity of psychopathology (Shahid et al. 2012). Evidently, there is a strong association between mood disorders and DSWPD; however, there is currently limited knowledge on the causative mechanisms or reciprocity of these relationships.

Studies have shown that about 30% of children and over 80% of adults with attention-deficit/hyperactivity disorder (ADHD) report difficulties falling asleep at a reasonable time (Van Veen et al. 2010; Corkum et al. 1999). Moreover, both children and adults with ADHD and sleep onset insomnia also demonstrate a delayed wake time and melatonin secretion, while sleep maintenance is similar to age-matched ADHD controls without sleep difficulties, demonstrating that this characteristic is due to DSWPD (Van Veen et al. 2010; Van der Heijden et al. 2005). Moreover, ADHD individuals of all ages are more often evening chronotypes and frequently score as extreme evening chronotypes, as compared to controls (Bijlenga et al. 2013; Baird et al. 2012). Therefore, individuals with ADHD are a particularly high-risk group for DSWPD.

11.2.3 History

A detailed history of an individual's sleep and activity pattern should be noted. Typically, sleep onset difficulty starts in the teenage years as the sleep propensity shifts later. Individuals with CRSWD describe that their peak of alertness and cognitive performance is in the evening and at night. If allowed to choose an ideal sleep period (e.g., on the weekends or in the summer break), those with CRSWD go to bed very late. In these situations, they do not have sleep onset insomnia and their sleep quality is good. With respect to differential diagnosis, delayed bedtime because of safety concerns in post-traumatic stress disorder, prolonged evening routines in obsessive compulsive disorder, diurnal improvement of mood in depression or social activities (communication with friends) at night should be considered.

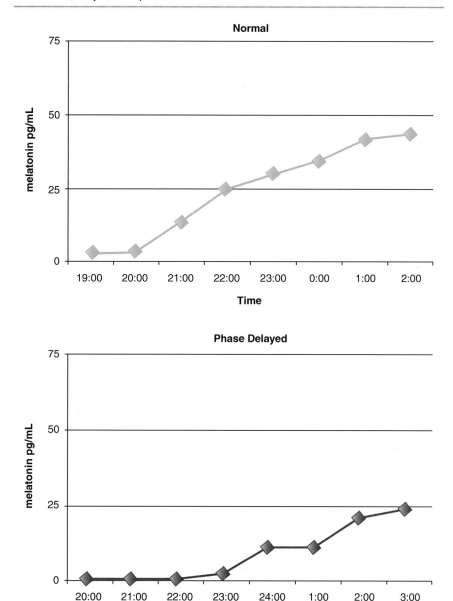

Fig. 11.1 Dim light melatonin onset (DLMO) test. The DLMO test involves sitting in a dark room (<30 lux, in order to avoid melatonin suppression by light) from approximately 7 pm to 3 am. Hourly samples (blood or, preferably from the patients' perspective, saliva) are collected. Additional samples may be needed for cases in which there may be extreme advanced or delayed melatonin rhythm. Samples are processed to determine melatonin levels, and an individual's melatonin profile is graphed. There are several methods to define DLMO, including when levels reach a fixed threshold of 3 or 4 pg/mL or when levels rise more than two standard deviations above at least three baseline values (or combinations of both). The graph below shows a normal pattern (DLMO at around 9 pm) and a delayed pattern of melatonin secretion in a DSWPD patient (DLMO at around 12 am)

11.2.4 Investigations

In addition to a detailed patient sleep history, current diagnostic tools assess both behavioural sleep-wake patterns and the endogenous timing of the circadian system. Sleep logs and actigraphy are recommended for at least 7 and preferably 14 days to discern patients' rest-activity schedules and patterns. Several questionnaires, including the Morningness-Eveningness Questionnaire (MEQ) (Appendix B) and the Munich Chronotype Questionnaire (MCQ), can also help determine an individual's preferred timing of various activities across a 24-h day (Zavada et al. 2005; Horne and Ostberg 1976). Similar questionnaires can be found for paediatric and adolescent populations (Werner et al. 2009). It is common for DSWPD patients to show extreme evening preference on questionnaires.

Most authorities state that overnight polysomnography (PSG) is typically not required. However, it may useful in assessing co-morbidity of other sleep disorders, such as sleep apnoea and periodic limb movement disorder (International Classification of Sleep Disorders 2014). If PSG is performed under a preferred or ad libitum schedule, sleep quantity and quality is generally normal for age; however, there may be a slight delay in sleep onset (Lack and Wright 2007; Saxvig et al. 2013).

We have shown that in a proportion of "phase delay" individuals, as described by self-report and sleep diaries or actigraphy, there may be a relatively easy sleep onset at what is viewed as a regular time if the person is put to sleep in a laboratory. If they are put to bed after a DLMO study (in our laboratory, shortly after 3 am), there may be a long sleep onset. Both of these patterns are somewhat paradoxical, suggesting that behavioural rather than biological factors are responsible for the late bedtime. Thus, these observations are clinically relevant and useful. We therefore feel that overnight sleep studies are beneficial in helping to clarify the diagnosis. Key body rhythm markers, including core body temperature and the nightly secretion of melatonin by the pineal gland, are important in revealing circadian timing abnormalities relative to the sleep-wake cycle. In normally entrained individuals, the rise in melatonin secretion during the biological night from nearly absent daytime levels occurs typically about 2–3 h before sleep onset, while the nadir of the core body temperature is about 2 h before sleep offset (Benloucif et al. 2005).

Determining the onset of melatonin secretion appears to be a more stable phase marker than core body temperature (Benloucif et al. 2005; Klerman et al. 2002) and is a more reliable, practical and more socially acceptable clinical measure to confirm the presence of a CRSWD (Sack et al. 2007). Melatonin can be measured in plasma and saliva or as its primary metabolite 6-sulfatoxymelatonin in urine.

One needs to recognize that, particularly amongst adolescents, some "choose" to go to bed late and others are "compelled" to go to bed late by virtue of their biology. It is nothing short of cruel to attempt to adjust the delayed phase in a teenager with a shifted biological clock by behavioural means as this invariably fails. Conversely, being persuaded by a change in sleep pattern that it must be a biological problem is naïve. This is the reason that DLMO testing needs to be more widely applied. There is no other hormonal disorder that would be treated without the relevant test.

Moreover, many treatments for CRSWD are phase dependent (as discussed later on); thus proper phase assessment not only helps with diagnostic specificity but also guides treatment.

11.2.5 Treatment

In order to properly realign the endogenous circadian system with environmental time, the management of DSWPD requires a comprehensive treatment approach involving environmental, behavioural and/or pharmacological factors. This may include chronotherapy, bright light therapy, exogenous melatonin administration and techniques to improve sleep hygiene.

Chronotherapy involves implementing a transient phase delaying regimen where sleep-wake times are progressively delayed by about 3 h every 2 days until sleep onset finally reaches the desired bedtime (Czeisler et al. 1981). Once an appropriate earlier bedtime is established, it is important for individuals to enforce a regular sleep-wake schedule and avoid delaying their circadian rhythms by staying up late on weekends or by being exposed to light late in the evening. Although a potentially successful treatment method, compliance is often difficult to maintain because of the daily restrictions placed on an individual's personal and societal lifestyle. Moreover, the long-term effectiveness of chronotherapy is variable, including common accounts of relapse (Ito et al. 1993). In reality, for most, this is only a textbook solution.

Bright light therapy is a common treatment method for CRSWD patients and involves appropriately timed bright light and darkness to adjust an individual's circadian phase and thus their sleep-wake cycle. As explained by the human PRC to light, exposure to light in the late subjective night or early morning phase advances circadian rhythms (resets pacemaker to an earlier time), whereas exposure to light in the early subjective night or late evening generates phase delays (resets pacemaker to a later time) (Czeisler et al. 1986; Khalsa et al. 2003). In DSWPD patients, a 2–3-h exposure to bright light at ~2500 lux given on awakening with limited light exposure in the evenings has been shown to phase advance body temperature, melatonin rhythms and sleep onset and to increase objective measures of daytime alertness (Rosenthal et al. 1990; Cole et al. 2002). Considering that the timing of light is crucial, caution should be taken to administer the morning light exposure after the core body temperature nadir (during the appropriate advance portion of the PRC), so as to avoid administering the bright light stimulus before the core body temperature nadir and inadvertently furthering the delayed circadian phase. Moreover, it is important to monitor and maintain treatment in order to keep the phase advancement of the sleep-wake schedule and prevent drifting back to a delayed pattern (Rosenthal et al. 1990; Wilhelmsen-Langeland et al. 2013). The theory behind this is good, but in clinical practice, it is often very difficult to do. Patients, particularly those with DSWPD who are liable to lie in in the morning, rarely have the time to sit in front of a light before rushing off to work or school. One of us (CS) has gone as far as admitting a patient to an inpatient ward (approximately 20 years ago) to try to ensure this was correctly done. However, on discharge the patient rapidly reverted to a delayed pattern. Exogenous melatonin can also phase shift the circadian pacemaker when given during the biological day, that is, when endogenous levels are nearly absent. As demonstrated by the human melatonin PRC, exogenous melatonin induces phase shifts opposite to light exposure; melatonin administration in the afternoon/evening generates phase advances, and melatonin administration in the morning generates phase delays (Lewy et al. 1998). In DSWPD patients, previous studies have shown that melatonin given during the afternoon or early evening can shift circadian rhythms (core body temperature and/or melatonin rhythms), as well as sleep-wake times to an earlier phase (Dahlitz et al. 1991; Nagtegaal et al. 1998; Kayumov et al. 2001; Mundey et al. 2005). These studies vary in terms of dosage and scheduling of melatonin administration. In one double-blind placebo-controlled crossover study, we showed that DSWPD subjects treated with 5 mg melatonin at 7 pm for 4 weeks led to a reduced PSG-determined sleep onset latency and normalization of urinary 6-sulfatoxymelatonin, as compared to placebo (Kayumov et al. 2001). A separate double-blind placebo-controlled study tested two different doses (0.3 mg vs. 3 mg) administered between 1.5 and 6.5 h prior to DLMO for 4 weeks (Mundey et al. 2005). Interestingly, both doses demonstrated comparable maximal phase advances, with a greater magnitude observed with earlier times of melatonin administration relative to DLMO. Similarly, in normally entrained individuals, the melatonin PRC to two different doses (0.5 mg vs. 3 mg) demonstrated comparable maximal magnitudes of phase delays and advances, with peak phase advancements occurring 3–5 h prior to DLMO (Lewy et al. 1998; Burgess et al. 2010). In our clinic, our standard procedure after obtaining the results of the DLMO showing a delayed rise is to give each patient two packets of pills marked "A" and "B" with the instruction to take one pill from "A" for a month and one pill from "B" for a month, both at 7 pm every night. This is a single-blind exercise using placebo and melatonin. The patient returns in 2 months, and 95% will have clearly identified the active treatment and wish to remain on the melatonin. Evidently, exogenous melatonin is an effective and recommended treatment of DSWPD; however, in order to establish more specific dose and scheduling guidelines, additional large-scale controlled trials are warranted (Morgenthaler et al. 2007).

Recent studies have also suggested that a combination of exogenous melatonin and bright light therapy has an additive effect on phase resetting (Wirz-Justice et al. 2004; Burke et al. 2013). When early evening melatonin is combined with morning bright light, a greater phase advance is observed than with either treatment alone, suggesting that this may be an efficient and effective treatment for DSWPD (Burke et al. 2013). Moreover, proper sleep hygiene is important for DSWPD patients in order to promote appropriate scheduling of social activities and regular sleep-wake schedules. Photic and non-photic treatments for DSWPD have been shown to improve symptoms of co-morbid psychiatric conditions, including depression (Rahman et al. 2010) and ADHD (Rybak et al. 2006). Nevertheless, DSWPD patients may require conventional treatments for these co-morbid conditions as well (see Clinical Vignette B).

11.3   Advanced Sleep-Wake Phase Disorder

11.3.1 Description

Advanced sleep-wake phase disorder (ASWPD) is a CRSWD in which the phase of the sleep-wake cycle is habitually advanced relative to conventional clock time. ASWPD is associated with difficulty staying asleep in the early morning and excessive evening sleepiness.

11.3.2 Risk Factors

The prevalence of ASWPD in the general population is unknown; however, an estimated prevalence of about 1% of middle-aged adults (40–64 years) has been reported (International Classification of Sleep Disorders 2014). Evidently, ASWPD is more common with advanced age and appears to be considerably less prevalent than DSWPD; however, an early sleep pattern is more acceptable for social and occupational obligations; therefore, ASWPD may also be under-reported.

The exact pathophysiology of ASWPD is unknown and remains perhaps more elusive than DSWPD; however, it likely involves multiple intrinsic and extrinsic factors. A shortened endogenous period has been reported amongst ASWPD individuals (Jones et al. 1999). ASWPD may also result from altered responsiveness to light, demonstrating a more dominant phase-advancing region and/or weakened phase-delaying region of the light PRC (International Classification of Sleep Disorders 2014; Rufiange et al. 2002). Changes in environmental light exposure, namely, increases in early morning light, may also contribute to and perpetuate ASWPD. ASWPD has a strong genetic predisposition, as most of its research is supported by cases with familial ASWPD. Genetic mutations which alter the function of casein kinase I (CKI) have been reported, including a missense mutation in the binding region of CKIε in a specific locus of the human PER2 gene (Toh et al. 2001) and a missense mutation in a different CKIδ gene (Xu et al. 2005).

11.3.3 History

ASWPD is characterized by chronic early sleep and rising, in which there is an involuntary sleep onset and wake time typically 2 or more hours earlier than the desired or required time (International Classification of Sleep Disorders 2014). Therefore, patients generally fall asleep between 6 pm and 9 pm and wake up at 2–5 am. ASWPD patients demonstrate a morning diurnal preference and may score as extreme morning types on chronotype questionnaires (e.g., Morningness-Eveningness Questionnaire and the Munich Chronotype Questionnaire); however, this should not serve as a primary diagnostic measure (Morgenthaler et al. 2007). There is a strong autosomal dominant familial ASWPD inheritance pattern, and therefore a good family history is extremely helpful.

11.3.4 Investigations

When allowed to follow usual sleep schedules, ASWPD patients may demonstrate an early sleep onset and awakening using PSG; however, sleep quality and duration is generally normal for age (Jones et al. 1999). When obligated to maintain conventional sleep-wake times, sleep onset can be delayed; however, ASWPD patients still awaken early which curtails sleep and results in partial sleep deprivation. Sleep logs and/or wrist actigraphy monitoring for a minimum of 1 week (including both working and nonworking days) displays a stable advance in sleep-wake patterns. Circadian phase markers, such as DLMO and core body temperature minimum, also indicate an advanced rhythm of greater than 2 h (Jones et al. 1999; Campbell et al. 1993; Lack and Wright 1993; Satoh et al. 2003).

11.3.5 Treatment

Treatment for ASWPD usually includes bright light therapy and chronotherapy; however, controlled trials of both are limited. Studies have demonstrated that exposure to bright light (~2500 lux for ~2–4 h) in the evening, typically between 7 pm and 9 pm, can appropriately delay circadian rhythms, sleep onset and awakening as well as improve sleep quality (Campbell et al. 1993; Lack and Wright 1993; Lack et al. 2005). There has been one case report demonstrating the successful treatment of ASWPD with chronotherapy (advancing 3 h every 2 days for 2 weeks) in which the appropriate alignment of sleep to an acceptable bedtime of 11 pm was maintained at 5-month follow-up (Moldofsky et al. 1986). Currently, there are no reports of clinical treatment of ASWPD with exogenous melatonin.

11.4   Non-24-H Sleep-Wake Rhythm Disorder

11.4.1 Description

The sleep propensity of individuals with non-24-h sleep-wake rhythm disorder (N24SWD) is continuously drifting "around the clock" because the normally longer-than-24-h endogenous circadian cycle is not entrained to the 24-h social and physical environmental rhythm. If allowed to sleep in their window of high sleep propensity, individuals with N24SWD report a progressive delay of their sleep period from night to morning, to midday, to early evening and back to night. When trying to maintain a socially desirable sleep period, those with N24SWD have a progressive difficulty with falling asleep at night, and they experience increasing daytime sleepiness as their sleep propensity is shifting around the clock. The daily increment of delay depends on the length of the endogenous circadian period and typically ranges from less than half an hour to more than an hour (International Classification of Sleep Disorders 2014). A number of individuals will describe going to bed an hour later on each successive night so that in a period of 3–4 weeks, they rotate fully around the clock. This causes an enormous social disjunction (see Clinical Vignette A). Some rotate in an even manner, but others find that at periods they will either rotate rapidly or even lose a night's sleep altogether. In this situation a differential of a bipolar illness needs to be considered.

11.4.2 Risk Factors

Total blindness is the main risk factor for N24SWD, because in blind individuals light signals are not transmitted to the SCN (Sack et al. 1992). N24SWD may also develop in sighted individuals with severe cognitive impairment due to suboptimal exposure to, or impaired cognitive processing of, environmental entrainment cues. Occasionally, individuals with normal intelligence and sight present with N24SWD. In these cases, psychiatric conditions (e.g., agoraphobia, severe depression) often precede or follow the onset of the circadian disorder. These psychiatric conditions perpetuate the sleep problem because these conditions impose confinement to the home environment. Head injury and, paradoxically, chronotherapy have also been described as triggering factors (International Classification of Sleep Disorders 2014) (Clinical Vignette A). It is noteworthy that lithium which is widely used as a mood stabilizer has an impact on circadian processes.

11.4.3 History

In addition to the usual sleep and particularly circadian rhythm history, for such individuals, an awareness of socialization and work history is particularly important. We have seen patients with this disorder who have elected to be permanent night shift workers or who, for example, could only maintain employment when they were free to come and go at the time they chose. Based on our observation, many such individuals have social anxiety, and one has to wonder whether it is a cause or a consequence.

11.4.4 Investigations

In addition to the usual investigations for general medical conditions, psychiatric conditions and other sleep disorders, particular emphasis should be placed on longer-term sleep diaries and actigraphy, preferably for a minimum of a month. There are cases where we have performed two DLMOs with a 2-week interval between them and obtained strikingly different results, emphasizing that for some there is a continuing shift in the actual melatonin production (in contradistinction to the pattern in phase delay syndrome when two such DLMO tests produce essentially identical results). Enquiring about neurological or cognitive problems as well as lifestyle and social rhythm should be part of the assessment. One of us (CS) has seen two such patients with pineal tumours, and if neurological symptoms are present, an MRI scan should be done.

11.4.5 Treatment

In general, the "recommended treatment" is low-dose melatonin just prior to bed-time. The bedtime recommendation of melatonin implies that it is used as a form of hypnotic, but there are better hypnotics. The real value of melatonin is to use it as a chronobiotic, and it should be prescribed to be taken a few hours before the desired bedtime. For example, we waited with a patient with N24SWD for his spontaneous sleep time to be at 11 pm. At this point we gave him 5 mg of melatonin every day at 7 pm. This locked his rhythm to an approximately 11 pm bedtime and resolved the free-running pattern. After more than 6 months on melatonin, the patient discontin-ued the medication and was able to maintain his rhythm until he travelled to his first-ever family function evolving a 3-h time change. He immediately became free-running again. He reapplied the melatonin with good effect at the point when his sleep propensity was high in the evening.

11.5   Irregular Sleep-Wake Rhythm Disorder

11.5.1 Description

The irregular sleep-wake rhythm disorder (ISWD) is characterized by a lack of predictable sleep pattern. If a regular, socially desirable sleep schedule is enforced, individuals with ISWD struggle with insomnia and excessive daytime sleepiness (International Classification of Sleep Disorders 2014). Typically, there are at least three, random, short (1–4 h) spontaneous sleep periods during the day.

11.5.2 Risk Factors

Older adults are at risk for ISWD because of the decreased sensitivity of the SCN to light and the decline in involvement with regular social and physical activities (Gibson et al. 2009). Those with dementia and elderly patients in nursing homes in particular are at increased risk for having ISWD, in part due to lack of exposure to outdoor light (Martin et al. 2006). Children with neurodevelopmental disorders and individuals with brain tumours or acquired brain injury can develop ISWD if the brain pathology affects melatonin secretion (Johnson and Malow 2008). It has also been seen in long-term hypnotic users and patients with a variety of addictions (Logan et al. 2014).

11.5.3 History

In practical terms, a history of napping at odd times across the day and significantly disrupted nocturnal sleep is the key to this diagnosis if other sleep disorders are ruled out. A history of being predominantly indoors and lack of regular physical and social activities as well as exposure to natural light are highly relevant. There may be a history of long-standing shift work which should be considered in the differential diagnosis.

11.5.4 Investigations

Actigraphy is likely to be the most constructive single investigation, particularly with a light sensor. An activity log should be done in parallel, recognizing that some individuals will not be able to do it themselves. The involvement of caregivers in recording activities is key.

11.5.5 Treatment

The first line of treatment is behavioural activation, but the judicious use of hypnotics to consolidate the sleep period can play a significant role. Light exposure during the day together with early evening melatonin will strengthen the circadian pattern as will social and physical activity during the daytime.

11.6   Shift Work Disorder

11.6.1 Description

Shift work disorder (SWD) occurs when the work hours overlap with the endogenous sleep window and the individual struggles with insomnia or excessive sleepiness. The sleep problem must be temporally related to the shift work and not be better explained by another sleep disorder. The prevalence of sleep disorders associated with shift work is at least 10% (International Classification of Sleep Disorders 2014). The insomnia develops because the individual attempts to sleep during the endogenous daytime when the SCN emits alerting signals. The excessive sleepiness during work hours is the result of the normally high sleep propensity at night and in the early morning. Additionally, sleep deprivation develops because the total sleep time is usually curtailed by 1–4 h. It should be noted that there is mounting evidence of an increase in cancer rates in shift workers as well as mood disorders and syndrome X with obesity (Wang et al. 2013; Itani et al. 2011).

11.6.2 Risk Factors

The individual's age (older individuals have more difficulties), circadian preference, the shift work schedule, concurrent sleep disorders and behavioural-social factors influence the capacity for adjustment to shift work. SWD is most commonly associated with early morning, night and rotating shift work schedules. Those with current sleep disorders (e.g., sleep apnoea) are at increased risk for SWD as the combination of the two insults (sleep disorder and shift work schedule) leads to an insurmountable fatigue (Hossain and Shapiro 1999). Exposure to light, a long commute to the workplace which effectively lengthens the shift, social demands and daytime activities may further curtail sleep opportunities and increase the risk for excessive sleepiness and insomnia.

11.6.3 History

The history is self-evident (Shen et al. 2006); however, there will be shift workers who claim significant disability as a route to trying to obtain a constant day shift pattern at the workplace or as a route to claiming disability. These situations are challenging for occupational health physicians, family health practitioners and psychiatrists.

11.6.4 Investigations

A detailed history of the evolution of sleep difficulties and concurrent psychosocial factors may provide clues to the underlying disorder. A formal sleep evaluation in these situations is well merited as a way to rule out other sleep disorders, and an in-depth medical assessment of the reasons and possible causes of fatigue and sleepiness should be conducted. An evaluation of mood and a consideration of the sleep markers suggestive of mood problems should be considered. Consideration of a temporary change in the shift schedule should be contemplated. A DLMO, particularly in older individuals, may reveal a lack of melatonin production (sometimes referred to as endopause) (Shin and Shapiro 2003).

11.6.5 Treatment

There has recently been the development of spectacles that eliminate blue light in a narrow bandwidth. The effect of the spectacles is to allow melatonin secretion to occur during the night in shift workers. The knee-jerk concern that the secretion of melatonin would cause sleepiness when doing the shift is not correct. There are studies in nurses and nuclear reactor workers showing that sleep patterns both on and off the shift period are better when using the spectacles; mood is improved and there are less errors made in the work environment (Kayumov et al. 2005).

For patient management, providing information is key. A highly illustrated booklet *Working the Shift* is available at no charge online (see sleepontario.com).

11.7   Jet Lag Disorder

11.7.1 Definition

Jet lag disorder is characterized by a desynchronization between the endogenous circadian system and the external environment as a result of trans-meridian travel. It occurs when crossing time zones but not when flying north-south. Jet lag disorder is associated with temporary symptoms of initial and maintenance insomnia, as well as excessive daytime sleepiness, fatigue and impaired functioning. Sleep disruption and sleep deprivation can trigger mania in those with bipolar disorder, and this can apply to jet leg as well.

11.7.2 History

The history of jet lag is self-evident in any situation in which people cross time zones in a short period. There is a substantial difference between travelling eastward and westward. The "internal day" is naturally slightly longer than 24 h, and therefore it is easier to go forward around the clock than to go backward. Thus, travelling eastward is associated with more severe jet lag than travelling west.

11.7.3 Investigations

The main diagnostic tool to identify jetlag is history. There are no specific investigations required.

11.7.4 Treatment

For most individuals, treatment is not required. For some, using a hypnotic for a couple of days to regularize their sleep cycle is possible. For others, prophylactic use of melatonin can be advantageous. The amount of jet lag depends on the number of time zones traversed. If melatonin is used, the simple instruction is to take melatonin at 7 pm (destination time) for 5 continuous days starting 2 days prior to departure. For example, if one travels from New York to Sydney, one would take the melatonin for 2 days in New York at 7 pm Sydney time, then once on the plane and for 2 days in Sydney at 7 pm. For the return trip, it is usually desirable to take the melatonin at 7 pm home time. This is best started the day that the traveller leaves the place that they had visited and to continue for a further 4 days. In the above example, the traveller would take the melatonin at 7 pm New York time the day before departure in Sydney and then for 4 days at 7 pm in New York. For most individuals, this will shorten the period of jet lag by half. As a rule of thumb, it naturally takes a day per hour of time change that one has travelled to accommodate.

Useful information about jet lag is provided in the booklet *Slam Jetlag*, which can be found on the website www.sleepontario.com. "SLAM" is an acronym for *sleep*, *light*, *action* and *medication/melatonin* as these are the key factors in treatment. Clinical Vignette C illustrates an innovative way to prevent jet lag.

Conclusion

Circadian rhythm disorders are often confused with psychiatric conditions. For example, patients with depression are sedentary in the evening and wake up early in the morning, and this pattern may mimic advanced sleep phase syndrome. Those with bipolar disorder stay up at night when in a manic phase and may sleep during the day when depressed. At first glance this sleep pattern is similar to the N24SWD pattern. At the same time, circadian sleep disorders can lead to mood problems. DSWPD, for example, is often associated with depression since individuals with this disorder are often sleep deprived and suffer from social judgement and self-blame (being "lazy" in the morning). Shift workers are also more likely to have depression than non-shift workers. In general, those with severe circadian disorders often suffer from the social consequences of their unusual sleep schedule which may cause anxiety or mood problems. Notably, circadian sleep problems are associated with insomnia if the individuals attempt to follow a socially desirable sleep schedule that is outside of their biological window of high sleep propensity. The differential diagnosis between insomnia and circadian sleep disorders is critically important because the two conditions require different treatment. Finally, it is important to note that behavioural factors (irregular schedule, indoor sedentary activities, inadequate exposure to natural light, going to bed outside of one's biologically preferred circadian sleep phase) can amplify both circadian and psychiatric problems. Therefore, the combination of medical and behavioural intervention is often merited.

Appendix

Clinical Vignette A

Mr. X heard a radio programme in which circadian sleep disorders were described. He contacted the sleep clinic and, when seen, described a long-standing pattern of non-24-h sleep-wake cycles.

Mr. X was adopted at age 2 and he had difficulties as a child. At school he was regularly caned for being late. He did not complete school, although a subsequent assessment showed that he had an IQ higher than 125. Mr. X claimed to have had "hundreds of jobs", most of which he has lost because of difficulties with timekeeping. The only job he kept for any length of time was in a photographic laboratory. As a technician he was allowed to come and go on his own schedule, provided a certain amount of work was done.

When seen initially he was living as a recluse, in a remote country cottage outside of Edinburgh. He made a number of statements suggesting a delusional disorder. For example, although he was unemployed, he believed that in the next few years, he would become a member of Margaret Thatcher's cabinet. He spoke of occasions when he did not sleep at all for a few days and instead worked "by the white heat of the night". Mr. X complained of difficulties making medical and dental appointments because of his rotating sleep pattern which caused him to go to bed and rise 1 h later every day. If an appointment was scheduled, he had to calculate whether he would be in a waking or sleeping phase during daytime hours.

Mr. X declined sleep a laboratory assessment. He was not heard of again until 3 years later when he had difficulties with the police. He had been writing and distributing malicious information about a senior civil servant. He telephoned the sleep clinic to request an intervention so that he would not have to appear in court the next day. He explained, "I will be sleeping in the middle of the day tomorrow". At this point, Mr. X agreed to hospital admission so that his circadian rhythm disorder could be monitored. Monitoring confirmed that he did go to bed 1 h later every day. This caused great inconveniences to the nurses who had to serve breakfast at 3 am one day, 4 am the next day and 4 pm 2 weeks later! Monitoring other circadian rhythms showed that they were synchronized with his sleep-wake rhythms.

A trial of lithium (this was before the days of melatonin availability) was decided upon in the belief that it would make his circadian rhythm worse, i.e. extend his rhythm to a 26-h rhythm, with a plan to follow that in a single-blind manner with sodium valproate which has the opposite effect on circadian rhythm. Immediately on commencing the lithium after being on placebo (single blind), he settled into an exactly 24-h rhythm. An MRI brain scan was done which showed a pineal tumour.

This clinical vignette highlights the interaction between the circadian rhythm problem and a possible mood-related issue and the impact of two well-known mood-stabilizing agents on circadian rhythms.

Clinical Vignette B

A 16-year-old boy presented to the sleep clinic with what appeared to be phase delay syndrome. A dim light melatonin onset study was done which confirmed the diagnosis. A single-blind treatment with one packet of melatonin and one packet of placebo was provided with the instruction to take one tablet from packet A for a month and one tablet from packet B for a month. He was to take the tablets at 7 pm on a regular basis. After showing the clear benefit of the active melatonin treatment (when he returned at the 2-month mark), he was placed on over-the-counter melatonin which did not produce the same effect. He returned a month later with his mother, and they requested that we provide them with the "pharmaceutical grade" melatonin that we import from a company in the United Kingdom.

At the return visit, his mother walked in with a piece of paper which had a series of Es heavily ringed. The physician's presumption was that this is a report card and that "E" is close to "F"—that is, the student has almost failed. The young man of 16 sat in the corner and smiled like a Cheshire cat. When asked what he was smiling about, his comment was "I am not stupid anymore, I am going to university". The 'Es were for "excellent" and his grade average had gone from 60 to 90% in a 3-month period. He entered university a year and a half later to a course that has only 24 slots and is the only course of its kind in the province.

This vividly illustrates the importance of detecting and treating circadian rhythm disorders as early as possible, particularly in adolescents who are in a very sensitive phase of their academic and social development.

Clinical Vignette C

A former professor at Harvard is travelling to Japan for a short trip. He uses the goggles that block out a narrow band of blue light during the day while he is in Japan. He takes a short nap each afternoon and sleeps during the night in Japan. Five days later he returns to Boston and has an immediate resumption of his normal circadian rhythm (unlike previous long trips to Australia or the Far East).

This vignette indicates the possibility of maintaining a set circadian period in the face of being in a different time zone. It is likely that the hour-long daytime naps were perceived as a "very short night" and the longer nocturnal sleeps in Japan were perceived as a "long nap". For travellers making short trips abroad, this may be a very useful strategy.

References

Archer SN, Robilliard DL, Skene DJ, Smits M, Williams A, Arendt J, et al. A length polymorphism in the circadian clock gene Per3 is linked to delayed sleep phase syndrome and extreme diurnal preference. Sleep. 2003;26(4):413–5. Epub 2003/07/05

Archer SN, Carpen JD, Gibson M, Lim GH, Johnston JD, Skene DJ, et al. Polymorphism in the PER3 promoter associates with diurnal preference and delayed sleep phase disorder. Sleep. 2010;33(5):695–701. Epub 2010/05/18

Baird AL, Coogan AN, Siddiqui A, Donev RM, Thome J. Adult attention-deficit hyperactivity disorder is associated with alterations in circadian rhythms at the behavioural, endocrine and molecular levels. Mol Psychiatry. 2012;17(10):988–95. Epub 2011/11/23

Benloucif S, Guico MJ, Reid KJ, Wolfe LF, L'Hermite-Baleriaux M, Zee PC. Stability of melatonin and temperature as circadian phase markers and their relation to sleep times in humans. J Biol Rhythm. 2005;20(2):178–88. Epub 2005/04/19

Bijlenga D, van der Heijden KB, Breuk M, van Someren EJ, Lie ME, Boonstra AM, et al. Associations between sleep characteristics, seasonal depressive symptoms, lifestyle, and ADHD symptoms in adults. J Atten Disord. 2013;17(3):261–75. Epub 2012/01/03

Borbely AA. A two process model of sleep regulation. Hum Neurobiol. 1982;1(3):195–204. Epub 1982/01/01

Buhr ED, Takahashi JS. Molecular components of the mammalian circadian clock. Handb Exp Pharmacol. 2013;217:3–27. Epub 2013/04/23

Burgess HJ, Revell VL, Molina TA, Eastman CI. Human phase response curves to three days of daily melatonin: 0.5 mg versus 3.0 mg. J Clin Endocrinol Metab. 2010;95(7):3325–31. Epub 2010/04/23

Burke TM, Markwald RR, Chinoy ED, Snider JA, Bessman SC, Jung CM, et al. Combination of light and melatonin time cues for phase advancing the human circadian clock. Sleep. 2013; 36(11):1617–24. Epub 2013/11/02

Campbell SS, Dawson D, Anderson MW. Alleviation of sleep maintenance insomnia with timed exposure to bright light. J Am Geriatr Soc. 1993;41(8):829–36. Epub 1993/08/01

Cole RJ, Smith JS, Alcala YC, Elliott JA, Kripke DF. Bright-light mask treatment of delayed sleep phase syndrome. J Biol Rhythm. 2002;17(1):89–101. Epub 2002/02/12

Corkum P, Moldofsky H, Hogg-Johnson S, Humphries T, Tannock R. Sleep problems in children with attention-deficit/hyperactivity disorder: impact of subtype, comorbidity, and stimulant medication. J Am Acad Child Adolesc Psychiatry. 1999;38(10):1285–93. Epub 1999/10/12

Crowley SJ, Acebo C, Carskadon MA. Sleep, circadian rhythms, and delayed phase in adolescence. Sleep Med. 2007;8(6):602–12. Epub 2007/03/27

Czeisler CA, Gooley JJ. Sleep and circadian rhythms in humans. Cold Spring Harb Symp Quant Biol. 2007;72:579–97. Epub 2008/04/19

Czeisler CA, Richardson GS, Coleman RM, Zimmerman JC, Moore-Ede MC, Dement WC, et al. Chronotherapy: resetting the circadian clocks of patients with delayed sleep phase insomnia. Sleep. 1981;4(1):1–21. Epub 1981/01/01

Czeisler CA, Allan JS, Strogatz SH, Ronda JM, Sanchez R, Rios CD, et al. Bright light resets the human circadian pacemaker independent of the timing of the sleep-wake cycle. Science. 1986;233(4764):667–71. Epub 1986/08/08

Czeisler CA, Duffy JF, Shanahan TL, Brown EN, Mitchell JF, Rimmer DW, et al. Stability, precision, and near-24-hour period of the human circadian pacemaker. Science. 1999;284(5423):2177–81. Epub 1999/06/26

Dagan Y, Stein D, Steinbock M, Yovel I, Hallis D. Frequency of delayed sleep phase syndrome among hospitalized adolescent psychiatric patients. J Psychosom Res. 1998;45(1):15–20. Epub 1998/08/28

Dahlitz M, Alvarez B, Vignau J, English J, Arendt J, Parkes JD. Delayed sleep phase syndrome response to melatonin. Lancet. 1991;337(8750):1121–4. Epub 1991/05/11

Dijk DJ, Czeisler CA. Paradoxical timing of the circadian rhythm of sleep propensity serves to consolidate sleep and wakefulness in humans. Neurosci Lett. 1994;166(1):63–8. Epub 1994/01/17

Dijk DJ, Czeisler CA. Contribution of the circadian pacemaker and the sleep homeostat to sleep propensity, sleep structure, electroencephalographic slow waves, and sleep spindle activity in humans. J Neurosci. 1995;15(5 Pt 1):3526–38. Epub 1995/05/01

Dijk DJ, Duffy JF, Czeisler CA. Circadian and sleep/wake dependent aspects of subjective alertness and cognitive performance. J Sleep Res. 1992;1(2):112–7. Epub 1992/06/01

Drennan MD, Klauber MR, Kripke DF, Goyette LM. The effects of depression and age on the Horne-Ostberg morningness-eveningness score. J Affect Disord. 1991;23(2):93–8. Epub 1991/10/01

Duffy JF, Cain SW, Chang AM, Phillips AJ, Munch MY, Gronfier C, et al. Sex difference in the near-24-hour intrinsic period of the human circadian timing system. Proc Natl Acad Sci U S A. 2011;108(Suppl 3):15602–8. Epub 2011/05/04

Ebisawa T, Uchiyama M, Kajimura N, Mishima K, Kamei Y, Katoh M, et al. Association of structural polymorphisms in the human period3 gene with delayed sleep phase syndrome. EMBO Rep. 2001;2(4):342–6. Epub 2001/04/18

Edgar DM, Dement WC, Fuller CA. Effect of SCN lesions on sleep in squirrel monkeys: evidence for opponent processes in sleep-wake regulation. J Neurosci. 1993;13(3):1065–79. Epub 1993/03/01

Gaspar-Barba E, Calati R, Cruz-Fuentes CS, Ontiveros-Uribe MP, Natale V, De Ronchi D, et al. Depressive symptomatology is influenced by chronotypes. J Affect Disord. 2009;119(1–3):100–6. Epub 2009/03/17

Gibson EM, Williams WP 3rd, Kriegsfeld LJ. Aging in the circadian system: considerations for health, disease prevention and longevity. Exp Gerontol. 2009;44(1–2):51–6. Epub 2008/06/27

Gooley JJ, Rajaratnam SM, Brainard GC, Kronauer RE, Czeisler CA, Lockley SW. Spectral responses of the human circadian system depend on the irradiance and duration of exposure to light. Sci Transl Med. 2010;2(31):31ra3. Epub 2010/05/14

Hohjoh H, Takahashi Y, Hatta Y, Tanaka H, Akaza T, Tokunaga K, et al. Possible association of human leucocyte antigen DR1 with delayed sleep phase syndrome. Psychiatry Clin Neurosci. 1999;53(4):527–9. Epub 1999/09/25

Hohjoh H, Takasu M, Shishikura K, Takahashi Y, Honda Y, Tokunaga K. Significant association of the arylalkylamine N-acetyltransferase (AA-NAT) gene with delayed sleep phase syndrome. Neurogenetics. 2003;4(3):151–3. Epub 2003/05/09

Horne JA, Ostberg O. A self-assessment questionnaire to determine morningness-eveningness in human circadian rhythms. Int J Chronobiol. 1976;4(2):97–110. Epub 1976/01/01

Hossain JL, Shapiro CM. Considerations and possible consequences of shift work. J Psychosom Res. 1999;47(4):293–6. Epub 2000/01/01

International Classification of Sleep Disorders. 3. Darien: American Academy of Sleep Med; 2014.

Itani O, Kaneita Y, Murata A, Yokoyama E, Ohida T. Association of onset of obesity with sleep duration and shift work among Japanese adults. Sleep Med. 2011;12(4):341–5. Epub 2011/ 03/08

Ito A, Ando K, Hayakawa T, Iwata T, Kayukawa Y, Ohta T, et al. Long-term course of adult patients with delayed sleep phase syndrome. Jpn J Psychiatry Neurol. 1993;47(3):563–7. Epub 1993/09/01

Johnson KP, Malow BA. Sleep in children with autism spectrum disorders. Curr Neurol Neurosci Rep. 2008;8(2):155–61. Epub 2008/05/08

Jones CR, Campbell SS, Zone SE, Cooper F, DeSano A, Murphy PJ, et al. Familial advanced sleep-phase syndrome: a short-period circadian rhythm variant in humans. Nat Med. 1999; 5(9):1062–5. Epub 1999/09/02

Jones KH, Ellis J, von Schantz M, Skene DJ, Dijk DJ, Archer SN. Age-related change in the association between a polymorphism in the PER3 gene and preferred timing of sleep and waking activities. J Sleep Res. 2007;16(1):12–6. Epub 2007/02/21

Kayumov L, Brown G, Jindal R, Buttoo K, Shapiro CM. A randomized, double-blind, placebo-controlled crossover study of the effect of exogenous melatonin on delayed sleep phase syndrome. Psychosom Med. 2001;63(1):40–8. Epub 2001/02/24

Kayumov L, Casper RF, Hawa RJ, Perelman B, Chung SA, Sokalsky S, et al. Blocking low-wavelength light prevents nocturnal melatonin suppression with no adverse effect on performance during simulated shift work. J Clin Endocrinol Metab. 2005;90(5):2755–61. Epub 2005/02/17

Khalsa SB, Jewett ME, Cajochen C, Czeisler CA. A phase response curve to single bright light pulses in human subjects. J Physiol. 2003;549(Pt 3):945–52. Epub 2003/04/30

Klerman EB, Gershengorn HB, Duffy JF, Kronauer RE. Comparisons of the variability of three markers of the human circadian pacemaker. J Biol Rhythm. 2002;17(2):181–93. Epub 2002/05/11

Lack L, Wright H. The effect of evening bright light in delaying the circadian rhythms and lengthening the sleep of early morning awakening insomniacs. Sleep. 1993;16(5):436–43. Epub 1993/08/01

Lack LC, Wright HR. Clinical management of delayed sleep phase disorder. Behav Sleep Med. 2007;5(1):57–76. Epub 2007/02/23

Lack L, Wright H, Kemp K, Gibbon S. The treatment of early-morning awakening insomnia with 2 evenings of bright light. Sleep. 2005;28(5):616–23. Epub 2005/09/21

Lazar AS, Slak A, Lo JC, Santhi N, von Schantz M, Archer SN, et al. Sleep, diurnal preference, health, and psychological well-being: a prospective single-allelic-variation study. Chronobiol Int. 2012;29(2):131–46. Epub 2012/02/14

Lee HJ, Rex KM, Nievergelt CM, Kelsoe JR, Kripke DF. Delayed sleep phase syndrome is related to seasonal affective disorder. J Affect Disord. 2011;133(3):573–9. Epub 2011/05/24

Lewy AJ, Bauer VK, Ahmed S, Thomas KH, Cutler NL, Singer CM, et al. The human phase response curve (PRC) to melatonin is about 12 hours out of phase with the PRC to light. Chronobiol Int. 1998;15(1):71–83. Epub 1998/03/11

Logan RW, Williams WP 3rd, McClung CA. Circadian rhythms and addiction: mechanistic insights and future directions. Behav Neurosci. 2014;128(3):387–412. Epub 2014/04/16

Mansour HA, Wood J, Chowdari KV, Dayal M, Thase ME, Kupfer DJ, et al. Circadian phase variation in bipolar I disorder. Chronobiol Int. 2005;22(3):571–84. Epub 2005/08/04

Martin JL, Webber AP, Alam T, Harker JO, Josephson KR, Alessi CA. Daytime sleeping, sleep disturbance, and circadian rhythms in the nursing home. Am J Geriatr Psychiatry. 2006;14(2): 121–9. Epub 2006/02/14

Merikanto I, Lahti T, Kronholm E, Peltonen M, Laatikainen T, Vartiainen E, et al. Evening types are prone to depression. Chronobiol Int. 2013;30(5):719–25. Epub 2013/05/22

Moldofsky H, Musisi S, Phillipson EA. Treatment of a case of advanced sleep phase syndrome by phase advance chronotherapy. Sleep. 1986;9(1):61–5. Epub 1986/01/01

Morgenthaler TI, Lee-Chiong T, Alessi C, Friedman L, Aurora RN, Boehlecke B, et al. Practice parameters for the clinical evaluation and treatment of circadian rhythm sleep disorders. An American Academy of sleep medicine report. Sleep. 2007;30(11):1445–59. Epub 2007/11/29

Mundey K, Benloucif S, Harsanyi K, Dubocovich ML, Zee PC. Phase-dependent treatment of delayed sleep phase syndrome with melatonin. Sleep. 2005;28(10):1271–8. Epub 2005/11/22

Nagtegaal JE, Kerkhof GA, Smits MG, Swart AC, Van Der Meer YG. Delayed sleep phase syndrome: a placebo-controlled cross-over study on the effects of melatonin administered five hours before the individual dim light melatonin onset. J Sleep Res. 1998;7(2):135–43. Epub 1998/07/31

Natale V, Adan A, Scapellato P. Are seasonality of mood and eveningness closely associated? Psychiatry Res. 2005;136(1):51–60. Epub 2005/07/19

Pereira DS, Tufik S, Louzada FM, Benedito-Silva AA, Lopez AR, Lemos NA, et al. Association of the length polymorphism in the human Per3 gene with the delayed sleep-phase syndrome: does latitude have an influence upon it? Sleep. 2005;28(1):29–32. Epub 2005/02/11

Rahman SA, Kayumov L, Shapiro CM. Antidepressant action of melatonin in the treatment of delayed sleep phase syndrome. Sleep Med. 2010;11(2):131–6. Epub 2010/01/02

Ralph MR, Foster RG, Davis FC, Menaker M. Transplanted suprachiasmatic nucleus determines circadian period. Science. 1990;247(4945):975–8. Epub 1990/02/23

Regestein QR, Pavlova M. Treatment of delayed sleep phase syndrome. Gen Hosp Psychiatry. 1995;17(5):335–45. Epub 1995/09/01

Reppert SM, Weaver DR. Coordination of circadian timing in mammals. Nature. 2002;418(6901): 935–41. Epub 2002/08/29

Robillard R, Naismith SL, Rogers NL, Ip TK, Hermens DF, Scott EM, et al. Delayed sleep phase in young people with unipolar or bipolar affective disorders. J Affect Disord. 2013a;145(2):260–3. Epub 2012/08/11

Robillard R, Naismith SL, Rogers NL, Scott EM, Ip TK, Hermens DF, et al. Sleep-wake cycle and melatonin rhythms in adolescents and young adults with mood disorders: comparison of unipolar and bipolar phenotypes. Eur Psychiatry. 2013b;28(7):412–6. Epub 2013/06/19

Robillard R, Naismith SL, Smith KL, Rogers NL, White D, Terpening Z, et al. Sleep-wake cycle in young and older persons with a lifetime history of mood disorders. PLoS One. 2014;9(2):e87763. Epub 2014/03/04

Rosenthal NE, Joseph-Vanderpool JR, Levendosky AA, Johnston SH, Allen R, Kelly KA, et al. Phase-shifting effects of bright morning light as treatment for delayed sleep phase syndrome. Sleep. 1990;13(4):354–61. Epub 1990/08/01

Rufiange M, Dumont M, Lachapelle P. Correlating retinal function with melatonin secretion in subjects with an early or late circadian phase. Invest Ophthalmol Vis Sci. 2002;43(7):2491–9. Epub 2002/07/02

Rybak YE, McNeely HE, Mackenzie BE, Jain UR, Levitan RD. An open trial of light therapy in adult attention-deficit/hyperactivity disorder. J Clin Psychiatry. 2006;67(10):1527–35. Epub 2006/11/17

Sack RL, Lewy AJ, Blood ML, Keith LD, Nakagawa H. Circadian rhythm abnormalities in totally blind people: incidence and clinical significance. J Clin Endocrinol Metab. 1992;75(1):127–34. Epub 1992/07/01

Sack RL, Auckley D, Auger RR, Carskadon MA, Wright KP Jr, Vitiello MV, et al. Circadian rhythm sleep disorders: part I, basic principles, shift work and jet lag disorders. An American Academy of sleep medicine review. Sleep. 2007;30(11):1460–83. Epub 2007/11/29

Satoh K, Mishima K, Inoue Y, Ebisawa T, Shimizu T. Two pedigrees of familial advanced sleep phase syndrome in Japan. Sleep. 2003;26(4):416–7. Epub 2003/07/05

Saxvig IW, Pallesen S, Wilhelmsen-Langeland A, Molde H, Bjorvatn B. Prevalence and correlates of delayed sleep phase in high school students. Sleep Med. 2012;13(2):193–9. Epub 2011/12/14

Saxvig IW, Wilhelmsen-Langeland A, Pallesen S, Vedaa O, Nordhus IH, Sorensen E, et al. Objective measures of sleep and dim light melatonin onset in adolescents and young adults with delayed sleep phase disorder compared to healthy controls. J Sleep Res. 2013;22(4): 365–72. Epub 2013/02/01

Schrader H, Bovim G, Sand T. The prevalence of delayed and advanced sleep phase syndromes. J Sleep Res. 1993;2(1):51–5. Epub 1993/03/01

Shahid A, Khairandish A, Gladanac B, Shapiro C. Peeking into the minds of troubled adolescents: the utility of polysomnography sleep studies in an inpatient psychiatric unit. J Affect Disord. 2012;139(1):66–74. Epub 2012/03/14

Shen J, Botly LC, Chung SA, Gibbs AL, Sabanadzovic S, Shapiro CM. Fatigue and shift work. J Sleep Res. 2006;15(1):1–5. Epub 2006/02/24

Shin K, Shapiro C. Menopause, sex hormones, and sleep. Bipolar Disord. 2003;5(2):106–9. Epub 2003/04/12

Sivertsen B, Pallesen S, Stormark KM, Boe T, Lundervold AJ, Hysing M. Delayed sleep phase syndrome in adolescents: prevalence and correlates in a large population based study. BMC Public Health. 2013;13:1163. Epub 2013/12/18

Stephan FK, Zucker I. Circadian rhythms in drinking behavior and locomotor activity of rats are eliminated by hypothalamic lesions. Proc Natl Acad Sci U S A. 1972;69(6):1583–6. Epub 1972/06/01

Takahashi Y, Hohjoh H, Matsuura K. Predisposing factors in delayed sleep phase syndrome. Psychiatry Clin Neurosci. 2000;54(3):356–8. Epub 2001/02/24

Takano A, Uchiyama M, Kajimura N, Mishima K, Inoue Y, Kamei Y, et al. A missense variation in human casein kinase I epsilon gene that induces functional alteration and shows an inverse association with circadian rhythm sleep disorders. Neuropsychopharmacology. 2004;29(10):1901–9. Epub 2004/06/10

Thorpy MJ, Korman E, Spielman AJ, Glovinsky PB. Delayed sleep phase syndrome in adolescents. J Adolesc Health Care. 1988;9(1):22–7. Epub 1988/01/01

Toh KL, Jones CR, He Y, Eide EJ, Hinz WA, Virshup DM, et al. An hPer2 phosphorylation site mutation in familial advanced sleep phase syndrome. Science. 2001;291(5506):1040–3. Epub 2001/03/10

Van der Heijden KB, Smits MG, Van Someren EJ, Gunning WB. Idiopathic chronic sleep onset insomnia in attention-deficit/hyperactivity disorder: a circadian rhythm sleep disorder. Chronobiol Int. 2005;22(3):559–70. Epub 2005/08/04

Van Veen MM, Kooij JJ, Boonstra AM, Gordijn MC, Van Someren EJ. Delayed circadian rhythm in adults with attention-deficit/hyperactivity disorder and chronic sleep-onset insomnia. Biol Psychiatry. 2010;67(11):1091–6. Epub 2010/02/19

Wang F, Yeung KL, Chan WC, Kwok CC, Leung SL, Wu C, et al. A meta-analysis on dose-response relationship between night shift work and the risk of breast cancer. Ann Oncol. 2013;24(11):2724–32. Epub 2013/08/27

Weitzman ED, Czeisler CA, Coleman RM, Spielman AJ, Zimmerman JC, Dement W, et al. Delayed sleep phase syndrome. A chronobiological disorder with sleep-onset insomnia. Arch Gen Psychiatry. 1981;38(7):737–46. Epub 1981/07/01

Werner H, Lebourgeois MK, Geiger A, Jenni OG. Assessment of chronotype in four- to eleven-year-old children: reliability and validity of the children's chronotype questionnaire (CCTQ). Chronobiol Int. 2009;26(5):992–1014. Epub 2009/07/29

Wilhelmsen-Langeland A, Saxvig IW, Pallesen S, Nordhus IH, Vedaa O, Lundervold AJ, et al. A randomized controlled trial with bright light and melatonin for the treatment of delayed sleep phase disorder: effects on subjective and objective sleepiness and cognitive function. J Biol Rhythm. 2013;28(5):306–21. Epub 2013/10/18

Wirz-Justice A, Krauchi K, Cajochen C, Danilenko KV, Renz C, Weber JM. Evening melatonin and bright light administration induce additive phase shifts in dim light melatonin onset. J Pineal Res. 2004;36(3):192–4. Epub 2004/03/11

Wood J, Birmaher B, Axelson D, Ehmann M, Kalas C, Monk K, et al. Replicable differences in preferred circadian phase between bipolar disorder patients and control individuals. Psychiatry Res. 2009;166(2–3):201–9. Epub 2009/03/13

Xu Y, Padiath QS, Shapiro RE, Jones CR, Wu SC, Saigoh N, et al. Functional consequences of a CKIdelta mutation causing familial advanced sleep phase syndrome. Nature. 2005;434(7033): 640–4. Epub 2005/04/01

Yazaki M, Shirakawa S, Okawa M, Takahashi K. Demography of sleep disturbances associated with circadian rhythm disorders in Japan. Psychiatry Clin Neurosci. 1999;53(2):267–8. Epub 1999/08/25

Zavada A, Gordijn MC, Beersma DG, Daan S, Roenneberg T. Comparison of the Munich chronotype questionnaire with the Horne-Ostberg's morningness-eveningness score. Chronobiol Int. 2005;22(2):267–78. Epub 2005/07/19

Obstructive Sleep Apnoea

12

Ruzica Jokic

12.1 Definitions of Obstructive Sleep Apnoea (OSA)

Obstructive sleep apnoea (OSA) is a common sleep disorder, characterized by complete or partial airway obstruction and caused by pharyngeal collapse during sleep. The resultant complete cessations of breathing are called apnoeas if their duration is 10 s or more. Hypopnoeas are a result of reduced inspiratory flow when the airway narrows but does not fully collapse (Strollo and Rogers 1996).

OSA syndrome is defined as (1) five or more episodes of apnoea or hypopnoea per hour of sleep (apnoea-hypopnoea index—AHI) with associated symptoms (e.g., excessive daytime sleepiness, fatigue or impaired cognition) or (2) AHI equal to or higher than 15, regardless of associated symptoms (Anon 1999).

12.2 Epidemiology and Risk Factors

Patients with severe OSA are often referred to sleep laboratories for investigations and confirmation of diagnosis. Epidemiological studies show that 4% of men and 2% of women aged 50 years or older suffer from symptomatic OSA. However, the prevalence of mild or moderate OSA in individuals who frequently do not present with typical symptoms of the disorder is estimated to be as high as 20–30% of the middle-aged population (Young et al. 1997). Thus, despite increased awareness over the last few decades, the availability of diagnostic tools as well as knowledge of its significant impact on daytime function and quality of life, OSA commonly remains an unrecognized and underdiagnosed disorder.

R. Jokic, M.D. F.R.C.P. (C), Ph.D.
Department of Psychiatry, Queen's University and Providence Care Hospital, Kingston, ON, Canada
e-mail: jokicr@providencecare.ca

© Springer-Verlag GmbH Germany, part of Springer Nature 2018
H. Selsick (ed.), *Sleep Disorders in Psychiatric Patients*,
https://doi.org/10.1007/978-3-642-54836-9_12

Table 12.1 Common risk factors for OSA	Obesity
	Male sex
	Middle age or older
	Micronagthia and retrognathia
	Large neck circumference
	Nasal allergies and stuffiness

Recent studies emphasize that the number of patients diagnosed as suffering from OSA has increased dramatically in the last few years and will continue to do so in the coming years (Leger et al. 2012).

The major risk factors for OSA are listed in Table 12.1.

Obesity is one of the most important risk factors for OSA. It has been determined that a 10% weight gain increases the risk of developing OSA sixfold. A recent longitudinal study that investigated the link between weight gain and OSA confirmed that increased adipose tissue in the region of the neck, fat infiltration and oedema in the soft palate associated with moderate weight change all had an impact on sleep-disordered breathing (Peppard et al. 2000).

The risk of OSA increases with age. Men have a higher prevalence of OSA than women, and abdominal fat and higher neck-to-waist ratios are significantly associated with the severity of OSA in men. Females are found to have less severe OSA at all ages. Menopause, pregnancy and polycystic ovarian syndrome increase the risk for OSA in women (Bixler et al. 1998).

12.3 Pathophysiology of OSA

Reduction of the expansion forces of the pharyngeal dilator muscles, genioglossal muscle dysfunction and discoordination between inspiratory activity of the muscle and respiratory effort all have an important influence on progression of the disease. Additional factors include altered upper airway anatomy in subjects with skeletal abnormalities, excessive or elongated tissues of the soft palate, macroglossia, tonsillar hypertrophy and a redundant pharyngeal mucosa (Fogel et al. 2004).

OSA is common in children with adenotonsillar hypertrophy and congenital craniofacial abnormalities (Gozal 1998). Children with Down syndrome often present with symptoms of sleep-disordered breathing, and 30–60% are diagnosed with OSA. Persistent anatomic causes and specific patterns of airway collapse explain the ongoing symptoms in many children despite surgical treatment (Guimaraes et al. 2008).

12.4 Symptoms of OSA

Symptoms of OSA are a consequence of oxyhaemoglobin desaturations and sleep fragmentation (arousals) due to associated respiratory effort during sleep. Table 12.2 lists some of the most common symptoms of OSA.

Table 12.2 Clinical features of OSA

Nocturnal symptoms:
Frequent awakenings, fragmented sleep
Gasping for air or choking
Loud snoring, dry mouthand sore throat
Nocturia
Daytime symptoms:
Excessive daytime sleepiness, fatigue
Insomnia, early morning awakening
Depression, anxiety, irritablility
Morning headache
Neurocognitive dysfunction

12.5 Course of OSA

The presentation of OSA typically changes over time and tends to be affected by the ageing process and weight gain. Transition to menopause has significant effect on the course of the illness in women (Jordan and McEvoy 2003).

In the early stages of the disease, fatigue is a common symptom, often attributed to sleep deprivation, stress or medical problems such as obesity or hypertension. Excessive daytime sleepiness (hypersomnolence) associated with fatigue begins insidiously and may be present for years before the patient is diagnosed with OSA. With the progression of the untreated disease, symptoms can become debilitating and have a significant impact on general health, daytime function and quality of life.

The typical clinical presentation in men involves loud snoring, fragmented sleep and daytime sleepiness. In women, insomnia, mood and anxiety symptoms and chronic pain are the most common symptoms. Some women report palpitations and ankle oedema (Gold et al. 2003).

Chronic fatigue syndrome, fibromyalgia, irritable bowel syndrome and migraine headaches are more commonly present in women and may be associated with milder forms of OSA.

12.6 Consequences of Untreated OSA

Table 12.3 lists the most common complications of untreated OSA.

Cardiovascular disease and OSA share several risk factors such as age, obesity and male gender. Untreated OSA is associated with additional cardiovascular and metabolic consequences, including hypertension, atherosclerosis and glucose intolerance. The prevalence of OSA in patients with hypertension, coronary artery disease, stroke and congestive heart failure (CHF) is much higher (approaching 30–50%) than in the general population. Repetitive hypoxia (due to intermittent airway obstruction that results in heightened sympathetic drive which persists even during wakefulness), endothelial dysfunction, chronic inflammation, metabolic dysregulation and repetitive intrathoracic pressure changes are all pathophysiological factors associated with cardiovascular abnormalities in OSA (Marin et al. 2005).

Table 12.3 Consequences of unrelated OSA

| Cardiovascular disorders: |
| Hypertension, |
| Coronary artery disease |
| Heart failure |
| Arrhythmias |
| Stroke |
| Increased mortality |
| Neurocognitive sequelae: Changes in attention and concentration, executive function and fine motor coordination |
| Motor vehicle accidents |
| Mood disorders |

Untreated OSA is related to increased mortality in patients with AHI > 20, as demonstrated in one longitudinal study (He et al. 1988). Absenteeism, disability and loss of work productivity are commonly associated with untreated OSA.

Excessive daytime sleepiness and fatigue in patients with untreated OSA is responsible for an increased prevalence of car accidents. This is a crucial public health issue as confirmed by a recent review, demonstrating a two- to threefold increased risk for accidents in patients with OSA (Ellen et al. 2006). It is important to evaluate accident-related risk factors in detecting OSA patients at risk of motor vehicle accidents, as further supported by results of a recent multicentre study in more than 8000 individuals with suspected OSA from the European OSA database (Karimi et al. 2014). Many countries require patients to inform their driving license authority about the diagnosis of OSA.

Decreased quality of life is one of the most important consequences of untreated OSA. Baldwin and colleagues investigated the effect of OSA on quality of life in the Sleep Heart Health Study of 5816 subjects with mean age of 63 years, 52.5% of whom were female (Baldwin et al. 2001). Subjects with OSA had significantly lower scores on all dimensions of the quality of life scale the 36-Item Short Form Health Survey (SF-36), as compared to the general population. Continuous positive airway pressure (CPAP) improved quality of life after 6 months of treatment. The benefit of treating patients with CPAP has been confirmed by several subsequent studies (Sin et al. 2002; Jing et al. 2008). Significant correlations have been demonstrated between severity of OSA, mood symptoms, sleepiness and quality of life (Akashiba et al. 2002).

12.7 Medical History and Physical Examination

Obtaining a thorough history is essential for diagnosing OSA. Partners, if available, can provide useful additional information about the patient's sleep.

Focused history should include:

- Daytime and night-time symptoms
- Medical history (cardiovascular diseases: systemic or pulmonary hypertension, metabolic syndrome, heart failure or arrhythmias, history of hypothyroidism, craniofacial abnormalities, acromegaly and Marfan's syndrome, history of tonsillectomy/adenoidectomy in childhood)

- Psychiatric history and use of psychotropic medications
- Substance use (alcohol intake and use of illicit drugs)
- Family history of OSA

Physical examination should focus on:

- Evaluation of BMI and obesity, neck circumference
- Examination of the upper airway (nose and throat)
- Assessment for the presence of anatomical abnormalities such as retrognathia, micrognathia, macroglossia and inferior displacement of the hyoid bone

12.8 Diagnosis of OSA

There are several questionnaires that can easily be used in primary care to screen patients for OSA, such as the Berlin Questionnaire (Netzer et al. 1999).

The American Thoracic Society and the American Academy of Sleep Medicine (AASM) recommend supervised polysomnography (PSG) in a sleep laboratory over two nights for the diagnosis of OSA, as well as for the initiation of CPAP therapy (Epstein et al. 2009). However, overnight PSG is not available in many hospitals, and it is associated with significant cost.

Continuous recording of oxygen desaturation during sleep is a common method for the detection of previously undiagnosed OSA. Only 20% of individuals required full PSG following oximetry to help with diagnostic uncertainty, as determined by a recent retrospective analysis in 30 patients referred to a sleep laboratory (Screening 2013). Another study evaluated the sensitivity and specificity of oximetry as a diagnostic screening tool for OSA syndrome as compared with PSG in 63 patients with possible OSA. The authors concluded that oximetry is a reliable screening tool for the diagnosis of OSA in patients without respiratory disease (Oliveira et al. 2007). Two hundred and eighty-eight patients referred to a sleep laboratory with suspicion of symptomatic OSA were randomized to have PSG or home oximetry after 4 weeks of treatment with an auto-adjusting CPAP device. The results of this study show that the ability of physicians to predict the outcome of CPAP in individual patients was not significantly better with PSG than with home oximeter-based monitoring (Whitelaw et al. 2005). Therefore, overnight oximetry is a simple diagnostic test that can be used for screening the at risk for OSA patient population.

The Epworth Sleepiness Scale (Appendix A) is a self-report questionnaire which measures an individual's likelihood of falling asleep during common life situations (Johns 1991).

Overnight PSG remains the gold standard for the diagnosis of OSA. PSG monitors sleeping stages, breathing during sleep, electrocardiogram, movements of the legs, oximetry and snoring. In addition, PSG records the distribution of the stages of sleep, the number of awakenings and apnoeas or hypopnoeas, the starting time of sleep, total sleep time and sleep efficiency (Kushida et al. 2005).

Ambulatory or home devices typically do not measure sleep but measure breathing and can be used for detecting OSA. Such devices have the potential advantage of reducing costs, improving convenience for the patient by avoiding

Table 12.4 Diagnostic criteria and classification of severity of OSA syndrome

A Excessive daytime sleepiness that is not better explained by other factors

B Two or more of the following that are not better explained by other factors:
  Choking or gasping during sleep
  Daytime fatigue
  Impaired concentration

C Overnight monitoring demonstrates ≥5 obstructed breathing events per hour during sleep Diagonosis of OSA syndrome is confirmed by the presence of criterion A or B, plus criterion C or by the presence of 15 or more obstructed breathing events per hour of sleep regardless of symptoms

Classification of severity of OSA on the basis of apnoea-hypopnoea index (AHI)		
Mild	**Moderate**	**Severe**
AHI 5–14	AHI 15–29	AHI ≥ 30

Reference: (Epstein et al. 2009)

an overnight trip to a sleep laboratory and improving access to care for those unable or unwilling to have in-lab PSG. The AASM published a classification that uses the term SCOPER which stands for Sleep, Cardiovascular, Oximetry, Position, Effort and Respiration to provide specificity to the type of signal that is used (Collop et al. 2011). Unattended home monitoring for the diagnosis of OSA should be performed only in conjunction with a comprehensive sleep evaluation. Negative or technically inadequate home tests in patients with a high pretest probability of moderate-to-severe OSA should prompt in-laboratory PSG (Collop et al. 2007).

The multiple sleep latency test and the maintenance of wakefulness test are complementary studies that can be used to measure daytime sleepiness and alertness, respectively (Carskadon et al. 1986; Sangal et al. 1992). Diagnostic criteria of OSA syndrome are summarized in Table 12.4.

12.9 OSA and Neurocognitive Functioning

The exact prevalence of cognitive dysfunction in adult patients with OSA is unknown; the literature reports considerable variability in prevalence of cognitive impairment (Quan et al. 2011).

One prospective observational study of 49 patients with OSA showed that 25% had at least some neurocognitive dysfunction. OSA was found to have a profound impact on psychomotor functioning as well as cognitive domains such as attention, memory and executive functioning. Global intelligence and language appear to be relatively spared (Antonelli et al. 2004).

Literature on cognitive function in OSA describes *a unique clinical syndrome* marked by impairment in attention/working memory, vigilance and executive functioning (Antonelli et al. 2004; Mazza et al. 2005; Naismith et al. 2004).

12.9.1 Risk Factors for Cognitive Impairment in OSA

OSA and neurocognitive decline share the same risk factors (e.g. obesity in men) independently associated with brain function abnormalities (Wong et al. 2006). Recent research has emphasized the association between OSA and neurocognitive decline in individuals with ApoE4 positivity (Elias et al. 2003). Smoking, hypertension, diabetes mellitus, congestive heart failure, cerebrovascular accidents, hypothyroidism, alcoholism and metabolic syndrome are all associated with high rates of cognitive decline. Therefore, pre-existing cognitive impairment due to different causes may be exacerbated by OSA.

Neuroimaging studies demonstrated an association between cognitive impairment and decrease of grey matter volume in specific cerebral regions (hippocampal and frontal brain regions). This can be reversed by treatment and is significantly correlated with improvement in specific neuropsychological tests (executive functioning and short-term memory), underlining the importance of early diagnosis and treatment of sleep apnoea. Emerging data suggest that neurochemical abnormalities in specific brain areas are associated with neurocognitive dysfunction in patients with OSA (Spira et al. 2008).

Nocturnal hypoxia seems to be the most important pathophysiological mechanism of cognitive dysfunction in OSA (Canessa et al. 2011). A multicentre randomized control trial of 1204 adults (mean age 51 years) with moderate-to-severe OSA who were treated for 6 months with either CPAP or sham CPAP found educational level to be the most significant factor explaining better neurocognitive performance (Quan et al. 2011). The prefrontal cortex, which is a primary regulator of executive function, is particularly susceptible to hypoxia, and this may explain the profound effect of untreated OSA on executive function (Yaffe et al. 2011; Beebe and Gozal 2002).

12.10 OSA and Mental Illness

OSA occurs more frequently in persons with psychiatric disorders, as compared to other medical conditions (Schroder and O'Hara 2005; Baran and Richert 2003). Nasr and colleagues recently published a study of 330 psychiatric outpatients and demonstrated that OSA was more prevalent in them compared to the general population (Nasr et al. 2010). In the largest cohort study of 4,060,504 subjects from the Veterans Health Administration databases, 2.9% of subjects were identified as suffering from OSA. Psychiatric comorbid diagnoses were common in individuals with OSA and included depression (21.8%), anxiety disorders (16.7%), PTSD (11.9%), psychosis (5.1%) and bipolar disorders (3.3%) (Sharafkhaneh et al. 2005).

Given the prevalence of mental disorders and OSA in the community, it is of great importance to adequately screen psychiatric patients for OSA.

12.10.1   Schizophrenia and OSA

Prevalence of OSA in patients with severe mental illness (SMI) has only recently become the focus of epidemiological research. One recent study of 100 patients with SMI attending a primary care clinic found 69% to be at high risk for OSA; 16% had a previously confirmed diagnosis of OSA (Alam et al. 2012).

Patients with SMI and OSA share several important risk factors, including high rates of obesity and smoking (Strassnig et al. 2003; George and Ziedonis 2009). Weight gain and obesity resulting from treatment of SMI, particularly with second-generation ("atypical") antipsychotics, are important risk factors for OSA (Wirshing et al. 2002).

OSA is found to be more common in patients with schizophrenia compared to other psychiatric disorders (Winkelman 2001). Prevalence of metabolic syndrome is common in schizophrenia (McEvoy et al. 2005). Results of a recently published longitudinal study indicate that sleep-disordered breathing is associated with metabolic syndrome in both men and women (Hall et al. 2012).

Common symptoms of OSA, such as daytime sleepiness, low motivation and depressed mood, are often difficult to distinguish from negative symptoms of schizophrenia and/or psychotropic medication-induced side effects. Despite the well-known relationship between OSA and cardiovascular morbidity and increased mortality in patients with OSA, the disorder remains underdiagnosed in patients with SMI.

Successful treatment of OSA in SMI can significantly improve unwanted daytime sedation, mood symptoms and psychotic symptoms such as aggressive outbursts (Karanti and Landen 2007). One case report described a schizophrenic patient with OSA who received CPAP therapy resulting in AHI reduction from 43.6 to 2.3. Negative symptoms such as blunted affect, psychomotor poverty and fatigue were all improved (Sugishita et al. 2010). For patients meeting the criteria for metabolic syndrome, the emphasis should be on healthy nutrition and exercise combined with CPAP treatment (Sharma et al. 2011).

In summary, OSA diagnosis and treatment can improve the mental and physical health of SMI patients.

12.10.2   Depression and OSA

The relationship between depression and OSA has been studied for many years, and researchers agree that this relationship is complex, bidirectional and still not well understood. There is significant variability in reports on the prevalence of depressive symptoms in OSA, likely because of the use of different questionnaires and diagnostic criteria. Objective measurements, such as overnight PSG, have been implemented in only a limited number of studies.

It is important to emphasize that OSA and depression share common symptoms such as sleepiness, fatigue, sleep disturbance, impaired cognitive function, mood and anxiety symptoms and irritability. As mentioned above, these symptoms are particularly common in patients with mild-to-moderate OSA.

One recently published literature review confirmed a wide range (from 5 to 63%) of major depressive disorder (MDD) prevalence in OSA (Ejaz et al. 2011), whereas a number of earlier studies had failed to demonstrate an association between the two disorders (Pillar and Lavie 1998) or a clinically significant level of depression in OSA (Lee 1990). The majority of studies confirm that the prevalence of MDD in OSA is higher than in the general population (Gall et al. 1993). A large telephone survey in five European countries of 18,980 subjects, representative of the general population, found that 17.6% of subjects with a breathing-related sleep disorder diagnosis (no sleep study performed) had MDD (Ohayon 2003). The risk of having a diagnosis of OSA based on clinical symptoms was five times higher in individuals with MDD as compared to nondepressed individuals; the association between the two conditions remained strong even when controlling for other factors, such as hypertension or diabetes (Ohayon 2003).

McCall and colleagues noted that 45% of subjects with OSA assessed by the Beck Depression Inventory (BDI) exhibited at least mild depressive symptoms, and depression was more common in women. Interestingly, the authors found no correlation between depressive symptoms, OSA severity, sleepiness and desaturation frequency (McCall et al. 2006). One recent study demonstrated the prevalence of depression was increased in patients with more severe OSA (Peppard et al. 2006).

The high rates of depressive symptoms, identified in a significant number of subjects with OSA, raised questions about the causal relationship between the two conditions (Schwartz et al. 2005; Mosko et al. 1989; Deldin et al. 2006). Recent studies attempted to address whether sleep fragmentation and hypoxia in OSA can cause depression. In a pilot study of 19 depressed patients, significant reduction in airflow and oxygen desaturations were identified, indicating a relationship between sleep fragmentation due to respiratory-related events during sleep (hypoxaemia) and depressive symptoms (Deldin et al. 2006). Furthermore, oxygen therapy was shown to improve depressive symptoms (Bardwell et al. 2007).

Persistent fatigue can explain depressive symptoms in OSA (Bardwell et al. 2003) and is the primary predictor of the level of depression in patients referred to a sleep laboratory, regardless of the level of severity of sleep-disordered breathing (Jackson et al. 2011). Furthermore, there is considerable evidence that depressive symptoms improve with CPAP treatment (Schwartz and Karatinos 2007; Kawahara et al. 2005; Habukawa et al. 2010). However, not all treated OSA patients experience a reduction in their daytime symptoms, such as sleepiness, and ongoing depressed mood may account for residual symptoms in these patients (Sánchez et al. 2009). Thus, study of the relationship between OSA and depression continues to be extremely important for clinical practice.

12.10.3 Bipolar Disorder and OSA

Studies addressing sleep-disordered breathing in patients with bipolar disorder are less common, and the findings are more conflicting, likely due to the complex presentation of mood disturbances in bipolar disorder and the fluctuating course of the illness (Peterson and Benca 2008). In one large cohort sample of patients with confirmed OSA, 4% were diagnosed with bipolar disorder, as compared to less than 2% in the non-apnoea sample (Sharafkhaneh et al. 2005).

Undiagnosed OSA in patients with bipolar disorder could be associated with poor response to treatment (Plante and Winkelman 2008; Bastiampillai et al. 2011). Bipolar disorder is a chronic mental illness that requires long-term treatment with psychotropic medications. Incidence of cardiovascular problems, metabolic syndrome and diabetes is high, independent of treatment with psychotropic medications. Common risk factors for bipolar disorder and OSA, as well as the high prevalence of both diseases in the community, point to the importance of further systematic studies of the prevalence and comorbidity of OSA and bipolar disorder.

12.10.4   Post-traumatic Stress Disorder (PTSD) and OSA

OSA is a common comorbid condition in patients with post-traumatic stress disorder (PTSD) (Krakow et al. 2004; Krakow et al. 2006; Spoormaker and Montgomery 2008). A high prevalence of OSA (69%) was reported in a study of 105 Vietnam-era veterans diagnosed with PTSD (Yesavage et al. 2012).

Comorbid OSA can worsen the typical night-time symptoms of PTSD, including insomnia and nightmares. CPAP therapy has been found to improve the symptoms of both disorders (Krakow et al. 2000). Several studies confirmed high rates of non-adherence to CPAP treatment in PTSD. In a retrospective study of 90 soldiers with OSA, comorbid PTSD was associated with significantly decreased CPAP adherence (El-Solh et al. 2010). Another study of 148 veterans, newly diagnosed with OSA, determined that CPAP usage and adherence were lower in veterans with PTSD (Collen et al. 2012). Although the reasons for such a high rate of non-adherence remain unclear, it is possible that, in addition to higher levels of anxiety, individuals with PTSD may experience difficulty initiating and maintaining sleep and the CPAP-related REM sleep rebound with increased nightmares could negatively impact CPAP use.

Given the potential for adverse clinical outcomes, treatment should focus on identifying potential barriers to CPAP adherence in patients with PTSD and comorbid OSA.

12.10.5   Anxiety Disorders and OSA

Anxiety symptoms are common in patients with OSA. Recently published studies focused on the role of oxidative stress states and their role in the frequent emergence of anxiety symptoms in OSA (Franco et al. 2012). Anxiety symptoms may have a significant impact on the level of adherence to CPAP treatment (Kjelsberga et al. 2005). Conversely, CPAP treatment can alleviate anxiety symptoms present in a substantial number of patients with OSA. Further research is needed to explain the complex relationship between insomnia, anxiety symptoms and OSA. (Kjelsberga et al. 2005; Einvik et al. 2011; Yang et al. 2011)

12.10.6   Panic Disorder (PD) and OSA

The comorbidity of OSA and PD has not been systematically addressed in the literature. One of the challenges in studying this relationship is due to the fact that arousals in OSA are often associated with panic symptoms, making it difficult to distinguish them from nocturnal panic attacks (Lopes et al. 2005). It has been demonstrated that more than 5% of OSA patients have panic attack symptoms (Freire et al. 2007).

Panic disorder can affect adherence to CPAP treatment. Judicious use of a hypnotic (which does not suppress respiratory drive) can be a very effective intervention for this problem, particularly in the first week of CPAP treatment (Dopp and Morgan 2010). Hypnotic agents can be considered in patients who might benefit from reduced awareness of the CPAP device and sleep consolidation. Several studies have demonstrated that acute use of zolpidem does not worsen severity of OSA or pressure requirements (Dopp and Morgan 2010).

Treatment of OSA can decrease the severity and frequency of panic symptoms and reduce the frequency of rescue medication use (Edlund et al. 1991; Takaesu et al. 2012). Therefore, it is important to identify underlying OSA in patients with PD.

12.10.7   Substance Use and OSA

Literature on OSA and the use of recreational drugs is lacking; however in recent years, there has been an increased interest. Studies in patients with current or previous substance abuse allow investigation of the role of different neurotransmitter systems in the pathophysiology of OSA. In a recent study of 30 recreational drug users, the majority reported symptoms consistent with OSA, insomnia or restless leg syndrome (Mahfoud et al. 2009).

Alcohol is the most commonly abused substance. It has a significant impact on sleep architecture and frequently worsens underlying OSA (Issa and Sullivan 1982). Alcohol use increases upper airway instability and the severity of OSA (Vitiello et al. 1990). Quality of life in individuals with alcohol dependence is significantly affected by cognitive deficits, particularly memory loss, impaired judgement and personality changes, and is further impacted by OSA.

Opioid-dependent patients often report subjective sleep complaints confirmed by disrupted sleep architecture. Sharkey and colleagues recently analysed at-home PSG in 71 patients undergoing methadone maintenance treatment for at least 3 months. They determined common breathing abnormalities during sleep and OSA were more prevalent than central sleep apnoea (CSA) (Sharkey et al. 2010). Interestingly, there seems to be a lack of association between OSA presence and severity of subjective sleep difficulties, indicating that factors other than OSA must account for disturbed sleep in opioid-dependent individuals. These findings confirm the importance of investigating for comorbid OSA and/or CSA in patients prescribed methadone (Wang et al. 2008).

Methylenedioxymethamphetamine (MDMA, "ecstasy"), is a popular recreational drug. Recent research has demonstrated increased OSA risk in individuals with a history of MDMA use (McCann et al. 2009). It is well known that MDMA abuse is associated with increased incidence of cardiovascular disease, stroke and death. Cognitive deficits and impulsivity identified in former MDMA users are thought to be related to comorbid OSA, suggesting the role of serotonergic neuron dysfunction in OSA pathogenesis (Chamberlin and Saper 2009).

Further research in patients with substance abuse and comorbid OSA will improve our understanding of cognitive deficits and psychiatric symptoms.

12.11 Treatment of OSA

12.11.1 Behavioural Modifications

Treatment of OSA starts with education about sleep hygiene and lifestyle modifications.

Patients with OSA should adhere to sleep hygiene principles, such as adoption of a regular sleep schedule, adequate environment for sleep, going to bed only when sleepy and avoidance of excessive time in bed.

Smoking cessation should be strongly encouraged as smoking increases inflammation of the upper airway.

Alcohol consumption should be avoided as it is associated with exacerbation of OSA.

Weight loss is an essential part of treatment. Weight loss is associated with decreased OSA disease severity in adults. In one meta-analysis of 342 adults, significant weight loss (mean BMI decreased by 17.9 kg/m^2 from a mean starting value of 55.3 kg/m^2) was followed by a significant reduction in OSA severity. However, a number of patients in this study continued to have moderate-to-severe OSA (Greenburg et al. 2009). Another study looked at the effect of low energy diet in obese patients with severe OSA and demonstrated a 67% AHI reduction with weight loss (Johansson et al. 2009). Physical exercise has a positive effect on respiratory drive and muscle tone in the upper airway and complements the effects of weight loss on OSA severity (Netzer et al. 1997).

12.11.2 Oral Appliances

One approach to the treatment of OSA is the use of oral appliances (mandible advancement appliances, lingual retainers and appliances that act upon the soft palate) (Liu et al. 2001). Mandible advancement appliances have been successful in eliminating snoring and apnoeas in patients with mild or moderate OSA scores (Rodríguez-Lozano et al. 2008). However, many patients experience difficulties with oral appliances such as pain, joint, dental or facial muscle discomfort, excessive salivation, dryness of the mouth, headaches and bruxism, which limits their use.

12.11.3 Surgical Techniques

In patients where standard treatments, such as CPAP or mandibular advancement, fail and/or are poorly tolerated, the following surgical procedures should be considered:

(a) Uvulopalatopharyngoplasty (UPPP) and laser-assisted uvulopalatoplasty (LA-UPP) reduce the uvula and the distal portion of the soft palate without total excision of the muscle of the uvula. Friedman et al. report a 41% success rate with this technique (Friedman et al. 2003).
(b) Tonsillectomy with the use of CO^2 laser or radiofrequency ablation.
(c) Maxillo-mandibular advancement is currently the first choice of surgical treatments for OSA, with a high success rate of 75–100% (Li 2007). This procedure should be considered in patients with severe OSA and excessive daytime sleepiness (Lye et al. 2008).
(d) Tracheotomy.

12.11.4 Pharmacological Treatments

Despite a number of clinical trials with various medications or topical agents, there is still insufficient evidence to recommend any specific pharmacological agents for the treatment of OSA (Smith et al. 2006). Decreased serotonin levels in the peripheral nervous system are postulated as one important mechanism associated with vulnerability of the upper airway towards collapse during sleep. One study examined the effect of mirtazapine (mixed 5HT2/5HT3 antagonist) in newly diagnosed OSA and found a 50% reduction of abnormal respiratory events during one night of sleep. However, there was no effect of mirtazapine on sleep quality, daytime alertness or oxygen saturation in this small group of patients (Carley et al. 2007).

12.11.5 CPAP

CPAP continues to be considered the gold standard for the treatment of OSA due to its efficacy, low risk associated with its use and relative ease of use (Basner 2007). CPAP acts as a physical pressure splint to prevent partial or complete collapse of the upper airway during sleep. Positive pressure is delivered using a mask connected to a flow generator.

Literature over many years has repeatedly demonstrated that CPAP use reduces daytime sleepiness and improves alertness (Marshall et al. 2006). Studies confirm a reduction in road traffic incident rates with regular use (George et al. 1997). One study of a cohort of patients, diagnosed between 1982 and 1992 and followed until 1996, found that the relative risk of mortality in patients with non-treated OSA would be at least in the order of two to three times that of the general population. CPAP use is associated with significantly decreased mortality rate, as compared with untreated patients in whom the mortality rate reaches 20% (Marti et al. 2002). Overall, quality of life is improved with CPAP treatment, not only for patients (Flemons 2002) but also their bed partners (Parish and Lyng 2003). CPAP use decreases costs associated with OSA (Albarrak et al. 2005). In addition, CPAP use lowers blood pressure and improves metabolic abnormalities (Dhillon et al. 2005) and overall cardiovascular function (McNicholas and Bonsigore 2007). As noted above, CPAP use is associated with improved neurocognitive function.

12.11.5.1   Adherence to CPAP Treatment

Definition of acceptable adherence to CPAP was previously debated in the literature. Most researchers and clinicians in recent years agree that longer CPAP use is associated with reduced daytime sleepiness and overall improvement in daily functioning (Weaver and Grunstein 2008; Olsen et al. 2008). CPAP use greater than 6 h a night is required to normalize daily function and levels of alertness (Weaver et al. 2003a). Patients who use CPAP every night, on average between 4 and 5 h per night at the prescribed pressure, are considered to be adherent with their treatment. It is important to emphasize that adequate CPAP adherence is important not only for patients with OSA but also in subjects with partial upper airway obstruction during sleep (Anttalainen et al. 2007).

Early CPAP use predicts long-term CPAP adherence (Collard et al. 1997). It has been demonstrated that 15–30% of patients have difficulty accepting CPAP during the titration study or the first week of treatment (Fletcher and Luckett 1991).

Poor adherence to CPAP is a major problem in the treatment of OSA. It has been demonstrated that the improvement in daytime function with CPAP use is reversed after only one night without treatment (Kribbs et al. 1993). Suboptimal adherence to CPAP treatment is associated with poor health and functional outcomes. Negative effects on mood and increased sleepiness or fatigue are frequently documented in patients with poor adherence to treatment.

Factors that impact on CPAP adherence include:

1. Subjective beliefs about the illness and judgements about the severity of its side effects; researchers have identified a positive correlation between higher internal locus of control (patients' belief they have control over their health, expectations for good or bad outcomes of treatment, values of their health and health outcomes) and adherence to treatment (Wallston 1992).
2. Increased risk perception and lower outcome expectancies—these tend to negatively affect CPAP use (Baron et al. 2011).
3. Self-efficacy or the belief that one can effectively overcome obstacles to adherence—this is a predictor of long-term CPAP use (Weaver et al. 2003b).
4. Nose stuffiness and air leaks around the mask.
5. Machine noise.
6. Spontaneous intimacy with the bed partner.
7. Insomnia (Pieh et al. 2013).

8. Disease severity; one recent study determined that only patients with very severe OSA use the CPAP device regularly. Interestingly, patients' subjective reported symptom severity and quality of life were not reliably correlated with objective OSA measures (Yetkin et al. 2008).

9. Personality style and motivation. Psychological factors such as elevated behavioural inhibition scores and neuroticism adversely affect CPAP usage. Motivation is an important additional factor (Moran et al. 2011).

10. Social support and marital satisfaction.

Strategies to Improve Adherence to CPAP Treatment

Identification of poor users early in treatment is important in order to deliver targeted interventions to patients who are experiencing difficulties accepting CPAP treatment.

Patient education about OSA and CPAP increases adherence to treatment. In addition to improving knowledge and beliefs about the risks of OSA, it is important to motivate patients to initiate and maintain CPAP treatment. Education programmes involve providing information to new CPAP users about how to appropriately use CPAP and overcome side effects related to treatment (Sawyer et al. 2011).

Management of CPAP side effects includes specific modifications to the device and interface. It is possible that the CPAP requirement changes over time, indicating a need for pressure readjustment.

Interventions aimed at improving treatment self-efficacy have the potential to reinforce adherence behaviour by creating a stronger link between CPAP use and subjective experience of the benefits of treatment. Recent literature emphasizes understanding individual differences in perceived treatment benefits (Stepnowsky Jr et al. 2006).

Motivational interviewing (MI) is another strategy used to enhance CPAP adherence. MI addresses the patient's ambivalence regarding CPAP use, outcome expectations, beliefs in ability to engage and readiness to engage in treatment (Miller and Rollnick 2002).

Cognitive Behavioural Therapy (CBT)

CBT is focused on education about the advantages and disadvantages of the treatment, troubleshooting, review of treatment goals and development of realistic expectations. Treatment focus is on the identification and modification of faulty beliefs regarding CPAP treatment. Simple relaxation techniques are implemented to minimize anxious reactions when patients use their masks. CBT is often delivered in group sessions.

Management of Claustrophobia

When present, claustrophobia (an abnormal dread or fear of closed spaces) can have a significant effect on adherence to CPAP therapy. One prospective study of 153 participants, followed for 3 months of treatment, described a number of subjects that experienced claustrophobia. In addition to the mask discomfort, the aversion to the CPAP mask and nasal discomfort, patients describe feelings of being closed in. Chasens and colleagues (2007) used the fear and avoidance scale to measure claustrophobic tendencies pre-CPAP treatment and again after 3 months. The authors found that poor CPAP adherence (< 2 h per night) was more than twice as high in participants with a high claustrophobia score, indicating that appropriate identification of individuals is essential in the initial stages of treatment. Prior to initiation of treatment, 49% of the participants in one study indicated that they would not use CPAP if it made them feel claustrophobic (Chasens et al. 2005).

Early recognition of patients with claustrophobia may identify those who might benefit more from other treatments such as surgery or oral appliances.

12.12 OSA in Special Populations

12.12.1 OSA in the Ageing Population

Epidemiological studies confirm that the risk of developing OSA increases with age. Sforza and colleagues demonstrated that a significant number of healthy older adults have breathing abnormalities during sleep, including subjects who have no symptoms of OSA or history of cardiac disease, dementia or stroke. AHI ≥ 15 was present in 53% of individuals in a large cross-sectional study of 827 subjects aged 68 ± 1.8 years (Sforza et al. 2010).

OSA is known to increase the risk of cardiovascular illnesses and stroke. It has been demonstrated that severe OSA increases the risk of dementia (Kim et al. 2011).

OSA has been associated with mild cognitive impairment (MCI) which is a strong risk factor for development of Alzheimer's disease (Caselli 2008; Petersen et al. 2010). Research studies show that comorbid OSA may have an additional impact on cognitive function in the ageing population, although the results fail to demonstrate consistent findings (Ayalon et al. 2010; Antonelli Incalzi et al. 2004; Mathieu et al. 2008).

One recent study pointed to the increased risk of cognitive impairment in older women with OSA due to intermittent hypoxia during sleep (Yaffe et al. 2011).

Risk factors for cognitive impairment in the elderly with OSA include:

1. Genetic factors (Kadotani et al. 2001).
2. Cigarette smoking, which is common in subjects with OSA (Peters et al. 2008).
3. Stroke, which is a common cause of cognitive impairment in patients with OSA (Tatemichi et al. 1990; Desmond et al. 2000).
4. Use of psychotropic medications such as benzodiazepines, narcotics and atypical antipsychotics, commonly prescribed to treat insomnia, pain syndromes and agitation in the elderly (Moore and O'Keeffe 1999; Shirani et al. 2011).
5. Circadian disruption, commonly identified in the elderly population; this is especially relevant to older women (Tranah et al. 2011).

Given the high prevalence of MCI and OSA in the ageing population, it is important to identify comorbid conditions and factors such as treatment with medications that could have an additional impact on cognitive function.

12.12.2   OSA in Children

Studies using PSG in the general paediatric population found that the prevalence of paediatric OSA ranges from 1.2% to 5.7%. Estimates of sleep-disordered breathing, which includes both OSA and snoring, are around 12% (Bixler et al. 2009). There is a predominance in boys and African American children (Redline et al. 1999; Ishman 2012; Rosen et al. 2003).

There are numerous factors that increase the risk of developing OSA in children. Comorbid factors such as obesity, craniofacial deformity, genetic syndrome status and metabolic disease have all been associated with an increased incidence of sleep-disordered breathing in children.

Epidemiologic risk factors for paediatric OSA syndrome include (Lumeng and Chervin 2008).

1. Adenotonsillar hypertrophy
2. Obesity (fatty infiltration of airway, abnormal ventilatory control)
3. Race (African American) (Sharma et al. 2011)
4. Gender (male)
5. Prematurity
6. Craniofacial dysmorphology (adverse craniofacial growth)
7. Neurologic disorders (abnormal ventilatory control)
8. Nasal/pharyngeal inflammation (increased airway resistance)
9. Socioeconomic/environmental factors
10. Family history of OSAS
11. Passive cigarette smoke or indoor allergens
12. Poor sleep quality (noise, stress)

There are several important differences in the presentation of OSA in children and adults. Children are more likely to present with partially obstructed breathing during sleep and hypopnoeas, whereas apnoeas, arousals and desaturations are less common than in adults.

12.12.2.1   Consequences of Untreated Paediatric Sleep Apnoea

Untreated OSA in children is associated with significant impairments, including cognitive deficits, hyperactivity, cardiovascular illness and inflammation (Peters et al. 2008). Studies of neuropsychiatric function show lower general intelligence, learning and memory impairment, decreased language and verbal skills and diminished attention in children with OSA (Gozal 2009; O'Brien et al. 2003; O'Brien et al. 2004).

Sleep fragmentation and intermittent hypoxia at critical periods in paediatric brain development (such as periods of brain myelination or peak acquisition of skills) are responsible for neurocognitive effects in children with OSA (Surratt et al. 2007).

Behavioural problems (aggression, oppositional behaviour) are commonly identified as accompanying symptoms in paediatric OSA (Surratt et al. 2007). There is increased incidence of attention deficit hyperactivity disorder (ADHD) and depression (Chervin et al. 2002). Impaired executive function in children with OSA is the likely cause of attention problems or behaviour dysregulation.

Comorbid medical conditions associated with paediatric OSA include cardiovascular disease, hypertension and autonomic dysfunction.

12.12.2.2 Treatment of Paediatric OSA

Adenotonsillectomy is the recommended initial treatment for OSA and sleep-disordered breathing for healthy children. There has been debate regarding the role of adenotonsillectomy in obese children who are more likely to have persistent paediatric OSA than nonobese children (Friedman et al. 2009; Baugh et al. 2011). School performance has been shown to improve after treatment of OSA with adenotonsillectomy (Baugh et al. 2011; Chervin et al. 2006).

Children who have their adenoids removed before age six, or who underwent partial tonsil removal, have a high risk for regrowth of adenoids or tonsils and recurrence of OSA symptoms (Chervin et al. 2006).

Additional surgical procedures can be used in children with neurological disease or complex craniofacial abnormalities. These include uvulopalatopharyngoplasty (UPPP), nasal turbinate reduction, lingual tonsillectomy, hyoid myotomy and suspension, genioglossal advancement, partial midline glossectomy and tongue suspension suture (James and Ma 1997; Wootten and Shott 2010).

There is limited information in the literature regarding the efficacy of weight loss on OSA in children. Most authors agree on the effectiveness of school-based programmes that include behavioural counselling, dietary counselling, nutrition education, scheduled physical activity and parental training and involvement (Epstein et al. 1990).

Short courses of oral and nasal steroids or montelukast therapy, as monotherapies or in combination with surgical treatments, all show modest improvements in children with mild OSA (Al-Ghamdi et al. 1997; Brouillette et al. 2001).

Oral appliance therapy has some efficacy in children with mild-to-moderate OSA, as does rapid maxillary expansion in children with maxillary constriction (Villa et al. 2011).

CPAP improves sleepiness and snoring, as demonstrated in a multicentre study of 29 children with a mean age of 10.5 years (Marcus et al. 2006). Adherence to treatment is the biggest challenge (Uong et al. 2007). Facial side effects such as skin injury, erythema and skin necrosis, global facial flattening and maxillary retrusion occurred with CPAP use. It is not clear if there are any effects on the bony facial structures (Fauroux et al. 2005).

References

Akashiba T, Kawahara S, Akahoshi T, Omori C, Saito O, Majima T, Horie T. Relationship between quality of life and mood or depression in patients with severe obstructive sleep apnea syndrome. Chest. 2002;122:861–5.

Alam A, Chengappa KNR, Ghinassi F. Screening for obstructive sleep apnea among individuals with severe mental illness at a primary care clinic. Gen Hosp Psychiatry. 2012;34(6):660–4.

Albarrak M, Banno K, Sabbagh AA, Delaive K, Walld R, Manfreda J, Kryger MH. Utilization of healthcare resources in obstructive sleep apnea syndrome: a 5-year follow-up study in men using CPAP. Sleep. 2005;28:1306–11.

Al-Ghamdi SA, Manoukian JJ, Morielli A, et al. Do systemic corticosteroids effectively treat obstructive sleep apnea secondary to adenotonsillar hypertrophy? Laryngoscope. 1997;107(10):1382–7.

Anon. Sleep-related breathing disorders in adults: recommendations for syndrome definition and measurement techniques in clinical research. The Report of an American Academy of Sleep Medicine. Sleep. 1999;22:667.

Antonelli Incalzi R, Marra C, Salvigni BL, et al. Does cognitive dysfunction conform to a distinctive pattern in obstructive sleep apnea syndrome? J Sleep Res. 2004;13(1):79–86.

Anttalainen U, Saaresranta T, Kalleinen N, Aittokallio J, Vahlberg T, Polo O. CPAP adherence and partial upper airway obstruction during sleep. Sleep Breath. 2007;11:171–6.

Ayalon L, Ancoli-Israel S, Drummond SP. Obstructive sleep apnea and age: a double insult to brain function? Am J Respir Crit Care Med. 2010;182(3):413–9.

Baldwin CM, Griffith KA, Nieto FJ, O'Connor GT, Walsleben JA, Redline S. The association of sleep-disordered breathing and sleep symptoms with quality of life in the sleep heart health study. Sleep. 2001;24:96–105.

Baran AS, Richert AC. Obstructive sleep apnea and depression. CNS Spectr. 2003;8(2):128–34.

Bardwell WA, Moore P, Ancoli-Israel S, Dimsdale JE. Fatigue in obstructive sleep apnea: driven by depressive symptoms instead of apnea severity? Am J Psychiatr. 2003;160:350–5.

Bardwell WA, Norma D, Ancoli-Israel S, Loredo JS, Lowery A, Lim W, Dimsdale JE. Effects of 2 week nocturnal oxygen supplementation and continuous positive airway pressure treatment on psychological symptoms in patients with obstructive sleep apnea: a randomized placebo-controlled study. Behav Sleep Med. 2007;5(1):21–38.

Baron KG, Berg CA, Czajkowski LA, Smith TW, et al. Self-efficacy contributes to individual differences in subjective improvements using CPAP. Sleep Breath. 2011;15:599–606.

Basner RC. Continuous positive airway pressure for obstructive sleep apnea. N Engl J Med. 2007;356:1751–8.

Bastiampillai T, Khor LJ, Dhillon R. Complicated management of mania in the setting of undiagnosed obstructive sleep apnea. J ECT. 2011;27:15–6.

Baugh RF, Archer SM, Mitchell RB, et al. Clinical practice guideline: tonsillectomy in children. American Academy of Otolaryngology-Head and Neck Surgery Foundation. J Otolaryngol Head Neck Surg. 2011;144(Suppl 1):S1–30.

Beebe DW, Gozal D. Obstructive sleep apnea and the prefrontal cortex: towards a comprehensive model linking nocturnal upper airway obstruction to daytime cognitive and behavioral deficits. J Sleep Res. 2002;11:1–16.

Bixler EO, Vgontzas AN, Ten Have T, Tyson K, Kales A. Effects of age on sleep apnoea in men: prevalence and severity. Am J Respir Crit Care Med. 1998;157:144.

Bixler EO, Vgontzas AN, Lin HM, et al. Sleep-disordered breathing in children in a general population sample: prevalence and risk factors. Sleep. 2009;32:731–6.

Brouillette RT, Manoukian JJ, Ducharme FM, et al. Efficacy of fluticasone nasal spray for pediatric obstructive sleep apnea. J Pediatr. 2001;138:838–44.

Canessa N, Castronovo V, Cappa SF, Aloia MS, Marelli S, Falini A, Alemanno F, Ferini-Strambi L. Obstructive sleep apnea: brain structural changes and neurocognitive function before and after treatment. Am J Respir Crit Care Med. 2011;183(10):1419–26.

Carley DW, Olopade C, Ruigt GS, Radulovacki M. Efficacy of mirtazapine in obstructive sleep apnea syndrome. Sleep. 2007;30(1):35.

Carskadon MA, Dement WC, Mitler MM, Roth T, Westbrook PR, Keenan S. Guidelines for the multiple sleep latency test (MSLT): a standard measure of sleepiness. Sleep. 1986;9:519–24.

Caselli RJ. Obstructive sleep apnea, apolipoprotein E e4, and mild cognitive impairment. Sleep Med. 2008;9(8):816–7.

Chamberlin NL, Saper CB. The agony of the ecstasy: serotonin and obstructive sleep apnea. Neurology. 2009;73:1947–8.

Chasens ER, Pack AI, Maislin G, Dinges FD, Weaver TE. Claustrophobia and adherence to CPAP treatment. West J Nurs Res. 2005;27(3):307–21.

Chervin RD, Archbold KH, Dillon JE, et al. Inattention, hyperactivity, and symptoms of sleep-disordered breathing. Pediatrics. 2002;109(3):449–56.

Chervin RD, Ruzicka DL, Giordani BJ, et al. Sleep-disordered breathing, behavior, and cognition in children before and after adenotonsillectomy. Pediatrics. 2006;117(4):769–78.

Collard P, Pieters T, Aubert G, Delguste P, Rodenstein DO. Compliance with nasal CPAP in obstructive sleep apnea patients. Sleep Med Rev. 1997;1(1):33–44.

Collen JF, Lettieri CJ, Hoffman M. The impact of posttraumatic stress disorder on CPAP adherence in patients with obstructive sleep apnea. J Clin Sleep Med. 2012;8(6):667–72.

Collop NA, Anderson WM, Boehlecke B, Claman D, Goldberg R, Gottlieb DJ, Hudgel D, Sateia M, Schwab R. Clinical guidelines for the use of unattended portable monitors in the diagnosis of obstructive sleep apnea in adult patients. J Clin Sleep Med. 2007;3(7):737–47.

Collop N, Tracy SL, Kapur V, Mehra R, Kuhlmann D, Fleishmann SA, Ojile JM. Obstructive sleep apnea devices for out-of-center (OOC) testing: technology evaluation. J Clin Sleep Med. 2011;7(5):531–48.

Deldin PJ, Phillips LK, Thomas RJ. A preliminary study of sleep-disordered breathing in major depressive disorder. Sleep Med. 2006;7:131–9.

Desmond DW, Moroney JT, Paik MC, et al. Frequency and clinical determinants of dementia after ischemic stroke. Neurology. 2000;54(5):1124–31.

Dhillon S, Chung SA, Fargher T, Huterer N, Shapiro CM. Sleep apnea, hypertension, and the effects of continuous positive airway pressure. Am J Hypertens. 2005;18:594–600.

Dopp JM, Morgan BJ. Pharmacologic approaches for the management of symptoms and cardiovascular consequences of obstructive sleep apnea in adults. Sleep Breath. 2010;14(4):307–15.

Edlund MJ, McNamara ME, Millman RP. Sleep apnea and panic attacks. Compr Psychiatry. 1991;32:130–2.

Einvik G, Hrubos-Strom H, Randby A, Nordhus IH, Somers VK, Omland T, et al. Major depressive disorder, anxiety disorders, and cardiac biomarkers in subjects at high risk of obstructive sleep apnea. Psychosom Med. 2011;73:378–84.

Ejaz SM, Khawaja IS, Bhatia S, Hurtwitz TD. Obstructive sleep apnea and depression: a review. Innov Clin Neurosci. 2011;8:17–25.

Elias MF, Elias PK, Sullivan LM, Wolf PA, D'Agostino RB. Lower cognitive function in the presence of obesity and hypertension: the Framingham heart study. Int J Obes Relat Metab Disord. 2003;27(2):260–8.

Ellen RL, Marshall SC, Palayew M, Molnar FJ, Wilson KG, Man-Son-Hing M. Systematic review of motor vehicle crash risk in persons with sleep apnea. J Clin Sleep Med. 2006;2:193–200.

El-Solh AA, Ayyar L, Akinnusi M, Relia S, Akinnusi O. Positive airway pressure adherence in veterans with posttraumatic stress disorder. Sleep. 2010;33:1495–500.

Epstein LH, Valoski A, Wing RR, et al. Ten-year follow-up of behavioral, family-based treatment for obese children. JAMA. 1990;264(19):2519–23.

Epstein LJ, Kristo D, Strollo PJ Jr, Friedman N, Malhotra A, Patil SP, et al. Clinical guideline for the evaluation, management and long-term care of obstructive sleep apnea in adults. J Clin Sleep Med. 2009;15:263–76.

Fauroux B, Lavis JF, Nicot F, et al. Facial side effects during noninvasive positive pressure ventilation in children. Intensive Care Med. 2005;31(7):965–9.

Flemons WW. Clinical practice. Obstructive sleep apnea. N Engl J Med. 2002;347:498–504.

Fletcher EC, Luckett RA. The effect of positive reinforcement on hourly compliance in nasal continuous positive airway pressure users with obstructive sleep apnea. Am Rev Respir Dis. 1991;143(5 Pt 1):936–41.

Fogel RB, Malhotra A, White DP. Sleep. 2: pathophysiology of obstructive sleep apnoea/hypopnoea syndrome. Thorax. 2004;59:159–63.

Franco CM, Lima AM, Ataide L Jr, Lins OG, Castro CM, Bezerra AA, et al. Obstructive sleep apnea severity correlates with cellular and plasma oxidative stress parameters and affective symptoms. J Mol Neurosci. 2012;47(2):300–10.

Freire RC, Valenca AM, Nascimento I, Lopes FL, Mezzasalma MA, Zin WA, et al. Clinical features of respiratory and nocturnal panic disorder subtypes. Psychiatry Res. 2007;152:287–91.

Friedman M, Ibrahim H, Lee G, Joseph NJ. Combined uvulopalatopharyngoplasty and radiofrequency tongue base reduction for treatment of obstructive sleep apnea/hypopnea syndrome. Otolaryngol Head Neck Surg. 2003;129:61.

Friedman M, Wilson M, Lin HC, et al. Updated systematic review of tonsillectomy and adenoidectomy for treatment of pediatric obstructive sleep apnea/hypopnea syndrome. J Otolaryngol Head Neck Surg. 2009;140(6):800–8.

Gall R, Isaac L, Kryger M. Quality of life in mild obstructive sleep apnea. Sleep. 1993;16(8 Suppl):S59–61.

George TP, Ziedonis DM. Addressing tobacco dependence in psychiatric practice: promises and pitfalls. Can J Psychiatr. 2009;54(6):353–5.

George CF, Boudreau AC, Smiley A. Effects of nasal CPAP on simulated driving performance in patients with obstructive sleep apnoea. Thorax. 1997;52:648–53.

Gold AR, Dipalo F, Gold MS, O'Hearn D. The symptoms and signs of upper airway resistance syndrome: a link to the functional somatic syndromes. Chest. 2003;123:87.

Gozal D. Sleep-disordered breathing and school performance in children. Pediatrics. 1998;102:616.

Gozal D. Sleep, sleep disorders and inflammation in children. Sleep Med. 2009;10(Suppl 1):S12–6.

Greenburg DL, Lettieri CJ, Eliasson AH. Effects of surgical weight loss on measures of obstructive sleep apnea: a meta-analysis. Am J Med. 2009;122(6):535–42.

Guimaraes CV, Donnelly LF, Shott SR, Amin RS, Kalra M. Relative rather than absolute macroglossia in patients with down syndrome: implications for treatment of obstructive sleep apnea. Pediatr Radiol. 2008;38(10):1062–7.

Habukawa M, Uchimura N, Kakuma T, et al. Effect of CPAP treatment on residual depressive symptoms in patients with major depression and coexisting sleep apnea: contribution of daytime sleepiness to residual depressive symptoms. Sleep Med. 2010;11(6):552–7.

Hall MH, Okun ML, Sowers M, Matthews KA, Kravitz HM, Hardin K, Buysse DJ, Bromberger JT, Owens JF, Karpoy I, Saunders MH. Sleep is associated with the metabolic syndrome in a multi-ethnic cohort of midlife women: the SWAN sleep study. Sleep. 2012;35:783–90.

He J, Kryger MH, Zorick FJ, Conway W, Roth T. Mortality and apnea index in obstructive sleep apnea. Experience in 385 male patients. Chest. 1988;94(1):9–14.

Ishman SL. Evidence-base practice: pediatric obstructive sleep apnea. Otolaryngol clinics of North America. Journal. 2012;45:1055–69.

Issa FG, Sullivan CE. Alcohol, snoring and sleep apnea. J Neurol Neurosurg Psychiatry. 1982;45:353–9.

Jackson ML, Stough C, Howard ME, Spong J, Downey LA, Thompson B. The contribution of fatigue and sleepiness to depression in patients attending the sleep laboratory for evaluation of obstructive sleep apnea. Sleep Breath. 2011;15(3):439–45.

James D, Ma L. Mandibular reconstruction in children with obstructive sleep due to micrognathia. PlastReconstr Surg. 1997;100:1131.

Jing J, Huang T, Cui W, Shen H. Effect on quality of life of continuous positive airway pressure in patients with obstructive sleep apnea syndrome: a meta-analysis. Lung. 2008;186:131–44.

Johansson K, Neovius M, Lagerros YT, Rossner S, Granath F, Hemmingsson E. Effect of a very low energy diet on moderate and severe obstructive sleep apnoea in obese men: a randomised controlled trial. BMJ. 2009;339:4609.

Johns MW. A new method for measuring daytime sleepiness: the Epworth sleepiness scale. Sleep. 1991;14:540–5.

Jordan AS, McEvoy RD. Gender differences in sleep apnea: epidemiology, clinical presentation and pathogenic mechanisms. Sleep Med Rev. 2003;7:377.

Kadotani H, Kadotani T, Young T, et al. Association between apolipoprotein E epsilon4 and sleep-disordered breathing in adults. J Am Med Assoc. 2001;285(22):2888–90.

Karanti A, Landen M. Treatment refractory psychosis remitted upon treatment with continuous positive airway pressure: a case report. Psychopharmacol Bull. 2007;40(1):113–7.

Karimi M, Hedner J, Lombardi C, Mcnicholas WT, Penzel T, Riha RL, Rodenstein D, Grote L, The Esada Study Group. Driving habits and risk factors for traffic accidents among sleep apnea patients – a European multi-centre cohort study. J Sleep Res. 2014;23(6):689–99.

Kawahara S, Akashiba T, Akahoshi T, Horie T. Nasal CPAP improves the quality of life and lessens the depressive symptoms in patients with obstructive sleep apnea syndrome. Intern Med. 2005;44:422–7.

Kim SJ, Lee JH, Lee DY, et al. Neurocognitive dysfunction associated with sleep quality and sleep apnea in patients with mild cognitive impairment. Am J Geriatr Psychiatry. 2011;19(4):374–81.

Kjelsberga FN, Ruud EA, Stavem K. Predictors of symptoms of anxiety and depression in obstructive sleep apnea. Sleep Med. 2005;6:341–6.

Krakow B, Lowry C, Germain A, Gaddy L, Hollifield M, Koss M, et al. A retrospective study on improvements in nightmares and post-traumatic stress disorder following treatment for comorbid sleep-disordered breathing. J Psychosom Res. 2000;49:291–8.

Krakow B, Haynes PL, Warner TD, Santana E, Melendrez D, Johnston L, et al. Nightmares, insomnia, and sleep-disordered breathing in fire evacuees seeking treatment for posttraumatic sleep disturbance. J Trauma Stress. 2004;17:257–68.

Krakow B, Melendrez D, Warner TD, Clark JO, Sisley BN, Dorin R, et al. Signs and symptoms of sleep-disordered breathing in trauma survivors: a matched comparison with classic sleep apnea patients. J Nerv Ment Dis. 2006;194:433–9.

Kribbs NB, Pack AI, Kline LR, Getsy JE, Schuett JS, Henry JN, et al. Effects of one night without nasal CPAP treatment on sleep and sleepiness in patients with obstructive sleep apnea. Am J Respir Crit Care Med. 1993;147:1162–8.

Kushida CA, Littner MR, Morgenthaler T, Alessi CA, Bailey D, Coleman J Jr. Practice parameters for the indications for polysomnography and related procedures: an update for 2005. Sleep. 2005;28:499.

Lee S. Depression in sleep apnea: a different view. J Clin Psychiatry. 1990;51:309–10.

Leger D, Bayon V, Laaban JP, Philip P. Impact of sleep apnea on economics. Sleep Med Rev. 2012;16:455–62.

Li KK. Hypopharyngeal airway surgery. Otolaryngol Clin N Am. 2007;40:845.

Liu Y, Lowe AA, Fleetham JA, Park YC. Cephalometric and physiologic predictors of the efficacy of an adjustable oral appliance for treating obstructive sleep apnea. Am J Orthod Dentofacial Orthop. 2001;120:639.

Lopes FL, Nardi AE, Nascimento I, Valenca AM, Mezzasalma MA, Freire RC, et al. Diurnal panic attacks with and without nocturnal panic attacks: are there some phenomenological differences? Rev Bras Psiquiatr. 2005;27:216–21.

Lumeng JC, Chervin RD. Epidemiology of pediatric obstructive sleep apnea. Proc Am Thorac Soc. 2008;5(2):242–52.

Lye KW, Waite PD, Meara D, Wang D. Quality of life evaluation of maxillomandibular advancement surgery for treatment of obstructive sleep apnea. J Oral Maxillofac Surg. 2008;66:968.

Mahfoud Y, Talih F, Streem D, Budur K. Sleep disorders in substance abusers: how common are they? Psychiatry (Edgmont). 2009;6:38–42.

Marcus CL, Rosen G, Ward SL, et al. Adherence to and effectiveness of positive airway pressure therapy in children with obstructive sleep apnea. Pediatrics. 2006;117:e4.

Marin JM, et al. Long-term cardiovascular outcomes in men with obstructive sleep apnoea-hypopnoea with or without treatment with continuous positive airway pressure: an observational study. Lancet. 2005;365:1046.

Marshall NS, Barnes M, Travier N, Campbell AJ, Pierce RJ, McEvoy RD, Neill AM, Gander PH. Continuous positive airway pressure reduces daytime sleepiness in mild to moderate obstructive sleep apnoea: a meta-analysis. Thorax. 2006;61:430–4.

Marti S, Sampol G, Munoz X, Torres F, Roca A, Lloberes P, Sagales T, Quesada P, Morell F. Mortality in severe sleep apnoea/hypopnoea syndrome patients: impact of treatment. Eur Respir J. 2002;20:1511–8.

Mathieu A, Mazza S, Decary A, et al. Effects of obstructive sleep apnea on cognitive function: a comparison between younger and older OSAS patients. Sleep Med. 2008;9:112–20.

Mazza S, Pépin JL, Naëgelé B, Plante J, Deschaux C, Lévy P. Most obstructive sleep apnoea patients exhibit vigilance and attention deficits on an extended battery of tests. Eur Respir J. 2005;25(1):75–80.

McCall WV, Harding D, O'Donovan C. Correlates of depressive symptoms in patients with obstructive sleep apnea. J Clin Sleep Med. 2006;2:424–6.

McCann UD, Sgambati FP, Schwartz AR, Ricaurte GA. Sleep apnea in young abstinent recreational MDMA ("ecstasy") consumers. Neurology. 2009;73:2011–7.

McEvoy JP, Meyer JM, Goff DC. Prevalence of the metabolic syndrome in patients with schizophrenia: baseline results from the clinical antipsychotic trials of intervention effectiveness (CATIE) schizophrenia trial and comparison with national estimates from NHANES III. Schizophr Res. 2005;80:19–32.

McNicholas WT, Bonsigore MR. Sleep apnoea as an independent risk factor for cardiovascular disease: current evidence, basic mechanisms and research priorities. Eur Respir J. 2007;29:156–78.

Miller W, Rollnick S. Motivational interviewing: preparing people for change. 2nd ed. New York: The Guilford Press; 2002.

Moore AR, O'Keeffe ST. Drug-induced cognitive impairment in the elderly. Drugs Aging. 1999;15(1):15–28.

Moran AM, Everhart DE, Davis CE, Wuensch KL, Lee DO, Demaree HA. Personality correlates of adherence with continuous positive airway pressure. Sleep Breath. 2011;15:687–94.

Mosko S, Zetin M, Glen S, et al. Self-reported depressive symptomatology, mood ratings, and treatment outcome in sleep disorders patients. J Clin Psychol. 1989;45:51–60.

Naismith S, Winter V, Gotsopoulos H, Hickie I, Cistulli P. Neurobehavioral functioning in obstructive sleep apnea: differential effects of sleep quality, hypoxemia and subjective sleepiness. J Clin Exp Neuropsychol. 2004;26(1):43–54.

Nasr S, Wendt B, Kora S. Increased incidence of sleep apnea in psychiatric outpatients. Ann Clin Psychiatry. 2010;22(1):29–32.

Netzer N, Lormes W, Giebelhaus V, Halle M, Keul J, Matthys H, et al. Physical training of patients with sleep apnea. Pneumologie. 1997;51:779.

Netzer NC, Stoohs RA, Netzer CM, Clark K, Strohl KP. Using the berlin questionnaire to identify patients at risk for the sleep apnea syndrome. Ann Intern Med. 1999;7:485–91.

O'Brien LM, Holbrook CR, Mervis CB, et al. Sleep and neurobehavioral characteristics of 5- to 7-year-old children with parentally reported symptoms of attention- deficit/hyperactivity disorder. Pediatrics. 2003;111(3):554–63.

O'Brien LM, Mervis CB, Holbrook CR, et al. Neurobehavioral implications of habitual snoring in children. Pediatrics. 2004;114(1):44–9.

Ohayon MM. The effects of breathing-related sleep disorders on mood disturbances in the general population. J Clin Psychiatry. 2003;64:1195–200. Quiz, 274–6

Oliveira VC, Dias AS, Teixeira R, Canhao J, Santos C, Pinto O, Barbara P, Revista Portuguesa C. The role of nocturnal oximetry in obstructive sleep apnoea-hypopnoea syndrome screening. Pneumologia. 2007;13(4):525–51.

Olsen SL, Smith SS, Oei T. Adherence to continuous positive airway pressure therapy in obstructive sleep apnoea suffers : a theoretical approach to treatment adherence and intervention. Clin Psychol Rev. 2008;28(8):1355–71.

Parish JM, Lyng PJ. Quality of life in bed partners of patients with obstructive sleep apnea or hypopnea after treatment with continuous positive airway pressure. Chest. 2003;124:942–7.

Peppard PE, Young T, Palta M, Dempsey J, Skarud J. Longitudinal study of moderate weight change and sleep-disordered breathing. J Am Med Assoc. 2000;284:3015.

Peppard PE, Szklo-Coxe M, Hla KM, Young T. Longitudinal association of sleep-related breathing disorder and depression. Arch Intern Med. 2006;166:1709–15.

Peters R, Poulter R, Warner J, Beckett N, Burch L, Bulpitt C. Smoking, dementia and cognitive decline in the elderly, a systematic review. BMC Geriatr. 2008;8:36.

Petersen RC, Roberts RO, Knopman DS, et al. Prevalence of mild cognitive impairment is higher in men. The Mayo Clinic study on aging. Neurology. 2010;75(10):889–97.

Peterson MJ, Benca RM. Sleep in mood disorders. Sleep Med Clin. 2008;3:231–49.

Pieh C, Bach M, Popp R, Jara C, et al. Insomnia symptoms influence CPAP compliance. Sleep Breath. 2013;17:99–104.

Pillar G, Lavie P. Psychiatric symptoms in sleep apnea syndrome: effects of gender and respiratory disturbance index. Chest. 1998;114:697–703.

Plante DT, Winkelman JW. Sleep disturbance in bipolar disorder: therapeutic implications. Am J Psychiatr. 2008;165:830–43.

Quan SF, Chan CS, Dement WC, Gevins A, Goodwin JL, Gottlieb DJ, Green S, Guilleminault C, Hirshkowitz M, Hyde PR, Kay GG, Leary EB, Nichols DA, Schweitzer PK, Simon RD, Walsh JK, Kushida CA. The association between obstructive sleep apnea and neurocognitive performance—the apnea positive pressure long-term efficacy study (APPLES). Sleep. 2011;34(3):303–314B.

Redline S, Tishler PV, Schluchter M, Aylor J, Clark K, Graham G. Risk factors for sleep-disordered breathing in children: associations with obesity, race, and respiratory problems. Am J Respir Crit Care Med. 1999;159(5):1527–32.

Rodríguez-Lozano FJ, Sáez-Yuguero R, Linares TE, Bermejo FA. Sleep apnea and mandibular advancement device. Revision of the literature. Med Oral Patol Oral Cir Bucal. 2008;13(9):E549–54.

Rosen CL, Larkin EK, Kirchner HL, et al. Prevalence and risk factors for sleep-disordered breathing in 8- to 11-year-old children: association with race and prematurity. J Pediatr. 2003;142(4):383–9.

Sánchez AI, Martínez P, Miró E, Bardwell WA, Buela-Casal G. CPAP and behavioral therapies in patients with obstructive sleep apnea: effects on daytime sleepiness, mood, and cognitive function. Sleep Med Rev. 2009;13(3):223–33.

Sangal RB, Thomas L, Miltler MM. Maintenance of wakefulness test and multiple sleep latency test. Measurement of different abilities in patients with sleep disorders. Chest. 1992;101:898–902.

Sawyer M, Canamucio MS, Moriarty H, Weaver TE, Richards K, Kuna ST. Do cognitive perceptions influence CPAP use? Patient Educ Couns. 2011;85(1):85–91.

Schroder CM, O'Hara R. Depression and obstructive sleep apnea (OSA). Ann Gen Psychiatry. 2005;4:13.

Schwartz DJ, Karatinos G. For individuals with obstructive sleep apnea, institution of CPAP therapy is associated with an amelioration of symptoms of depression which is sustained long term. J Clin Sleep Med. 2007;3:631–5.

Schwartz DJ, Kohler WC, Karatinos G. Symptoms of depression in individuals with obstructive sleep apnea may be amenable to treatment with continuous positive airway pressure. Chest. 2005;128(3):1304–9.

Screening MA. For obstructive sleep apnea: is the best solution? Letters to the editor. Sleep Med. 2013;14:695–7.

Sforza E, Roche F, Thomas-Anterion C, et al. Cognitive function and sleep related breathing disorders in a healthy elderly population: the SYNAPSE study. Sleep. 2010;33:515–21.

Sharafkhaneh A, Giray N, Richardson P, Young T, Hirshkowitz M. Association of psychiatric disorders and sleep apnea in a large cohort. Sleep. 2005;28:1405–11.

Sharkey KM, Kurth ME, Anderson BJ, Corso RP, Millman RP, Stein MD. Obstructive sleep apnea is more common than central sleep apnea in methadone maintenance patients with subjective sleep complaints. Drug Alcohol Depend. 2010;108(1–2):77–83.

Sharma SK, Agrawal S, Damodaran D, Sreenivas V, Kadhiravan T, Lakshmy R, Jagia P, Kumar A. CPAP for the metabolic syndrome in patients with obstructive sleep apnea. N Engl J Med. 2011;365:2277–86.

Shirani A, Paradiso S, Dyken ME. The impact of atypical antipsychotic use on obstructive sleep apnea: a pilot study and literature review. Sleep Med. 2011;12(6):591–7.

Sin DD, Mayers I, Man GC, Ghahary A, Pawluk L. Can continuous positive airway pressure therapy improve the general health status of patients with obstructive sleep apnea? a clinical effectiveness study. Chest. 2002;122:1679–85.

Smith I, Lasserston TJ, Wright J. Drug therapy for obstructive sleep apnoea in adults. Cochrane Database Syst Rev. 2006;5:CD003002.

Spira AP, Blackwell T, Stone KL, Redline S, Cauley JA, Ancoli-Israel S, Yaffe K. Sleep-disordered breathing and cognition in older women. J Am Geriatr Soc. 2008;56(1):45–50.

Spoormaker VI, Montgomery P. Disturbed sleep in post- traumatic stress disorder: secondary symptom or core feature? Sleep Med Rev. 2008;12:169–84.

Stepnowsky CJ Jr, Marler MR, Palau J, Annette Brooks J. Social-cognitive correlates of CPAP adherence in experienced users. Sleep Med. 2006;7(4):350–6.

Strassnig M, Brar JS, Ganguli R. Nutritional assessment of patients with schizophrenia: a preliminary study. Schizophr Bull. 2003;29(2):393–7.

Strollo PJ, Rogers RM. Obstructive sleep apnea. N Engl J Med. 1996;334:99.

Sugishita K, Yamasue H, Kasai K. Continuous positive airway pressure for obstructive sleep apnea improved negative symptoms in a patient with schizophrenia. Psychiatry Clin Neurosci. 2010;64:665.

Surratt PM, Barth JT, Diamond R, et al. Reduced time in bed and obstructive sleep-disordered breathing in children are associated with cognitive impairment. Pediatrics. 2007;119(2):320–9.

Takaesu Y, Inoue Y, Komada Y, Kagimura T, Iimori M. Effects of nasal continuous airway pressure on panic disorder comorbid with obstructive sleep apnea syndrome. Sleep Med. 2012;13:156–60.

Tatemichi TK, Foulkes MA, Mohr JP, et al. Dementia in stroke survivors in the stroke data bank cohort. Prevalence, incidence, risk factors, and computed tomographic findings. Stroke. 1990;21(6):858–66.

Tranah GJ, Blackwell T, Stone KL, et al. Circadian activity rhythms and risk of incident dementia and mild cognitive impairment in older women. Ann Neurol. 2011;70:722–32.

Uong EC, Epperson M, Bathon SA, et al. Adherence to nasal positive airway pres- sure therapy among school-aged children and adolescents with obstructive sleep apnea syndrome. Pediatrics. 2007;120(5):e1203–11.

Villa MP, Rizzoli A, Miano S, et al. Efficacy of rapid maxillary expansion in children with obstructive sleep apnea syndrome: 36 months of follow-up. Sleep Breath. 2011;15(2):179–84.

Vitiello MV, Prinz PN, Personius JP, Vitaliano PP, Nuccio MA, Koerker R. Relationship of alcohol abuse history to nighttime hypoxemia in abstaining chronic alcoholic men. J Stud Alcohol Drugs. 1990;51:29–33.

Wallston K. Hocus-pocus, the focus isn't strictly on locus: Rotter's social learning theory modified for health. Cogn Ther Res. 1992;16(2):183–99.

Wang D, Teichtahl H, Goodman C, Drummer O, Grunstein RR, Kronborg I. Subjective daytime sleepiness and daytime function in patients on stable methadone maintenance treatment: possible mechanisms. J Clin Sleep Med. 2008;4:557–62.

Weaver TE, Grunstein RR. Adherence to continuous positive airway pressure therapy: the challenge to effective treatment. Proc Am Thorac Soc. 2008;5(2):173–8.

Weaver T, Maislin G, Venditti L, Mahowald M, Kader G, Bloxham T, et al. CPAP dose duration for effective outcome response. Am J Res Crit Care Med. 2003a;167:A324.

Weaver TE, Maislin G, Dinges D, Younger J, Cantor C, McCloskey S, Pack A. Self-efficacy in sleep apnea: instrument development and patient perceptions of OSA risk, treatment benefit, and volition to use CPAP. Sleep. 2003b;26:727–32.

Whitelaw WA, Brant RF, Ward Flemons W. Clinical usefulness of home Oximetry compared with Polysomnography for assessment of sleep apnea. Am J Respir Crit Care Med. 2005;171:188–93.

Winkelman JW. Schizophrenia, obesity, and obstructive sleep apnea. J Clin Psychiatry. 2001;62(1):8–11.

Wirshing DA, Pierre JM, Wirshing WC. Sleep apnea associated with antipsychotic-induced obesity. J Clin Psychiatry. 2002;63:369–70.

Wong KK, Grunstein RR, Bartlett DJ, Gordon E. Brain function in obstructive sleep apnea: results from the brain resource international database. J Integr Neurosci. 2006;5(1):111–21.

Wootten CT, Shott SR. Evolving therapies to treat retroglossal and base-of-tongue obstruction in pediatric obstructive sleep apnea. Arch Otolaryngol Head Neck Surg. 2010;136(10):983–7.

Yaffe K, Laffan AM, Harrison SL, Redline S, Spira AP, Ensrud KE, Alcoli-Isreael S, Stone KL. Sleep-disordered breathing, hypoxia, and risk of mild cognitive impairment and dementia in older women. J Am Med Assoc. 2011;306:613–9.

Yang CM, Liao YS, Lin CM, Chou SL, Wang EN. Psychological and behavioral factors in patients with comorbid obstructive sleep apnea and insomnia. J Psychosom Res. 2011;70:355–61.

Yesavage JA, Kinoshita LM, Kimball T, Zeitzer J, Friedman L, Noda A, et al. Sleep-disordered breathing in Vietnam veterans with posttraumatic stress disorder. Am J Geriatr Psychiatr. 2012;20:199–204.

Yetkin O, Kunter E, Gunen H. CPAP compliance in patients with obstructive sleep apnea syndrome. Sleep Breath. 2008;12:365–7.

Young T, et al. Estimation of the clinically diagnosed proportion of sleep apnea syndrome in middle-aged men and women. Sleep. 1997;20:705.

Central Hypersomnias

13

Azmeh Shahid, Jianhua Shen, and Colin M. Shapiro

13.1 Introduction

Hypersomnia refers to a large group of disorders. Excessive daytime sleepiness (EDS) is the main characteristic of hypersomnia. In the *International Classification of Sleep Disorder* (American Academy of Sleep Medicine 2001), narcolepsy, recurrent hypersomnia, idiopathic hypersomnia and post-traumatic hypersomnia are independently listed in the section of dyssomnia, while in the revised *International Classification of Sleep Disorders* (American Academy of Sleep Medicine 2005), hypersomnia includes primary hypersomnia (narcolepsy, idiopathic hypersomnia and recurrent hypersomnia) and secondary hypersomnia (such as hypersomnia induced by sleep apnoea). However, in the recently published 5th edition of the *Diagnostic and Statistical Manual of Mental Disorders* (DSM-V, American Psychiatric Association 2013), hypersomnia is described as 'hypersomnolence disorder', while narcolepsy is separately listed as an independent sleep disorder. Both hypersomnolence disorder and narcolepsy are under the category of sleep-wake disorders. In this chapter, hypersomnia disorders including narcolepsy, recurrent hypersomnia, idiopathic hypersomnia and post-traumatic hypersomnia are discussed.

A. Shahid · C. M. Shapiro (✉)
Youthdale Child and Adolescent Sleep Centre, Toronto, ON, Canada

Youthdale Treatment Centre, Toronto, ON, Canada

University of Toronto, Toronto, ON, Canada

Department of Psychiatry, University Health Network, Toronto, ON, Canada

Sleep Research Unit University Health Network, Toronto, ON, Canada

J. Shen
Sleep Research Unit University Health Network, Toronto, ON, Canada

© Springer-Verlag GmbH Germany, part of Springer Nature 2018
H. Selsick (ed.), *Sleep Disorders in Psychiatric Patients*,
https://doi.org/10.1007/978-3-642-54836-9_13

Although hypersomnia has been described and researched for more than 200 years, significant insight about these conditions has only occurred recently. The use of overnight polysomnographic sleep studies and the multiple sleep latency test (MSLT) has greatly improved the accuracy of the diagnosis and differential diagnosis. Neurophysiological findings in this field, such as hypocretin changes in narcoleptic patients, have added new knowledge and enhanced our understanding of the causes and genetics of the disorders. The interplay between hypersomnia-related disorders and psychiatric disease has increasingly received attention.

In order to recognize the symptomatology and presentation of sleep disorders and their interdigitation with psychiatric illness, it is important to familiarize oneself with the relationship between psychiatric conditions and sleep. This can help in not only identifying sleep problems but also in treating them and thus preventing their perpetuation into symptoms mimicking a psychiatric disorder or indeed triggering one (commonly a mood disorder). Hypersomnia can have many different presentations, and it is associated with psychiatric illness both in adults and children. It is accompanied by significant distress in all areas of functioning.

13.2 Prevalence and Investigations of Hypersomnia

Hypersomnia is a common symptom in the general population and in sleep disorder clinics. No clear consensus has been reached as to when sleepiness is considered 'excessive sleepiness' or hypersomnia, thus accounting, in part, for the 100-fold difference in prevalence estimates of daytime sleepiness, with a range of 0.3–35.8% found in various population studies (Partinen and Hublin 2000). In a randomly selected large number of subjects in five European countries (the UK, Germany, Italy, Portugal and Spain), 15% reported excessive daytime sleepiness. There is no significant difference between the prevalence rate in males and females. Of those individuals with daytime sleepiness as their primary reason for coming to the sleep disorder clinics for assessment, approximately 5–10% are diagnosed with hypersomnia/hypersomnolence disorder (Ohayon et al. 2002). Reported prevalence rates of daytime sleepiness in children and adolescents vary, ranging from 4% in young children to almost 20% in high school seniors (Kotagal 2009).

In polysomnographic studies, each hypersomnia disorder has its own criteria. Generally, hypersomnia patients have normal or prolonged sleep duration. Their sleep latency is short, their sleep efficiency is usually increased, and their sleep continuity is normal or increased. Some individuals evince a slow-wave sleep increase, while their rapid eye movement (REM) sleep is usually normal. Daytime sleepiness in hypersomnia may be objectively measured by using the multiple sleep latency test (MSLT). A criterion of a mean sleep latency <10 min (American Psychiatric Association 2013) or <8 min (Vernet and Arnulf 2009) is used to indicate excessive daytime sleepiness. A limitation of this approach is that the MSLT (which takes a day to complete) is collapsed into a single number, i.e. the average duration it takes to fall asleep. Two individuals may score very differently to arrive at this same average figure. For example, one may fall asleep in 10, 11, 10 and

11 min on the four tests to produce an average result of 10.5 min. Another person may fall asleep in 1 min in the first two sessions and stay awake in the other two tests to produce the same result of 10.5 min. These two results are likely to be very different, but the summary of the MSLT is the same. Daytime sleepiness may also be evaluated by using subjective tools, such as the Epworth Sleepiness Scale (ESS) (Johns 1991) (see Appendix 1).

The terms 'sleepiness', 'fatigue' and 'tiredness' are commonly used and interpreted as being the same. Sixty percent of individuals with sleep complaints report being fatigued, and this increases to 75% when a mental disorder is concomitant with the sleep complaints (Ohayon and Shapiro 2000). Sleepiness and fatigue are two separate terms and have different neuropsychiatric implications (Shapiro and Kayumov 2000). It should be noted that sleepiness is not necessarily the opposite of wakefulness (Shapiro and Kayumov 2000). For example, sleepiness and fatigue are commonly associated with psychiatric disorders, especially depression, and have separate effects on the quality of life. There are a number of questionnaires and objective tools to measure these 'brain state' effects (Shahid et al. 2012a, b), but it is still difficult to distinguish between these constructs (Shen et al. 2011).

13.3 Relationship Between Hypersomnia and Psychiatric Disorders

There is a close relationship between hypersomnia and psychiatric disorders. This applies particularly to major depressive disorder (MDD), including seasonal affective disorder (SAD) and the depressive phase of bipolar mood disorder. Other reported psychiatric disorders in which hypersomnia occurs include anxiety disorders, eating disorders and psychotic disorders. Conversely, each 'sleep-related' hypersomnia problem, such as narcolepsy, has specific connections with certain psychiatric disorders.

Vignette
A 51-year-old married gentleman, working as a director of a firm, had a history of difficulty with falling asleep, nightmares, daytime sleepiness and fatigue for the previous 2 years. He felt 'tired' and 'fatigued'. He reported difficulty in concentration, and he felt 'his memory was not as sharp' as it had been. He would forget names, and he was worried that he was developing dementia as there was a family history of it. He had decreased motivation, was sleepy during the day and would fall asleep at meetings. He reported becoming agitated easily and he was irritable. Five months previously, he was diagnosed with depression, and he was started on 100 mg of sertraline (an SSRI) and 7.5 mg of zopiclone to help with sleep. He discontinued the sertraline 4 weeks prior to presenting. He continued the zopiclone as it helped him to fall asleep. However, he did not feel rested. On the ESS, he scored 18/24 which indicates severe daytime sleepiness. On the fatigue severity scale, he scored 4.3, which suggests that he was fatigued, and on the Center for Epidemiologic Studies Depression Scale (CES-D), he scored 12; a score of 16 or more is suggestive of depression.

He snored in his sleep, and he was told by his partner that he stops breathing in his sleep. He was overweight and he had hypertension. On the STOP questionnaire (used to screen for obstructive sleep apnoea), he scored 4/4 which is highly suggestive of sleep apnoea (see Shahid et al. 2012a, b for details of these questionnaires).

He had an MSLT to assess his daytime sleepiness. The results of the sleep study showed rapid sleep-onset latency of 3.7 min, early REM sleep onset of 68 min and decreased slow-wave sleep. He had severe sleep apnoea with breathing stops 72 times per hour and frequent oxygen desaturation events. He had 41.2 arousals per hour, the majority being respiratory related. On the MSLT, the mean sleep latency was 2.7 min which indicates severe daytime sleepiness. There were no sleep-onset REM periods.

He had some sleep markers of depression: early onset REM, decreased slow-wave sleep and sleep fragmentation. The most prominent issues were sleep apnoea and daytime sleepiness. Treatment with continuous positive airway pressure (CPAP) was initiated.

He reported dramatic improvement on the CPAP and stated 'I have a new life on the machine'. He felt rested and he reported that his cognitive ability was back to normal. He was happy and was not getting frustrated. He felt relaxed and was sleeping well and was no longer using zopiclone. He was alert in meetings. Subsequently, the maintenance of wakefulness test (MWT) (Doghramji et al. 1997) was performed which showed that he was able to remain awake throughout all four sessions. He commented, 'I could be a poster patient for your clinic'. Recently, another patient of (CS) told him that 'CPAP was better than using crack cocaine'.

There is a high chance of misinterpreting the symptoms of sleep apnoea as depression (see above), dementia (Bradley and Shapiro 1993) or laziness. The chances of misdiagnosis and self-medication or misdirected psychiatric treatment are high. Many people are treated for depression while the underlying sleep apnoea is not treated.

13.3.1 Hypersomnia and Depression: General Information

Depressive disorders are associated with hypersomnia. Approximately 15% of depressed patients complain of hypersomnia. Compared to subjects without sleep difficulties, individuals with hypersomnia have a 2.9-fold risk of suffering from depression (Abad and Guilleminault 2005). Some hypersomnia individuals meet diagnostic criteria for MDD, while other hypersomnia patients may have prodromal features of a mental disorder. This raises the possibility of early intervention to prevent or decrease the severity of a full episode (American Psychiatric Association 2013; Ohayon et al. 2012). The potential of screening depression and sleep apnoea in the home is emerging and is expected to be a significant development in psychiatry in the next few years.

MDD patients with significant sleep disruptions (including hypersomnia) are more likely to attempt suicide than those without a complaint of sleep problems (Agargun and Beisoglu 2005; Bernert 2007). Furthermore, hypersomnia is more common in suicidal patients (Agargun and Beisoglu 2005). We have recently shown that with increasing sleep disruptions, adolescents have increased suicidal behaviour (Shahid et al. 2012a, b). One proposed mechanism for the association between suicidal behaviours and sleep problems is related to the role of serotonin. Low serotonergic function has been seen in patients who have a suicide attempt and in those who have completed suicide (Ursin 2002). Serotonin deficiency may decrease the amount of slow-wave sleep and exacerbate hypersomnia. This may also weaken control of aggression, which is frequently related to suicidal behaviours (Singareddy and Balon 2001).

Excessive daytime sleepiness may increase the risk of developing depression in the elderly. In a study investigating 3824 subjects aged 65 or older, the Center for Epidemiologic Studies Depression Scale (CES-D) was used to measure mood at baseline and at 2 and 4 years later. The results of this study showed that excessive daytime sleepiness doubled the risk of developing depression in this population (odds ratio = 2.05; confidence interval = 1.30–3.23) (Jaussent et al. 2011).

13.3.1.1 Pathophysiology of Excessive Daytime Sleepiness (EDS) and Depression

EDS is a common presentation in depression. The exact mechanism is not clear; however one of the theories is the association of depression with circadian rhythm deregulation and imbalance of the neurotransmitters, especially the cholinergic and aminergic systems (Reiman et al. 2001). These hypotheses are still under investigation, and more information about the circadian system and the role of neurotransmitters is needed to help in the management of EDS in patients with depression (Chellappa and Cajochen 2011).

13.3.2 Narcolepsy

13.3.2.1 Prevalence

Narcolepsy is a lifelong disabling sleep disorder. It is reported that the prevalence rates are between 0.02% and 0.05% (Choo and Guilleminault 1998; Kotagal 2009). A survey of a large population (n = 18,980) by Ohayon et al. (2002) found that the prevalence of narcolepsy was 0.047%. Prevalence rates of narcolepsy are almost equal in male and female populations. In about one-third of patients, the onset of symptoms occurs before the age of 16 years. The peak age of onset is around 14 years of age (American Academy of Sleep Medicine 2001; Kotagal 2009).

13.3.2.2 Essential Features

The essential feature of narcolepsy is that REM sleep 'segments' intrude into wakefulness. Irresistible EDS is the most common clinical symptom. Repeated episodic daytime naps are the characteristic feature of the EDS in narcoleptic patients. The duration of such a nap is usually between 10 and 20 min; it is rarely an hour. After napping, the patient typically feels refreshed for a short time. In the next couple of hours, the patient begins to feel sleepy again. At the onset of symptoms, the patient may fall asleep in boring situations, such as sitting in a car as a passenger or attending a lecture. During this period, the patient may succeed in staying awake. Subsequently, sudden sleep attacks may occur (American Academy of Sleep Medicine 2001).

Cataplexy is one of the symptoms of narcolepsy. An episode of cataplexy is a sudden loss of muscle tone. The severity of cataplexy can be variable, from a mild sensation of weakness to complete collapse with the person falling to the ground. The duration of a cataplectic episode is usually short, lasting several seconds to a few minutes. During cataplexy, consciousness and memory are not impaired. Cataplexy is often triggered by emotion, such as laughter, surprise and anger. The frequency of cataplexy is very variable, from a few events per year to multiple attacks in a single day. Based on the presence or absence of cataplexy, narcolepsy may be divided into two clinical subtypes: narcolepsy with cataplexy and narcolepsy without cataplexy (American Academy of Sleep Medicine 2001; Dauvilliers et al. 2007; Kotagal 2009). *The International Classification of Sleep Disorders 3* (IDCS-3) divides narcolepsy into Type 1 with either cataplexy or low hypocretin and Type 2 with no cataplexy and either a hypocretin level which is normal or has not been measured (American Academy of Sleep Medicine 2014).

Other clinical symptoms include hypnagogic and hypnopompic hallucinations, sleep paralysis and nocturnal sleep disruption. Hypnagogic and hypnopompic hallucinations are vivid wakeful hallucinations; hypnagogic hallucinations are experienced when one is falling asleep, and hypnopompic is when one is waking up. The commonly reported examples are seeing a cat sitting on the bed, spiders or shadows. These hallucinations can be misdiagnosed, and patients may be treated for schizophrenia with antipsychotics which can exacerbate the symptoms (Douglass et al. 1993).

During sleep paralysis, the patient feels awake and aware of their surroundings, but they are not able to move or speak. Some patients may feel unable to breathe even though the diaphragm is functioning and respiration is preserved, which is a very frightening experience (sometimes leading to lasting anxiety).

Some patients may report mild impairments of consciousness and memory. They report feeling confused but they are awake. Patients may describe the experience of, for example, going from place A to place B but, on arrival, not knowing why or how they got there (Dauvilliers et al. 2007; Dyken and Yamada 2005; Kotagal 2009). This may lead to concerns about memory.

13.3.2.3   Investigations

A nocturnal polysomnographic sleep study combined with an MSLT is used to confirm a diagnosis of narcolepsy. When performing these tests, patients need to be free of the medications which may affect sleep and alertness; specifically, drugs that suppress REM sleep (most antidepressants and antipsychotics) should be stopped at least 2 weeks before the test to overcome the phenomenon of REM rebound. Other medications such as stimulants should not be taken the day of the test as they can bias the test results. A nocturnal polysomnographic sleep study includes sleep electroencephalogram (measuring brain activity), electro-oculography (measuring eye movements), electromyogram (measuring chin and leg muscle activity), electrocardiography (measuring heart rhythm and activity), nasal airflow, thoracic and abdominal respiratory movement bands and oxygen saturation measurements. Characteristic findings in an overnight polysomnographic sleep study in a patient with narcolepsy are short sleep latency ($\leq$10 min) and early onset REM period (REM appearing $\leq$20 min after sleep onset) (American Academy of Sleep Medicine 2001; Dauvilliers et al. 2007). The MSLT provides an objective measure of excessive sleepiness and demonstrates the presence of sleep-onset REM periods. During the MSLT, patients are scheduled to have four nap periods. Each nap is for 20 min, and patients are asked to go to the room and sleep. The nap intervals are approximately 2 h apart, and during this time, patients can read a book or listen to music or walk around the clinic.

The MSLT measures the speed of falling asleep and sleepiness level. Short REM sleep latency ($\leq$15 min) has important diagnostic value. Similarly, the MSLT results must show a mean sleep latency of $\leq$10 min, and typically $\leq$5 min, and $\geq$2 sleep-onset REM periods over four or five naps in order to confirm the diagnosis of narcolepsy (American Academy of Sleep Medicine 2001; Dauvilliers et al. 2007) where clinical suspicion led to the test. Two sleep-onset REM periods were thought to be the pathognomonic of narcolepsy, but we have shown that this may occur in other conditions such as obstructive sleep apnoea, depression or anxiety (Kim et al. 2012).

It has recently been shown that narcolepsy is caused by the loss of neurons in the hypothalamus that produce hypocretin. Hypocretin (also called orexin) is a neurotransmitter associated with wakefulness. Some narcolepsy patients may have a low level of hypocretin in the cerebrospinal fluid. The loss of hypocretin-secreting neurons could be caused by an autoimmune response. Most (99%) narcolepsy with cataplexy patients, in comparison with 12–38% of normal controls, are HLA DQB1*0602 positive. These patients may have hypocretin deficiency, defined as being either in the lower one-third of control values or $\leq$110 pg/ml in the cerebrospinal fluid. Cerebrospinal fluid hypocretin-1 measurement may become a reliable method for diagnosing narcolepsy, especially when a patient has clinical narcoleptic symptoms but the MSLT results are normal, or the results are equivocal (American Academy of Sleep Medicine 2001; American Psychiatric Association 2013; Bourgin et al. 2008; Dauvilliers et al. 2007; Kotagal 2009). In the study by Mignot et al. (2002), they reported that measuring hypocretin level was a definitive differentiator for patients with narcolepsy-cataplexy subtype.

The mechanism of hypocretin deficiency has not been clearly documented. A popular opinion is that a loss of hypocretin-secreting neurons occurs in the dorsolateral hypothalamus of narcolepsy with cataplexy patients. Hypocretin has the function of promoting alertness. Hypocretin neurons project widely to the forebrain and the brainstem. In the process of maintaining wakefulness, several brain locations, including the tuberomammillary nucleus (histaminergic), the locus coeruleus (noradrenergic), the raphe system (serotonergic) and the hypothalamic hypocretin system, are involved. These locations have a reciprocal connection with sleep-promoting neurons of the ventrolateral preoptic nucleus. Some ventrolateral preoptic nuclei facilitate non-REM sleep, while others promote REM sleep. Decreased hypocretin neurons and several other conditions, such as inflammation and trauma, may disturb the balance between wakefulness and sleepiness and induce hypersomnia (Kotagal 2009).

13.3.2.4 Narcolepsy and Psychiatric Disorders

Narcolepsy is associated with psychiatric disorders, including mood disorders (MDD and bipolar disorder), anxiety disorders, eating disorders and psychotic disorders (Fortuyn et al. 2010; Kishi et al. 2004; Mamelak 2009; Walterfang et al. 2005). Limited publications have reported a possible connection between narcolepsy, personality disorders and sexual difficulties (Fortuyn et al. 2011).

Depression

It is well documented that many narcoleptic patients concurrently suffer from a depressive disorder. Investigators have found that, compared with normal controls, a higher percentage of narcoleptic patients are depressed (Fortuyn et al. 2011; Vignatelli et al. 2010). Using the Beck Depression Inventory, the Zung Self-Rating Depression Scale, the Global Impression of Severity of Depression and the Profile of Mood States, a study investigated 70 narcoleptic patients and normal controls and found that patients with narcolepsy were more depressed than age- and sex-matched normal controls (Jara et al. 2011). Another study, using the Schedule for Clinical Assessment in Neuropsychiatry, compared depressive symptoms in a large group of narcoleptic patients with those in an age- and sex-matched control group. The results of this study showed that the symptoms of depressive mood (30%), pathological guilt feelings (22%), crying spells (25%) and anhedonia (27%) were significantly higher in the narcoleptic group than in the normal controls (Fortuyn et al. 2010). It is found that the risk of depression was associated with some specific narcoleptic symptoms, with a 2.0-fold increase in those having hypnagogic hallucinations, 2.1-fold increase in those with sleep paralysis and 1.3-fold increase in cataplexy (Abad and Guilleminault 2005).

In children and adolescents, depression is more common in those with narcolepsy. A study of 42 narcoleptic children and 23 age-matched normal controls found that, compared with normal children, narcolepsy patients had more depressive symptoms with higher scores on the Child Depression Inventory ($P < 0.01$). The authors advised that when treating narcolepsy patients, a physician should provide both pharmacologic therapy and emotional support (Kotagal 2009).

There are similarities between overnight sleep study features of depression and those of narcolepsy. Polysomnographic features of depression typically include decreased REM sleep latency, increased wakefulness and increased arousals. These features are also seen in the polysomnograms of narcoleptic patients. Depressed patients may have shortened REM sleep latency, which may be induced by a combined effect of monoaminergic deficiency and cholinergic oversensitivity. Interestingly, this combined effect is also seen in narcolepsy patients (Mamelak 2009).

Anxiety Disorder

Compared to depression, anxiety disorders in narcolepsy have received much less attention. In a case-control study, 60 narcolepsy patients and 120 age- and sex-matched normal controls were evaluated. The Schedule for Clinical Assessment in Neuropsychiatry was used to measure symptoms of mood and anxiety disorders. The results of this study showed that more than half of the patients had anxiety and panic attacks; 35% of them were diagnosed with anxiety disorders (odds ratio = 15.6). Of the anxiety disorders, social phobia was the most common diagnosis. The study reported that there was no significant difference in the prevalence of anxiety or mood symptoms and disorders between this group of narcolepsy patients and the normal controls in terms of age, sex, illness duration or medication use. Anxiety disorder may be induced by the long-standing symptoms of narcolepsy and decreased hypocretin signalling. Patients with chronic narcolepsy thus have difficulties regulating stress (Fortuyn et al. 2010). Patients also may feel anxious of experiencing a cataplexy episode in public as it is reported to be very distressing for most individuals.

Eating Disorder

Although eating disorders in narcolepsy patients were described more than 80 years ago, it was confirmed recently by a few publications. Using a case-control design, a study compared the body mass index (BMI) of 31 narcoleptic children at the time of diagnosis with that of age- and sex-matched healthy controls and found that childhood narcolepsy had an intrinsic tendency to body weight gain (Kotagal et al. 2004). Another study compared energy balance between 13 narcoleptic patients with age-, sex- and ethnicity-matched normal controls. Among the 13 narcoleptic patients, seven were 'typical', being HLA DQB1*0602 positive, and they had clear cataplexy attacks; they therefore probably had hypocretin deficiency. The other patients ($n = 6$) were 'atypical', i.e. they were HLA DQB1*0602 negative or did not have cataplexy. The results showed that, as a group, the narcoleptic patients had a tendency to be overweight and had a lower basal metabolism, but only the 'typical' narcoleptic patients tended to eat less. These overweight narcoleptic patients only ate half as much as others. The prolactin level in narcoleptic patients was twice as high as that in the controls. These patients had higher scores on the EAT-40 questionnaire and had more clear features of bulimia nervosa than controls, suggesting that they had a mild eating disorder (Chabas et al. 2007). Using the Schedule for Clinical Assessment in Neuropsychiatry and the Eating Disorder Examination Questionnaire, a study compared 60 narcolepsy with cataplexy patients with 32 BMI-matched normal controls. It was found that 23.3% of the patients met the clinical criteria for eating disorders, mainly atypical binge eating disorder. In comparison, no eating disorder was found in the control group (Fortuyn et al. 2008). A case-control study (Fortuyn et al. 2008) looked into the prevalence of eating disorders in patients with narcolepsy. There were 60 patients with narcolepsy/cataplexy, recruited from specialized sleep centres, and 120 healthy controls. The authors concluded that the majority of patients with narcolepsy had not only craving for certain types of food but also binge eating. Most of them met criteria for 'eating disorder not otherwise specified'. However, there was a contrary report which did not find any difference between narcoleptic patients ($n = 116$) and the normal controls ($n = 80$) in the prevalence of bulimia nervosa, binge eating disorder, anorexia nervosa or the frequency of eating attacks (Dahmen et al. 2008).

When one of us (CS) first saw narcoleptic patients with unusual eating patterns, for example, 'only eating broccoli and chicken liver for breakfast everyday', he thought the patient was odd. In the light of the above studies and subsequent knowledge, it was perhaps not so unusual at all.

Psychotic Disorder

Opinions on the relationship between narcolepsy and schizophrenia are controversial. Some researchers support the idea that psychotic symptoms, such as hallucinations, are frequently seen in narcoleptic patients and, therefore, there is a relationship between narcolepsy and schizophrenia (Kishi et al. 2004). However, other authors disagree; they do not accept the above-mentioned opinion because of differences between these two conditions in clinical symptoms, human leukocyte measurements, REM sleep distribution, dopamine D2-receptor sensitivity and hypocretin level and function (Walterfang et al. 2005; Douglass et al. 1993). Studies have suggested that the hypocretin peptide system is affected in many disease processes and not just in narcolepsy. Figure 13.1 illustrates that the hypocretin peptide has a role in many different areas and not only in sleep regulation (Ganjavi and Shapiro 2007).

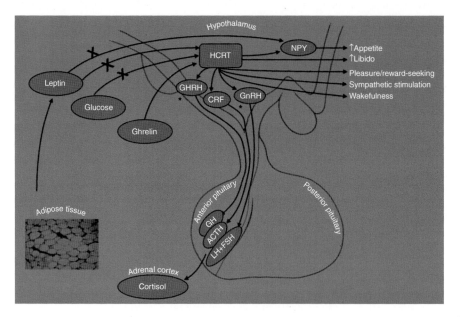

Fig. 13.1 The regulation and functions of hypocretin. Hypocretin (Hcrt) neurons are present in the dorsal and lateral hypothalamus. Hcrt excretion is inhibited by leptin and glucose and increased by ghrelin. Increased Hcrt promotes wakefulness, increases appetite, is involved in reward/pleasure-seeking behaviours and stimulates sympathetic activity. Hcrt also promotes corticotropin-releasing factor (CRF) release from the hypothalamus which causes adrenocorticotrophic hormone (ACTH) release from the anterior pituitary. In vitro and in vivo studies have shown that Hcrt increased growth hormone-releasing hormone (GHRH) and growth hormone (GH) release from the hypothalamus and anterior pituitary, respectively. Increased gonadotropin-releasing hormone (GnRH) release from the hypothalamus and follicle-stimulating hormone (FSH) and luteinising hormone (LH) from the anterior pituitary have also been shown, but the physiological relevance of these interactions remains unclear. As an illustrative example, an individual who consumes large quantities of sweets will have elevated blood glucose levels which would downregulate Hcrt levels. Decreased Hcrt levels would decrease appetite and libido and cause sleepiness. Over time, if the individual continues on such a diet, increased body fat would cause the downregulation of Hcrt via leptin (Ganjavi and Shapiro 2007)

Vignette

A 26-year-old male presents with a history of daytime sleepiness and difficulty waking up in the morning for the last year. He had missed university or been late to class most of the year. He was irritable, and he became easily frustrated. When he woke up after sleep attacks, he was confused and agitated, and he would often experience hallucinations. He was given a diagnosis of bipolar disorder and started on antipsychotic medication, which was not helpful.

He was referred to the sleep clinic. He not only had a history of sleep attacks (including one episode where he had fallen asleep in the shower) but he also had symptoms of cataplexy, experiencing weakness in the muscles in response to emotion. Cataplexy is often misdiagnosed as a conversion reaction or a seizure. His hallucinations were hypnopompic, occurring on waking from sleep at night or after a nap. He would see a male figure in his room staring at him. On the ESS he scored 24/24 which indicates very severe daytime sleepiness. On the Center for Epidemiological Studies Depression Scale for children (CESD-C), he scored 22 which is suggestive of depression.

He had an overnight sleep study and MSLT. At night he fell asleep in 5 min, REM latency was very short at 20 min. The MSLT confirmed severe daytime sleepiness with a mean sleep-onset latency of 1.1 min. REM was observed on three of the naps which is strongly suggestive of narcolepsy.

He was diagnosed with narcolepsy and was treated with the stimulant modafinil. There was not only a significant improvement in his sleepiness, but his psychiatric symptoms also abated. This case report in the literature indicates that narcolepsy is usually not recognized and thus may not be treated for many years after the presentation. The excessive daytime sleepiness is often interpreted as 'laziness' or a feature of depression. Cataplexy and sleep paralysis may be mistaken for attention seeking, a conversion disorder or seizures. Some cases are not diagnosed (as in the case above) and are treated as a psychotic disorder. In the paper by Kryger et al. (2002), it was reported that psychiatrists made the correct diagnosis in only 11% of the cases seen and paediatricians in 0% of cases.

13.3.3 Recurrent Hypersomnia

Recurrent hypersomnia is a group of disorders characterized by recurrent episodes of hypersomnia. The interval between two episodes of hypersomnia is typically a few weeks or several months. The best known and most typical recurrent hypersomnia is Kleine-Levin syndrome. Other forms of recurrent hypersomnia include Kleine-Levin syndrome without compulsive eating, menstrual-related hypersomnia and recurrent hypersomnia with co-morbidity (Billiard et al. 2011). Menstrual-related hypersomnia was first described by Billiard et al. (1975) as a distinct disorder different form Kleine-Levin syndrome. It is described as 'excessive daytime sleepiness a few days before the onset of menstrual flow and disappears shortly after the onset of menstruation.'

13.3.3.1 Prevalence

Kleine-Levin syndrome occurs in about 1–2 cases per million people (Geoffroy et al. 2013). The prevalence in people whose first-degree relatives suffer from the syndrome is much higher than in the general population. The ratio of male to female is 4.08 in Kleine-Levin syndrome, 2.85 in Kleine-Levin syndrome without compulsive eating and 2.50 in recurrent hypersomnia with co-morbidity. Peak onset of Kleine-Levin syndrome is in adolescence (around the age of 15) and occasionally in early adulthood; however the age onset can be between the age of 4 and 82 years (Arnulf et al. 2005; Billiard et al. 2011; Kotagal 2009).

13.3.3.2 Essential Features

In addition to hypersomnia, the most frequent symptoms of hypersomnia disorders are hyperphagia (66%), hypersexuality (53%) and depressed mood (53%) (Geoffroy et al. 2013). Another study reported that in 186 Kleine-Levin syndrome patients, the common symptoms of these patients were hypersomnia (100%), derealization and other cognitive changes (96%), eating disturbances (80%), depressed mood (48%), hypersexuality (43%) and compulsions (29%) (Arnulf et al. 2005). In Kleine-Levin syndrome, a typical episode of hypersomnia lasts several days to several weeks. On average, the frequency of the hypersomnia episode is twice a year, but it can be more than ten times yearly. During hypersomnolent episodes, patients may sleep 18–20 h a day. They may give an unclear verbal response when they receive a strong stimulus. An acute febrile episode and severe somatic stresses often precipitate a somnolent episode. Immediately following the episode of hypersomnolence, patients may completely recover to their normal behaviour and alertness for several months. A similar episode of hypersomnolence may repeat subsequently (Billiard et al. 2011; Kotagal 2009).

The other common symptom of recurrent hypersomnia is hyperphagia (compulsive or binge eating), where patients consume a large amount of food in a short time. Consequently, they often gain 2–5 kg of body weight during an episode. However, weight loss may be seen in some forms of recurrent hypersomnia, such as Kleine-Levin syndrome without compulsive eating (Billiard et al. 2011; Kotagal 2009).

Following a period of somnolence, patients may have transitional cognitive and behavioural abnormalities, such as confusion, amnesia, depersonalization, insomnia, impulsive behaviour, aggression, restlessness and odd behaviours. Emotionally, they are likely to come across as blunted, unstable and having elated or irritable mood. These cognitive and behavioural abnormalities are most likely expressions of cerebral cortex function impairments, especially inhibitory functions, which may be related to excessive sleepiness (Billiard et al. 2011; Kotagal 2009).

Hypersomnia, hyperphagia, hypersexuality and mental status changes in Kleine-Levin syndrome suggest that the possible pathological impairments are in the hypothalamic and limbic function, but magnetic resonance scans are invariably normal. No evidence of structural impairment has been established.

Symptoms of other forms of hypersomnia disorders are similar to, but not as common in their presentation as, those of the Kleine-Levin syndrome (Billiard et al. 2011; Kotagal 2009).

Reported data suggest that recurrent hypersomnia has a benign course. In most patients, the episodic hypersomnia gradually decreases in severity; final resolution is usually over several years. Between episodes, patients can sleep normally, and their medical condition and mental status are normal (Billiard et al. 2011; Kotagal 2009).

13.3.3.3 Investigation

During the somnolent episode, the polysomnographic features of Kleine-Levin syndrome are shortened sleep latency, diffuse alpha activity, reduced percentage of slow-wave sleep, shortened REM latency and decreased REM sleep. The MSLT of patients with Kleine-Levin syndrome may show moderately shortened mean sleep latency. REM sleep occurs in one or more naps. Neurological tests such as brain imaging may be necessary to exclude some types of central nervous system pathology (American Academy of Sleep Medicine 2001; Kotagal 2009). Recurrent hypersomnia has an association with histocompatibility antigen DQB*0201. It is occasionally induced by systemic infections, and its features of relapsing and remitting course raise the possibility of autoimmune aetiology (Kotagal 2009).

13.3.3.4 Recurrent Hypersomnia and Mood Disorders

Although anxiety and psychotic symptoms may be seen in Kleine-Levin syndrome and other recurrent hypersomnia disorder patients, mood disorders are much more frequently reported (Billiard et al. 2011). These mood problems include MDD, SAD, bipolar disorder and dysthymia. In these patients, episodic hypersomnia usually diminishes over time and may totally disappear after several years. However, in some patients, hypersomnia does not disappear but evolves into typical depression. The majority of these depressed patients are females (Kotagal 2009; Billiard et al. 2011). A small number of patients report a positive familial or personal psychiatric history. A systematic study of 399 recurrent hypersomnia patients was compared in the four clinical forms: (1) Kleine-Levin syndrome (239 cases), (2) Kleine-Levin syndrome without compulsive eating (54 cases), (3) menstrual-related hypersomnia (18 cases) and recurrent hypersomnia with co-morbidity (27 cases). In those patients with a family psychiatric history, mood disorder history was reported in 6.4% ($n = 16$) and schizophrenia or any other psychotic disorder in 1.6% ($n = 5$) of cases with Kleine-Levin syndrome. Mood disorder was seen in 11.9% ($n = 5$) of Kleine-Levin syndrome without compulsive eating, in 6% ($n = 1$) of menstrual-related hypersomnia and 10.6% ($n = 3$) of recurrent hypersomnia with co-morbidity.

In those patients with a positive past psychiatric history, mood disorders were even less common. Mood disorder history was reported in 2.0% of Kleine-Levin syndrome patients and schizophrenia and other psychotic disorders in 1.6% of patients with Kleine-Levin syndrome (Billiard et al. 2011).

Among recurrent hypersomnia with bipolar mood disorder patients, rates of suicidal ideation were high, occurring in 40.4% of women with Kleine-Levin syndrome and 35.3% of women with menstrual recurrent hypersomnia. Elevated mood occurs in 13.5% of men with bipolar disorder during hypersomniac episodes (Billiard et al. 2011). In Kleine-Levin syndrome patients who concurrently suffer from bipolar disorder, these two conditions may obscure the natural course of the other condition. Consequently, they may be underestimated. Kleine-Levin syndrome and bipolar disorder may have common risk factors, such as sharing similar immune-inflammatory processes. This has raised the question as to whether recurrent hypersomnia is a variant of depression (Geoffroy et al. 2013; Masi et al. 2000). One of us (CS) would take the view based on clinical experience that the affect is characteristically different and that the hypersomnia is not a form of mood disorder. However we have seen some patients with excessive rapid cycling mood on a 48-h schedule in which the patient is manic for 48 h and then extremely sleepy and depressed for 48 h. The cycle then repeats itself. Hence the association between sleep and mood is unquestionable.

13.3.4 Idiopathic Hypersomnia

Idiopathic hypersomnia is deemed to be a central nervous system disorder. There are two forms of idiopathic hypersomnia: one with lengthened major sleep duration (10 h or longer) and the other is with relatively normal sleep duration. Patients with longer sleep durations are usually younger than those with shorter sleep durations (Kotagal 2009; Vernet and Arnulf 2009).

13.3.4.1   Epidemiology
Idiopathic hypersomnia is a rare disease. Its prevalence is approximately 0.005%. Due to the fact that the criteria used for diagnosing excessive sleepiness are inconsistent, this estimate may vary significantly. No gender differences were found in this condition (Kotagal 2009; Vernet and Arnulf 2009).

The age of onset is often difficult to determine. At presentation, many patients have already suffered the disorder for years. Due to a possibility of being confused with other forms of excessive sleepiness, idiopathic hypersomnia is difficult to diagnose at an early stage. By the time idiopathic hypersomnia is diagnosed, it may have already affected many facets of the patient's life and induced multiple stresses. A study reported that in 77 idiopathic hypersomnia patients, the mean onset age was 16.6 years with a range between 0 and 46 years (Anderson et al. 2007). Another study ($n = 75$) reported that the average age of diagnosis was 34.0 years (Vernet and Arnulf 2009).

13.3.4.2   Essential Features
Idiopathic hypersomnia is characterized by excessive daytime sleepiness and daytime naps. After experiencing a long period of drowsiness, patients may have a sleep attack, which may be confused with narcolepsy (Anderson et al. 2007; Kotagal 2009; Vernet and Arnulf 2009). Other symptoms, such as hypnagogic hallucinations, sleep paralysis and unrefreshing naps, may also appear in these patients with a rate of 24%, 28% and 36%, respectively; in normal controls, they occur at rates of 8.7%, 4.3% and 5.0%, respectively. The frequencies of these symptoms are much

lower than those in narcolepsy patients. Interestingly, these symptoms may also be seen in children. In some children, idiopathic hypersomnia may be an intermediate stage before they develop typical narcolepsy (Anderson et al. 2007; Kotagal 2009; Vernet and Arnulf 2009).

The duration of a typical daytime nap is 1 h or longer. Short naps usually have little refreshing effect. Specific situations, such as reading a book or watching television, may make it easier for patients to feel sleepy or fall asleep. Some patients may have difficulty waking up and experience disorientation (sleep inertia/drunkenness) on awakening. Peripheral vascular problems, headaches, orthostatic hypotension and fainting attacks may also occur; these symptoms suggest the possibility of autonomic nervous system malfunctions (Anderson et al. 2007; Kotagal 2009; Vernet and Arnulf 2009).

Idiopathic hypersomnia is a lifelong disorder for the majority of patients, although a few studies suggest that 14–25% of them may spontaneously recover. At an early stage, hypersomnia tends to be progressive, but it usually stabilizes (Vernet and Arnulf 2009).

13.3.4.3 Investigations

Nocturnal polysomnographic studies often demonstrate normal sleep quality. Sleep-onset latency may be shortened, and sleep efficiency may be increased. Total sleep time is normal or extended. Slow-wave sleep may be normal or slightly increased. Percentage of REM sleep in idiopathic hypersomnia patients is higher than that in normal people. Overnight polysomnographic recordings usually do not have sleep-onset REM periods (Anderson et al. 2007; Kotagal 2009; Vernet and Arnulf 2009).

On the MSLT, the mean sleep latency is frequently 8 min or shorter. Sleep-onset REM periods are not seen or only occur in a single nap. Clinically, the severity of idiopathic hypersomnia may not closely correlate with the mean latency of the MSLT, and thus some clinically severe idiopathic hypersomnia patients may not have a short mean MSLT sleep-onset latency (Kotagal 2009; Vernet and Arnulf 2009).

Other laboratory tests include human leukocyte antigen (HLA) examination. Idiopathic hypersomnia populations may have elevated HLA-Cw2, while the level of HLA-DR2 is found to be either normal or decreased. This differs from narcolepsy as most narcoleptic patients are HLA-DR2 positive (American Academy of Sleep Medicine 2001).

Before making a diagnosis of idiopathic hypersomnia, two other causes of sleepiness syndromes—hydrocephalus and post-traumatic hypersomnia—need to be ruled out. At an early stage of progressive hydrocephalus, excessive sleepiness may be the preeminent early symptom when other clinical features of hydrocephalus may be absent. Computer tomography, skull radiography and electroencephalography may be necessary to clarify the differential diagnosis. Six to 18 months after receiving a head trauma, patients may gradually develop post-traumatic hypersomnia symptoms, which may possess all features of primary form idiopathic hypersomnia (American Academy of Sleep Medicine 2001; Watson et al. 2007).

13.3.4.4   Idiopathic Hypersomnia and Psychiatric Disorders

Mood and anxiety disorders are commonly seen in idiopathic hypersomnia patients. Using the Hospital Depression and Anxiety Rating Scale, a study compared 75 idiopathic hypersomnia patients with 30 age- and sex-matched normal controls and found that scores of depression (7.1 ± 5.0) and anxiety (8.7 ± 4.0) were higher in idiopathic hypersomnia patients than in normal controls (4.0 ± 3.0 and 6.1 ± 3.6, respectively) (both P values < 0.01) (Anderson et al. 2007; Vernet and Arnulf 2009).

In those with mood disorders, dysthymia is the predominating diagnostic item. Their depressed mood is usually induced by daytime sleepiness. Patients with idiopathic hypersomnia often deny subjective symptoms of mood changes. Therefore, evaluating clinical symptoms, such as decreased interests and anhedonia, is an important ancillary feature. Observation of clinical signs, such as depressed facial expression and posture, and exploration of a family history of mood disorders may also be useful (American Academy of Sleep Medicine 2001; Anderson et al. 2007; Vernet and Arnulf 2009). Patients with idiopathic hypersomnia, on objective assessments such as polysomnography and MSLT, have different characteristics from patients who would have hypersomnia in the context of depression. It is important to take a thorough history to rule out other sleep disorders such as sleep apnoea, which may be the underlying cause of EDS but was not detected in patients with depression.

13.3.5 Post-traumatic Hypersomnia

13.3.5.1   Prevalence

Hypersomnia is a common symptom after a traumatic brain injury. Reported prevalence rates range from 9% to 42% (Baumann et al. 2007; Hou et al. 2013; Kempf et al. 2010; Sommerauer et al. 2013). In a systematic study of 98 patients with traumatic brain injuries, nine (9%) had post-traumatic hypersomnia. All nine patients were male, with a mean age of 42 years; in five (56%) of the patients, brain injury was the result of a vehicle accident. Traumatic brain injury was severe in nature in 14 (15%) members of the sample (Hou et al. 2013).

13.3.5.2   Essential Features

Post-traumatic hypersomnia is characterized by frequent daytime sleepiness. The sleep duration of patients is usually lengthened, in comparison with both their prior sleep and that of normal people. A study compared the sleep logs of 36 traumatic brain injury patients with those of 36 age- and sex-matched normal controls and found that the mean sleep duration of patients was 9.4 h, while that of controls was 7.5 h (Sommerauer et al. 2013). Excessive daytime sleepiness may be accompanied with other post-traumatic encephalopathic symptoms, such as loss of consciousness, fatigue, headaches, lack of concentration and memory impairment (American Academy of Sleep Medicine 2001; Hou et al. 2013; Kempf et al. 2010). The sleepiness typically appears immediately following the traumatic event and diminishes over weeks to months. However, residual sleepiness may persist or gradually worsen for 3 years or longer following an injury (Kempf et al. 2010).

Multiple brain locations may be related to post-traumatic hypersomnia. The most frequently implicated locations are the posterior hypothalamus, the pineal region, the midbrain and the pons (American Academy of Sleep Medicine 2001).

13.3.5.3 Investigations

Objective sleep measurements, mainly polysomnography and the MSLT, and questionnaires, such as the ESS, have been used to investigate daytime sleepiness in post-traumatic hypersomnia patients. A case-control study of 36 post-traumatic patients found that, in comparison with a control group ($n = 36$), their mean sleep-onset latency was shorter (8.7 min vs. 12.4 min; $P < 0.001$) and the percentage of slow-wave sleep was increased (20.4% vs. 13.8%; $P = 0.009$). In the MSLT, the mean sleep latency of 15 (42%) of the patients was 8 min or shorter, while the mean sleep latency of all the controls was longer than 8 min. The scores on the ESS of 13 (36%) patients were 10 or higher, indicating excessive daytime sleepiness, but all those of normal controls were lower than 10. Actigraphy measurement found that 21 (58%) patients had 10 h or more sleep per 24 h, while all the normal controls had <10 h of sleep per day (Sommerauer et al. 2013).

13.3.5.4 Post-traumatic Hypersomnia and Psychiatric Disorders

Psychiatric sequelae are common in traumatic brain injury patients. A large prospective cohort study reported that 31% of patients had psychiatric disorders in the 12 months following their traumatic brain injury (Bryant et al. 2010).

Mood Disorder

Within 1 year of a traumatic brain injury, 17–61% of patients suffer from depression. Two out of three of these patients are affected by depression within 7 years (Hou et al. 2013). Several factors are related to developing depression after traumatic brain injury, especially in those with post-traumatic hypersomnia. Traumatic brain injury may impair or damage brain areas of emotional control, such as the frontal lobe, hypothalamus and other areas of the limbic system. Changes in certain neurotransmitters, such as serotonin and noradrenaline, may play an important role. After brain injury, patients need to face their physical, mental and social changes; this may induce a depressed mood or make depression worse. Genetic predisposition, past psychiatric history and family function disturbances may be involved in the development of depression (Hou et al. 2013; Rapoport 2012).

Anxiety Disorder

Anxiety disorder is another common psychiatric problem following traumatic brain injury. Several subtypes of anxiety disorder such as generalized anxiety disorder, social phobia, post-traumatic stress disorder and agoraphobia are seen in these patients. A study reported that in 1084 brain injury patients, 9% had generalized anxiety disorder, 6% had post-traumatic stress disorder and 6% had agoraphobia. Mild traumatic brain injury patients were more likely to develop anxiety problems; in these patients, the odds ratio of social phobia was 2.07, that of panic disorder was

2.01, that of agoraphobia was 1.94 and that of generalized anxiety disorder was 1.92 (Bryant et al. 2010).

Psychotic Disorder

It is reported that between 1.35% and 9.2% of traumatic brain injury patients develop a psychotic disorder. There are some reports at the higher end of this range. This is approximately threefold more than in the general population. Patients may have positive and negative symptoms, such as hallucinations, delusions, language and behaviour disorganization, speech poverty, emotional apathy, lack of motivation, impairments of memory and absence of insight. About half of the patients experience hallucinations; the most common hallucinations are auditory (43.3%) and visual (15%). These symptoms may occur at almost any time, from 2 days to 48 years following brain injury (Batty et al. 2013; Guerreiro et al. 2009).

13.4 Treatment of Hypersomnia Disorders
(Tables 13.1 and 13.2)

Several medications, including modafinil, armodafinil, sodium oxybate, amphetamine, methamphetamine, dextroamphetamine, methylphenidate and selegiline hydrochloride, have been used to treat excessive daytime sleepiness in narcolepsy and idiopathic hypersomnia patients (Mignot 2012). Although all these medications are more or less effective, modafinil is far more frequently used. Modafinil 200–400 mg daily is usually well-tolerated, and it increases alertness. In narcolepsy, it reduces the number and duration of sleep attacks and naps, increases mean sleep latency and decreases the likelihood of falling asleep during the daytime (Choo and Guilleminault 1998; Freedom 2011; Melamed et al. 2009). Modafinil is also used to treat excessive daytime sleepiness in children (Ivanenko et al. 2003). Side effects include insomnia, back pain, diarrhoea, dizziness, hypertension, flu-like symptoms and headache. Some patients may feel nauseous and nervous (Melamed et al. 2009).

Table 13.1 Medication used to treat hypersomnia

Medication for hypersomnia	Mean total daily dose
Modafinil	100–400 mg/day
Methylphenidate	20–40 mg/day
Dextroamphetamine	20–40 mg/day
Methamphetamine	36 ± 17.1 mg
Sodium oxybate	4.5 g/day
Selegiline HCl	10–30 mg/day
Monoamine oxidase B inhibitor	15–30 mg/day
Lithium (mEq/ml)	Dose adjusted until adequate blood levels (0.8–1.2 mEq/ml)

Table 13.2 Medications for cataplexy, hypnagogic and hypnopompic hallucinations and sleep paralysis

Name of medication	Mean total dose
Clomipramine	150 mg/day
Fluoxetine	20–60 mg/day
Venlafaxine	37.5–300 mg/day
Duloxetine	20–60 mg/day
Atomoxetine	10–80 mg/day
Sodium oxybate	Taken as a split dose with the first half taken at bedtime and the second dose in the middle of the night. Start with a total of 4.5 g per night for 2 weeks; if needed, increase in increments of 1.5 g a night every 2 weeks up to a maximum of 9 g per night

Selective serotonin reuptake inhibitors (SSRIs), specifically fluoxetine, and tricyclic antidepressants, particularly clomipramine, are effectively used to treat cataplexy, hypnagogic hallucinations and sleep paralysis (Freedom 2011).

Modafinil has been considered for improving alertness in depressed patients (Kotagal 2009).

A case report suggests that a narcoleptic patient with psychotic disorder can have significant improvement of symptoms with a combination of treatments using medications such as modafinil 200 mg daily and risperidone 6 mg daily. The authors suggest that a combination of stimulant, SSRI and antipsychotic medication may be indicated in narcolepsy with cataplexy and vivid psychotic presentations (Melamed et al. 2009).

Lithium and valproic acid have been reported to be effective in treating recurrent hypersomnia (Kotagal 2009). A study treated Kleine-Levin syndrome patients ($n = 75$) with stimulants (mainly amphetamines) and found that 40% of the cases showed benefit vis-a-vis excessive sleepiness, but antipsychotic medications and antidepressants have little benefit. Only lithium had a higher reported response rate for decreasing relapses, while carbamazepine or other antiepileptics did not show significant benefit (Arnulf et al. 2005).

An article systematically reviewed 108 Kleine-Levin syndrome patients and reported that amantadine, an antiviral medication with dopamine reuptake-inhibiting function, had significant effect. However, its effect was typically seen in the first trial but was often lost in subsequent episodes in this population. Modafinil, methylphenidate and amphetamine had limited effects on improving alertness. Antidepressants had no effect in improving most Kleine-Levin syndrome symptoms, but venlafaxine and fluoxetine were occasionally effective in improving the depressed mood of these patients. Among antipsychotic medications, only risperidone partially decreased delusions. Lithium and valproate equally and partially reduced further episodes in 25% of the patients. The impact of mood stabilizers was disappointing. Lithium was reported to be effective in only 24% of cases. It is important to raise the dose until adequate blood levels (0.8–1.2 mEq/ml) are attained (Arnulf et al. 2012). Carbamazepine and benzodiazepines had little benefit in this population. Intravenous immunoglobulins lengthened the interval between episodes in one-third of the patients. No non-medical therapies were effective (Arnulf et al. 2008). Some clinicians used mood stabilizers, such as carbamazepine, lithium and valproate, to prevent the recurrence of the episodes (Billiard et al. 2011).

Treatment of depressed post-traumatic hypersomniac patients includes (1) regular management of hypersomnia, (2) antidepressants, (3) psychological treatment and (4) other treatments. Among antidepressant medications, SSRIs, specifically sertraline and citalopram, and serotonin-norepinephrine reuptake inhibitors, such as venlafaxine, are effective (Table 13.1). Because of the potential for serious side effects, monoamine oxidase inhibitors and high-dose tricyclic antidepressants should be avoided. Among the medications commonly used to treat traumatic brain injury with psychotic disorder, antipsychotic medication is the most effective (Guerreiro et al. 2009).

Conclusion

Hypersomnia includes a large group of disorders. Among these, narcolepsy has attracted much attention. Although tremendous efforts have been made regarding the clinical observations and laboratory-based investigations, such as polysomnographic studies, MSLT measurements and quantitative analysis of hypocretin-1, many questions remain unanswered. Better understanding of the pathogenesis and the development of new therapies are critically needed. Randomized clinical trials with large sample sizes should be performed to provide more knowledge in this field, especially for improving management in children and geriatric populations. The difficulties are that these conditions are relatively rare, but they have profound effects on the quality of life both directly and through the psychiatric co-morbidities.

Summary

History
- Ascertain the different types of hypersomnia and the diagnostic criteria.
    - Relationship of hypersomnia and psychiatric disorders
    - The symptoms, causes, pathways and ways of presentation and duration of the symptoms
    - Case vignette highlighting the complexity of presentation with these symptoms and ways to investigate and treat them
- Look for supporting diagnostic criteria.
    - A thorough screening for sleep disorders and psychiatric history
    - Importance of objective test such as overnight polysomnography and mean sleep latency test (MSLT)
- Establish the diagnosis and rule out other sleep disorders such as sleep apnoea.
    - Exclude an alternative explanation for the symptoms such as history of head injury, trauma, etc.

- – Rule out other medical problems such as thyroid disease, anaemia and other neurological causes.
- Seek to identify exacerbating or triggering factors.
  - – Sleep deprivation and excessive alcohol, caffeine or tobacco or other substances used
  - – Past medications used and other investigations such as MRI and blood work to be done
  - – Family history of sleep disorders, especially narcolepsy and depression, as they have a strong genetic association

Examination
- General examination for evidence of anaemia or other predisposing disorders such as thyroid disease

Investigations
- Polysomnography with MSLT
- Cerebrospinal fluid (CSF) hypocretin level (if available)
- Genetic testing
- Full blood count, electrolytes, thyroid profile, serum ferritin level, blood sugar, EKG, renal function

Management
- Rectify any reversible causes such as thyroid disease, anaemia, etc.
- If possible, stop medication that might be exacerbating symptoms.
- Avoid sleep deprivation and ensure good sleep hygiene.
- Reduce caffeine, alcohol and tobacco usage.

If medication is required, they should be used based on the diagnosis and the symptoms (refer to Tables 13.1 and 13.2 in the chapter).

References

Abad V, Guilleminault C. Sleep and psychiatry. Dialogues Clin Neurosci. 2005;7:291–303.

Agargun MY, Beisoglu L. Sleep and suicidality: do sleep disturbances predict suicide risk? Sleep. 2005;28:1039–40.

American Academy of Sleep Medicine. International classification of sleep disorders: diagnostic & coding manual. Darien, IL: American Academy of Sleep Medicine; 2001.

American Academy of Sleep Medicine. International classification of sleep disorders, revised: diagnostic & coding manual. Darien, IL: American Academy of Sleep Medicine; 2005.

American Academy of Sleep Medicine. International classification of sleep disorders. 3rd ed. Darien, IL: American Academy of Sleep Medicine; 2014.

American Psychiatric Association. Diagnostic and statistical manual of mental disorders. 5th ed. Washington, DC: American Psychiatric Association; 2013.

Anderson KN, Pilworth D, Sharples LD, Smith IE, Shneerson JA. Idiopathic hypersomnia: a study of 77 cases. Sleep. 2007;30:1274–81.

Arnulf I, Zeitzer JM, File J, Farber N, Mignot E. Kleine-Levin syndrome: a systematic review of 186 cases in the literature. Brain. 2005;128:2763–76.

Arnulf I, Lin L, Gadoth N, File J, Lecendreux M, Franco P, Zeitzer J, Lo B, Faraco JH, Mignot E. Kline-Levin syndrome: a systematic study of 108 patients. Ann Neurol. 2008;63:482–92.

Arnulf I, Rico T, Mignot E. Diagnosis, disease course and management of patient's with Kleine–Levin syndrome. Lancet Neurol. 2012;11:918–28.

Batty RA, Rossell SL, Francis AJP, Ponsford J. Psychosis following traumatic brain injury. Brain Impair. 2013;14:21–41.

Baumann CR, Werth E, Stocker R, Ludwig S, Bassetti CL. Sleep-wake disturbances 6 months after traumatic brain injury: a prospective study. Brain. 2007;130:1873–83.

Bernert RA, Joiner TE. Sleep disturbances and suicide risk: a review of the literature. Neuropsychiatr Dis Treat. 2007;3:735–43.

Billiard M, Guilleminault C, Dement WC. A menstruation linked periodic hypersomnia. Klien Levin syndrome or new clinical entity. Neurology. 1975;25:436–43.

Billiard M, Jaussent I, Dauvilliers Y, Besset A. Recurrent hypersomnia: a review of 339 cases. Sleep Med Rev. 2011;15:247–57.

Bourgin P, Zeitzer JM, Mignot E. CSF hypocretin-1 assessment in sleep and neurological disorders. Lancet Neurol. 2008;7:649–62.

Bradley DT, Shapiro CM. Unexpected presentations of sleep apnea: use of CPAP in treatment. BMJ. 1993;36:1260–2.

Breslau N, Roth T, Rosenthal L, Andreski P. Hypersomnia and psychiatric disorder: a longitudinal epidemiological study of young adults. Biol Psychiatry. 1996;39:411–8.

Bryant RA, O'Donnell ML, Creamer M, McFarlane AC, Clark CR, Silove D. The psychiatric sequelae of traumatic injury. Am J Psychiatry. 2010;167:312–20.

Chabas D, Foulon C, Gonzalez J, Masr M, Lyon-Caen O, Willer JC, Derenne JP, Arnulf I. Eating disorder and metabolism in narcoleptic patients. Sleep. 2007;30:1267–73.

Chellappa SL, Cajochen C. Depression and sleepiness: a chronological approach. In: Thorpy MJ, Billiard M, editors. Sleepiness causes, consequences and treatment. Cambridge: Cambridge University press; 2011. p. 279–91.

Choo KL, Guilleminault C. Narcolepsy and idiopathic hypersomnolence. Clin Chest Med. 1998;19:169–81.

Dahmen N, Becht J, Engel A, Thommes M, Tonn P. Prevalence of eating disorders and eating attacks in narcolepsy. Neuropsychiatr Dis Treat. 2008;4:257–61.

Dauvilliers Y, Arnulf I, Mignot E. Narcolepsy with cataplexy. Lancet. 2007;369:499–511.

Doghramji K, Mitler M, Sangal RB, Shapiro C, Taylor S, Walslebenr J, Belisle C, Erman MK, Hayduk R, Hosn R, O'Malley EB, Sangal JM, Schutte SL, Youakim JM. A normative study of the maintenance of wakefulness test (MWT). Electroencephalogr Clin Neurophysiol. 1997;103:554–62.

Douglass AB, Shipley JE, Haines RF, Scholten RC, Dudley E, Tapp A. Schizophrenia, narcolepsy, and HLA-DR15, DQ6. Biol Psychiatry. 1993;34:773–80.

Dyken ME, Yamada T. Narcolepsy and disorders of excessive somnolence. Prim Care. 2005;32:389–413.

Fortuyn HA, Swinkels S, Buitelaar J, Renier WO, Furer JW, Rijnders CA, Hodiamon PP, Overeem S. High prevalence of eating disorders in narcolepsy with cataplexy: a case-control study. Sleep. 2008;31(3):335–41.

Fortuyn HA, Lappenschaar MA, Furer JW, Hodiamont PP, Rijnders CA, Renier WO, Buitelaar JK. Anxiety and mood disorders in narcolepsy: a case-control study. Gen Hosp Psychiatry. 2010;32:49–56.

Fortuyn HA, Mulders PC, Renier WO, Buitelaar JK, Overeem S. Narcolepsy and psychiatry: an evolving association of increasing interest. Sleep Med. 2011;12:714–9.

Freedom T. Hypersomnia. Disease-a-Month. 2011;57(7):353–63. https://doi.org/10.1016/j.disamonth.2011.04.008.

Ganjavi H, Shapiro CM. Hypocretin/orexin: a molecular link between sleep, energy regulation, and pleasure. J Neuropsychiatry Clin Neurosci. 2007;19:413–9.

Geoffroy PA, Arnulf I, Etain B, Henry C. Kleine–Levin syndrome and bipolar disorder: a differential diagnosis of recurrent and resistant depression. Bipolar Disorders. 2013;15(8):899–902.

Guerreiro DF, et al. Psychosis secondary to traumatic brain injury. Brain Injury. 2009;23(4):358–61. https://doi.org/10.1080/02699050902800918.

Hou L, Han X, Sheng P, Tong W, Li Z, Xu D, Yu D, Huang L, Zhao Z, Lu Y, Dong Y. Risk factors associated with sleep disturbance following traumatic brain injury: clinical findings and questionnaire based study. PLoS One. 2013;8:1–8.

Ivanenko A, Tauman R, Gozal D. Modafinil in the treatment of excessive daytime sleepiness in children. Sleep Med. 2003;4:579–82.

Jara CO, Popp R, Zulley J, Hajak G, Geisler P. Determinants of depressive symptoms in narcoleptic patients with and without cataplexy. J Nerv Ment Dis. 2011;199:329–34.

Jaussent I, Bouyer J, Ancelin ML, Akbaraly T, Peres K, Ritchie K. Insomnia and daytime sleepiness are risk factors for depression symptoms. Sleep. 2011;34:1103–10.

Johns MW. A new method for measuring daytime sleepiness: the Epworth Sleepiness Scale. Sleep. 1991;14:540–5.

Kempf J, Werth E, Kaiser PR, Bassetti CL, Baumann CR. Sleep-wake disturbances 3 years after traumatic brain injury. J Neurol Neurosurg Psychiatry. 2010;81:1402–5.

Kim YC, Ong A, Chung SA, Shapiro CM. SOREMs in sleep clinic patients: association with sleepiness, alertness and fatigue. Sleep Hypn. 2012;14:1–2.

Kishi Y, Konishi S, Koizumi S, Kudo Y, Kurosawa H, Kathol RG. Schizophrenia and narcolepsy: a review with a case report. Psychiatry Clin Neurosci. 2004;58:117–24.

Kotagal S. Hypersomnia in children: interface with psychiatric disorders. Child Adolesc Psychiatr Clin N Am. 2009;18:967–77.

Kotagal S, Krahn LE, Slocumb N. A putative link between childhood narcolepsy and obesity. Sleep Med. 2004;5:147–50.

Kryger MH, Walid R, Manfreda J. Diagnoses received by narcolepsy patients in the year prior to diagnosis by a sleep specialist. Sleep. 2002;25:36–41.

Mamelak M. Narcolepsy and depression and the neurobiology of gamma hydroxybutyrate. Prog Neurobiol. 2009;89:193–219.

Masi G, Favilla L, Millepiedi S. The Kleine-Levin syndrome as a neuropsychiatric disorder: a case report. Psychiatry. 2000;63(1):93–100. https://doi.org/10.1080/00332747.2000.11024898.

Melamed Y, Daliahu Y, Paleacu D. Narcolepsy and psychotic states-a case report. Isr J Psychiatry Relat Sci. 2009;46:70–3.

Mignot E. A practical guide to the therapy of narcolepsy and hypersomnia syndromes. Neurotherapeutics. 2012;9(4):739–52. https://doi.org/10.1007/s13311-012-0150-9.

Mignot E, Lammers GJ, Ripley B, et al. The role of cerebrospinal fluid hypocretin measurement in the diagnosis of narcolepsy and other hypersomnias. Arch Neurol. 2002;59:1553–62.

Ohayon MM, Dauvilliers Y, Reynolds CF 3rd. Operational definitions and algorithms for excessive sleepiness in the general population: implications for DSM-5 nosology. Arch Gen Psychiatry. 2012;69:71–9.

Ohayon MM, Shapiro CM. Sleep and fatigue. Semin Clin Neuropsychiatry. 2000;5:56–7.

Ohayon MM, Priest RG, Zulley J, Smirne S, Paiva T. Prevalence of narcolepsy symptomatology and diagnosis in the European general population. Neurology. 2002;58:1826–33.

Partinen M, Hublin C. Epidemiology of sleep disorders. In: Kryger MH, Roth T, Dement WC, editors. Principles and practice of sleep medicine. 3rd ed. Philadelphia, PA: Saunders; 2000. p. 558–79.

Rapoport MJ. Depression following traumatic brain injury: epidemiology, risk factors and management. CNS Drugs. 2012;26:111. https://doi.org/10.2165/11599560-000000000-00000.

Reiman D, Berger M, Voderholzer U. Sleep and depression –results from psychobiological studies: an overview. Biol Psychol. 2001;57:67–103.

Shahid A, Wilinson K, Marcu S, Shapiro CM. STOP-THAT, One hundred other sleep scales. New York, NY: Springer Science Publication Inc.; 2012a.

Shahid A, Gladanac B, Khairandish A, Shapiro CM. Peeking into the mind of disturbed adolescents? The utility of Polysomnography in an inpatient psychiatric unit. J Affect Disord. 2012b;139(1):66–74.

Shapiro CM, Kayumov L. Sleepiness, fatigue, and impaired alertness. Semin Clin Neuropsychiatry. 2000;5:2–5.

Shen J, Hossain N, Streine DL, Ravindran AV, Wang X, Deb P, Huang X, Sun F, Shapiro CM. Excessive daytime sleepiness and fatigue in depressed patients and therapeutic response of a sedating antidepressant. J Affect Disord. 2011;134:421–6.

Singareddy RK, Balon R. Sleep and suicide in psychiatric patients. Ann Clin Psychiatry. 2001;13:93–101.

Sommerauer M, Valko PO, Werth E, Baumann CR. Excessive sleep need following traumatic brain injury: a case-control study of 36 patients. J Sleep Res. 2013;22:634–9.

Ursin R. Serotonin and sleep. Sleep Med Rev. 2002;6:57–69.

Vernet C, Arnulf I. Idiopathic hypersomnia with and without long sleep time: a controlled series of 75 patients. Sleep. 2009;32:753–9.

Vignatelli L, Plazzi G, Peschechera F, Delaj L, D'Alessandro R. A 5-year prospective cohort study on health-related quality of life in patients with narcolepsy. Sleep Med. 2010;12:19–23.

Walterfang M, Upjohn E, Velakoulis D. Is schizophrenia associated with narcolepsy? Cogn Behav Neurol. 2005;18:113–8.

Watson NF, Dikmen S, Machamer J, Doherty M, Temkin N. Hypersomnia following traumatic brain injury. J Clin Sleep Med. 2007;3:363–8.

Zai C, Wigg KG, Barr CL. Genetics and sleep disorders. Semin Clin Neuropsychiatry. 2000;5:33–43.

Non-REM Parasomnias and REM Sleep Behaviour Disorder

14

Sofia Eriksson and Matthew Walker

14.1 Introduction

Parasomnias are undesirable physical events or experiences associated with sleep. Episodes are usually classified according to the stage of sleep during or from which they occur. Parasomnias frequently involve complex behaviours that may appear purposeful but are not conscious or under deliberate control. Patients are often unaware of episodes that may, however, result in injury and sleep disruption with subsequent daytime symptoms such as excessive daytime somnolence. The consequences of parasomnias are not limited to the patient but often affect the bed partner as well. People are often amnesic for their parasomnia but, with both non-REM parasomnias and REM sleep behaviour disorder (RBD), patients may recall some dream mentation.

Onset of non-REM (NREM) parasomnias usually occurs in childhood and can be seen in up to 20% of children. The majority grow out of this parasomnia in their teens, but up to 25% of patients continue to have episodes, and over 2–3% of the population may still have events in adulthood (Ohayon et al. 2012). NREM parasomnias may also first manifest in adulthood.

In contrast to NREM parasomnias that are more common in childhood, RBD is more common in older patients, and there is a male predominance (Boeve et al. 2007). RBD results from the loss of normal muscle atonia during REM sleep, resulting in dream enactment. This loss of REM atonia can result from degeneration affecting brainstem nuclei, and thus RBD is strongly associated with certain neurodegenerative conditions, such as Parkinson's disease or multisystem atrophy (Boeve et al. 2007). However, RBD may develop months or years before the onset of any

S. Eriksson (✉) · M. Walker
National Hospital for Neurology and Neurosurgery, London, UK

UCL Institute of Neurology, London, UK
e-mail: sofia.eriksson@ucl.ac.uk

© Springer-Verlag GmbH Germany, part of Springer Nature 2018
H. Selsick (ed.), *Sleep Disorders in Psychiatric Patients*,
https://doi.org/10.1007/978-3-642-54836-9_14

underlying neurological disorder. RBD is less common than NREM parasomnia but may affect up to 0.5% of the population (Ohayon et al. 1997) and is more prevalent in the elderly with a mean onset of 50–65 years.

14.2 Description of Sleep Disorders

The *International Classification of Sleep Disorders* (ICSD-3) divides parasomnias into NREM-related parasomnias, REM-related parasomnias, other parasomnias and isolated symptoms and normal variants (American Academy of Sleep Medicine 2014). This chapter will focus on NREM parasomnias and RBD.

14.2.1 NREM Parasomnias

NREM parasomnias usually arise from deep NREM sleep (slow-wave sleep, N3 or NIII-IV), and episodes typically take place during the first third of the night when slow-wave sleep is most predominant. There are several different types of NREM parasomnias; the most common are night terrors, sleepwalking (somnambulism) and confusional arousal, occasionally with violent or aggressive behaviour. Abnormal sexual behaviour and sleep-related eating disorders are less common. It is not uncommon for a person to have more than one type of disorder with overlapping features. Overall, the four 'basic drives' (sleep, sex, feeding and aggression) can manifest during NREM parasomnia episodes. NREM parasomnia episodes vary greatly in complexity and can range from simple gesturing or walking to remarkably complex behaviour requiring high-level planning and motor control such as cooking and driving. Events can last from a few seconds to up to 30 min, most commonly a few minutes.

During a confusional arousal, the person may just sit up in bed and look around in a confused manner, sometimes appearing frightened, before rapidly returning to sleep. Some events may be longer in duration and can then be associated with more complex behaviours.

Night terrors (pavor nocturnus) are typically described in children who may sit up in bed, appear extremely frightened, yet are unresponsive to external stimuli and often cry or scream inconsolably. This is generally associated with an increased autonomic drive resulting in rapid breathing, tachycardia, sweating, dilated pupils and increased muscle tone. The child is usually amnesic for the events which are often more traumatic for the parent.

During sleepwalking episodes, the patient will get up and walk around and may walk out of the bedroom and occasionally also leave the house. The patient may display complex behaviour and appear awake, but there is reduced responsiveness, and tasks are usually performed more clumsily than when awake. This increases the risk of injury.

Atypical sexual behaviour during sleep ('sleep sex' or 'sexsomnia') can occur both during confusional arousals and sleepwalking (Shapiro et al. 2003). This includes masturbation and intercourse in a way that is often unlike the person's sexual behaviour during wakefulness. This can lead to assault or molestation and can have significant forensic consequences. The majority of patients with the condition also have other types of NREM parasomnia events such as confusional arousals and sleepwalking.

Sleep-related eating disorder (SRED) constitutes recurrent episodes of involuntary eating and drinking during arousals from sleep. Eating is usually 'out of control' and can pose dangers to the patients who may eat excessively resulting in obesity or even eat inedible or toxic substances. Cooking during events may also be dangerous, particularly as judgement during events is affected. SRED may be more common in patients with daytime eating disorders but does also frequently occur in patients without daytime symptoms. As with the sexsomnias, there is often a history of other types of NREM parasomnias.

The patients are often said to be amnesic for events. However, some recall of the events is reported in up to 71% of patients (Oudiette et al. 2009b), and this often relates to perceived threat or unpleasant experiences such as feeling chased or cornered or 'seeing' people or animals in the room. This may be due to misperception of external stimuli (i.e. a dressing gown on a hanger mistaken for an intruder) or confusion. Eyes are usually open during sleepwalking episodes, and patients can interact with people and the environment, although judgement may be impaired. Further, dreamlike mentation is not confined to REM sleep but may also occur during NREM sleep, and many patients are able to recall short, unpleasant dream contents relating to the events, although these are usually more basic than the complex dreams we generally associate with REM sleep (Oudiette et al. 2009b). Patients often describe a sense of urgency during the events, and the strong feeling of threat may lead to protective or violent behaviour that may in turn lead to injurious behaviour.

NREM parasomnias are often referred to as disorders of arousal or incomplete arousals from deep sleep. This is supported by post-arousal patterns seen on EEG (Fig. 14.1) with frontal delta activity recorded in about half of patients with somnambulism and night terrors, whilst more posterior EEG rhythms are more typical for the waking state (i.e. a state in which only parts of the brain are roused and importantly the frontal cortex remains 'asleep'). Cerebral blood flow visualized using SPECT during a sleepwalking episode supports this, as it shows an increase in cerebellum and posterior cingulate cortex blood flow but a reduced blood flow in large areas of the frontal and parietal association cortices, suggesting a 'dissociation between mental and motor arousal' (Bassetti et al. 2000). More recently it has been suggested that NREM parasomnias may not only be a disorder of arousal but a disorder of slow-wave sleep. Altered slow-wave activity with a different time course for decay of slow-wave activity during the night, more hyper-synchronous delta waves during NREM sleep and increased cyclic alternating pattern (CAP) rate suggest NREM instability in patients who sleepwalk (see Zadra et al. 2013 for review). Further, the increase in slow-wave sleep and slow-wave sleep consolidation normally seen after sleep deprivation is not seen in patients who sleepwalk. This appears to be limited to deep NREM sleep only, and there is a reduction of arousals from light and REM sleep after sleep deprivation.

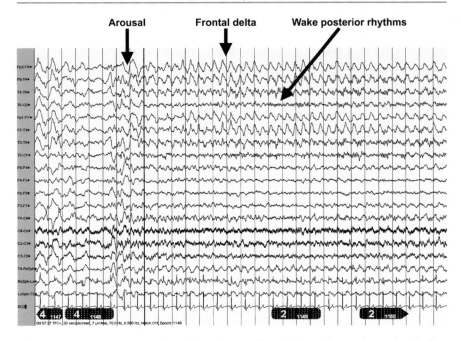

Fig. 14.1 EEG demonstrating dissociation between frontal slow and normal posterior rhythms (alpha) during a NREM parasomnia episode

14.2.2 REM Sleep Behaviour Disorder

REM sleep behaviour disorder (RBD) is characterized by a loss of atonia during REM sleep resulting in motor activity and 'dream enactment' (Fig. 14.2). The reported movements are usually brief, variable and violent, e.g. flailing arms, punching, kicking and even lunging from the bed (Schenck et al. 1986). However, it is rare for people to leave the bed during RBD, and the eyes are usually closed during events. The enactment of violent dreams can result in self-injury or injury to the bed partner. The duration of these episodes varies from seconds to minutes. People with RBD have more frequent violent dreams than those without, but this is not reflected in increased daytime aggressiveness (Fantini et al. 2005).

Less commonly, non-violent behaviours occur during RBD including masturbating, urinating and defecating, laughing, singing and dancing (Oudiette et al. 2009a). Associated sleep-talking commonly occurs and is often mumbled with logical sentence structure but nonsensical content.

The person does not show any awareness of their environment (in contrast to non-REM parasomnias), which may contribute to the injuries that occur from hitting, for example, a wall or bedstead. Also, the lack of awareness of the environment means that people may mime eating or more violent behaviours, such as stabbing, but do not actually eat or seek a weapon. Strangulation can, however, occur.

More recently, SPECT imaging during RBD has demonstrated similar pathways involved irrespective of the underlying cause. Interestingly, the basal ganglia are not involved during REM sleep-related movements, which may explain why patients

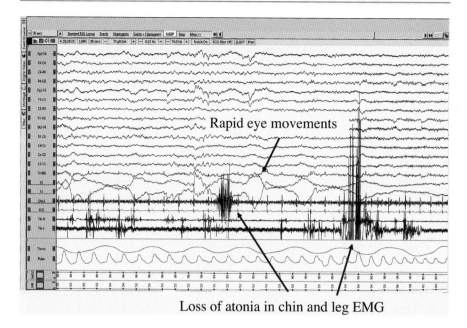

Fig. 14.2 Polysomnogram demonstrating typical rapid eye movement and desynchronised EEG during REM sleep. However, there are bursts of EMG activity indicative of loss of REM sleep atonia, typical for RBD

with Parkinson's disease and RBD do not have hypokinesia or tremor during the episodes (Mayer et al. 2015).

In addition, there are people without overt REM behaviour disorders who have loss of REM sleep atonia. This is usually identified incidentally in patients during polysomnography. The loss of REM atonia is an electrophysiological finding without accompanying abnormal motor behaviour during REM sleep. Overall, there is less REM sleep-associated electromyogram (EMG) activity in isolated loss of REM sleep atonia than in RBD (Khalil et al. 2013), indicating that this may represent 'subclinical' or 'preclinical' RBD in some cases. However, there are no longitudinal studies of isolated loss of REM sleep atonia to enable prognostication.

In young people (<50 years old), RBD not uncommonly coexists with NREM parasomnias as an overlap disorder (Schenck et al. 1997; Bonakis et al. 2009).

14.3   Risk Factors

14.3.1 NREM Parasomnias

There is often a family history of NREM parasomnias; up to 80% of patients who sleepwalk have at least one affected family member, particularly in cases where the disorder continues into adulthood. There is also a tenfold risk of sleepwalking in first-degree relatives of patients who sleepwalk. In a twin study, monozygotic twins had a five times higher concordance rate for adult sleepwalking than dizygotic twins (Hublin et al. 1997). Recently a locus for sleepwalking has been described in a large family at chromosome 20q12-q13.12 with suggested autosomal dominant inheritance pattern with reduced penetrance (Licis et al. 2011). More research is needed to identify specific genes and to evaluate if the same genes are implicated in other families.

In susceptible patients there may be a number of precipitating factors for events. Factors that may cause sleep deprivation or increase the number of arousals can trigger episodes. For most people with NREM parasomnias, sleep deprivation is a common trigger. Increased emotional stress is often associated with a deterioration of symptoms, with more frequent and more severe NREM parasomnia episodes during stressful times. Alcohol overuse may be associated with NREM parasomnias, but the forensic implication of alcohol as a trigger for episodes remains controversial, as discussed further below. Other concomitant sleep disorders such as obstructive sleep apnoea (OSA) and periodic limb movements of sleep (PLMS) can precipitate NREM parasomnias, both by causing arousals and by disrupting sleep, thereby causing sleep deprivation. In a recent audit, we found OSA or PLMS deemed to be severe enough to be of clinical significance in up to 20% of patients with polysomnography-confirmed NREM parasomnias (Fois et al. 2015).

There are case reports linking specific antidepressants to different NREM parasomnias, but there are also case series of NREM parasomnias improving with antidepressant medication (Wilson et al. 1997). There are currently no clear guidelines to suggest that antidepressants should be avoided in this group of patients, but careful monitoring of treatment effects and side effects is recommended.

Z-drugs, in particular zolpidem, have been associated with increased frequency of abnormal nocturnal behaviour, including driving, eating and sleepwalking (Ben-Hamou et al. 2011). This particularly appears to be the case if zolpidem is combined with alcohol, and it has been suggested that this is due to an enhancement of slow-wave activity from which episodes may occur (Dolder and Nelson 2008). Although the risk is likely to be low, zolpidem is a commonly prescribed drug, and patients should be informed about the potential risk of emergence of complex nocturnal behaviours and warned of the possible potentiation of combining the drug with alcohol.

Many patients with NREM parasomnias have a history of, or ongoing, depression, and some studies have suggested that NREM parasomnias such as sleepwalking are more common in patients with depressive disorder or obsessive-compulsive disorder (Ohayon et al. 2012). However, this remains debated, and others have proposed that the psychiatric symptoms are a consequence of the NREM parasomnia (Lopez et al. 2013). Further, successful treatment of the psychiatric symptoms often does not control the parasomnia, suggesting that the disorders are not necessarily linked.

14.3.2 REM Sleep Behaviour Disorder

RBD in older adults is very commonly associated with neurodegenerative disorders (parkinsonism, multisystem atrophy, Lewy body dementia), cerebrovascular disease, multiple sclerosis or Guillain-Barré syndrome (Postuma et al. 2013a). RBD may develop months or years before the onset of other signs or symptoms of the underlying neurological disorder, and with prolonged follow-up, the proportion of patients developing some neurodegenerative disorder is over 80% (Schenck et al. 2013).

In younger adults, there is a stronger association with narcolepsy, depression, post-traumatic stress disorder and medication. RBD may also emerge during withdrawal from alcohol or sedative-hypnotic abuse and with anticholinergic and other drug intoxication states leading to loss of REM atonia (Bonakis et al. 2009; Ju 2013). Antidepressant medication, in particular serotonin reuptake inhibitors, can also cause or unmask RBD and may need to be discontinued, if possible (Lam et al. 2008). The association of depression with neurodegenerative disease (depression often preceding other symptoms) and the prescription of antidepressants for depression mean that there is a complex association between neurodegeneration, depression and antidepressant medication. However, the chance of developing a neurodegenerative condition is less in those who develop RBD on antidepressants than in those not on antidepressants. This is possibly because the antidepressants are causing the RBD or uncovering an RBD earlier in the course of the disease (Postuma et al. 2013b).

14.4 History

Paroxysmal nocturnal events often pose a differential diagnostic dilemma as patients commonly have limited recollection of events. Even if there is a witness, the person may not see the onset of the episode, is often woken from sleep and may not be entirely awake to provide a good description of the course of events. Non-REM parasomnias and RBD usually have very different semiologies; night terrors characteristically result in a fearful arousal with eyes open and some response to the environment. In extreme cases of night terrors and in many sleepwalking events, the person may leave the bed, whilst RBD usually occurs in bed with sudden violent movements and with eyes shut. Whilst people will often be amnesic for the episodes, when described, the dream mentation is usually very different with non-REM parasomnias being associated with a vague description of a perceived threat or fear, whilst RBD is often associated with dreams with more of a narrative structure.

Differential diagnoses include panic attacks and dissociative disorders or confusion due to other conditions, but nocturnal epileptic seizures may be particularly difficult to distinguish from parasomnias. Several scales and scores have been devised to facilitate the differential diagnosis between epilepsy and parasomnias. The most commonly used is the Frontal Lobe Epilepsy and Parasomnias (FLEP) scale (Table 14.1) that comprises specific questions reflecting the clinical features of nocturnal frontal lobe epilepsy and parasomnias (Derry et al. 2006). Derry and co-workers have further developed a diagnostic decision tree to further facilitate differentiation between the epilepsy and parasomnia (Derry et al. 2009). Features strongly favouring parasomnia include interactive behaviour, failure to wake after event and indistinct offset. The sensitivity for the FLEP scale to correctly identify, in particular, RBD has been questioned, raising a note of caution for its use (Manni et al. 2008).

Table 14.1 FLEP score (after Derry et al. 2006)

Clinical features		Score
Age at onset		
What age did the patient have their first event?	<55 years	0
	>55 years	−1
Duration		
What is the duration of a typical event?	<2 min	+1
	2–10 min	0
	>10 min	−1
Clustering		
What is the typical number of events to occur in a single night?	1 or 2	0
	3–5	+1
	>5	+2
Timing		
At what time of night do the events most commonly occur?	Within 30 min of sleep onset	+1
	Other times (including if no clear pattern identified)	0
Symptoms		
Are events associated with definite aura?	Yes	+2
	No	0
Does the patient wander outside the bedroom during the events?	Yes	−2
	No (or uncertain)	0
Does the patient perform complex, directed behaviours (e.g. picking up objects, dressing) during event?	Yes	−2
	No (or uncertain)	0
Is there a clear history of prominent dystonic posturing, tonic limb extension or cramping during events?	Yes	+1
	No (or uncertain)	0
Stereotypy		
Are the events stereotyped or variable in nature?	Highly stereotyped	+1
	Some variability/uncertain	0
	Highly variable	−1
Recall		
Does the patient recall the events?	Yes, lucid recall	+1
	No or vague recollection only	0
Vocalization		
Does the patient speak during the event, and if so, is there subsequent recollection of speech?	No	0
	Yes, sounds only or single words	0
	Yes, coherent speech with incomplete or no recall	−2
	Yes, coherent speech with recall	+2

Scores: <0 very unlikely to have epilepsy, >3 very likely to have epilepsy, +1 to +3 relatively high chances of epilepsy and further investigation would be required in these individuals

In clinical practice, where using the full FLEP scale may be cumbersome and clinicians may not always have the scale at hand, there are a number of clinical features that may be useful for the differential diagnosis.

1. Timing of events during sleep—i.e. soon after sleep onset or later, towards morning?

   NREM parasomnias usually occur in the first third of the night where deep, slow-wave sleep is most prominent, whereas RBD is more likely to occur later during sleep where there is in general more REM sleep. These are general rules and may not apply in patients who have disrupted or disorganized sleep architecture.

2. How often during the night—i.e. how many events each night?

   There are often one to three episodes of NREM parasomnias per night, and although this can vary, episodes are rarely as frequent as epileptic seizures that can occur many times per night and may cluster. RBD events are usually reported to occur one to two times per night. However, this most likely only takes into account bigger episodes that may wake the patient or bed partner as much more frequent subtle episodes can be seen in many patients throughout REM sleep during polysomnography.

3. Frequency of events—i.e. do events occur every night, once per week, once per month or less frequently, and does the frequency vary over time?

   The frequency of NREM parasomnias often varies and may be influenced by, for example, overall stress levels where a patient may have nightly episodes during stressful times followed by times with no episodes when stressors are reduced. The frequency of epileptic seizures also varies although it is generally less affected by stress. RBD usually occurs every night, but the severity of episodes may vary.

4. Lifetime duration—i.e. what age did events start and has there been any change in frequency/severity over time?

   NREM parasomnias usually start in childhood, and the majority of patients grow out of the parasomnia in their teens. Adult onset does, however, not exclude a diagnosis of an NREM parasomnia. Epilepsy can start any time of life, but RBD usually starts later in life unless it is associated with other disorders.

Information regarding possible triggers for episodes (e.g. sleep deprivation, stress), alcohol habits and family history of similar episodes are important parts of the history, as is a detailed drug history including recreational and prescribed drugs. Moreover, psychiatric diseases including depression, anxiety and post-traumatic stress disorder are important associations. If RBD is considered, a neurological examination to look for extrapyramidal symptoms should be performed.

14.5 Forensic Implications of Parasomnias

Parasomnias are increasingly being used as a defence for serious crime including murder and rape, especially in the setting of excessive alcohol. An act committed during a parasomnia would be defined legally as an automatism and may consequently lack both actus reus and mens rea (i.e. the guilty act and the guilty mind) (Morrison et al. 2014). Demonstrating that someone has parasomnias is not sufficient for a defence, as parasomnias are common in people and their occurrence may be coincidental. It therefore needs to be shown that someone was having a parasomnia at the time of the act.

Since people with RBD are not aware of their environment, then clearly the hitting out and injury would also lack actus reus. The problem is more difficult with non-REM parasomnias during which people interact with their environment. In this circumstance it may also be difficult to differentiate a non-REM parasomnia from a factitious account and an alcohol-fuelled event. Usually non-REM parasomnias involve the dissociation between arousal of the limbic system and dysfunction of the frontal cortex (Bassetti et al. 2000), so that acts lack planning and social context.

14.6 Investigations

Overnight polysomnography (PSG) is often used to assist in the diagnosis of NREM parasomnia. However, the diagnostic value of the test has not been established. The American Academy of Sleep Medicine (AASM) published practice parameters for the indications for polysomnography for different sleep disorders, including parasomnia (Chesson et al. 1997; Kushida et al. 2005). According to their recommendations, PSG should be performed when evaluating patients with sleep behaviours suggestive of unusual or atypical parasomnias, when nocturnal events are thought to be seizure-related and the clinical evaluation and EEG are inconclusive and when the sleep disorder does not respond to conventional therapy. Conversely the guidelines state that polysomnography is not routinely indicated in cases of typical, uncomplicated and non-injurious parasomnias when the diagnosis is clearly delineated from the history. A recent audit at our own centre is in agreement with these suggestions.

A proportion of patients with paroxysmal nocturnal events do not have any events during their polysomnography. To increase the diagnostic yield, a protocol combining sleep deprivation before admission and auditory stimulus during the polysomnography with recovery sleep has been proposed to trigger forced arousals with NREM parasomnia episodes (Pilon et al. 2008). This protocol has not been tested for the differentiation between, for example, NREM parasomnias and nocturnal epilepsy and is currently not in general use, nor is it proposed in the AASM practice parameters.

Polysomnography should hence be performed in patients with an atypical history or with suspected epilepsy. In view of the frequently encountered concomitant sleep disorders, the recording should include leg electrodes and respiratory measurements and benzodiazepine and antidepressant medication should be withdrawn if at all possible. However, differential diagnosis may be a challenge even with access to good-quality video-EEG telemetry, and there is often disagreement between experts who are shown the same videos (Vignatelli et al. 2007).

In the forensic setting, polysomnography is rarely helpful as it cannot exclude the diagnosis of a non-REM parasomnia, and demonstrating a non-REM parasomnia does not mean that one took place at the time of the crime. Nevertheless, demonstrating a predisposition to non-REM parasomnias may be helpful to the defence.

RBD can be diagnosed with polysomnography. However, the criteria for pathological loss of REM atonia vary from unit to unit, partly due to differences in the criteria used to define loss of REM atonia and partly due to different methods used to measure muscle activity (conventionally submental EMG electrodes are used) (Khalil et al. 2013; McCarter et al. 2014).

14.7 Treatment

For the majority of patients with NREM parasomnias, there is no need for medical treatment, but reassurance and advice to avoiding trigger factors such as sleep deprivation are sufficient to control the symptoms. For example, for patients in whom alcohol has been identified as a trigger, avoiding excess alcohol will be part of the treatment. Basic sleep hygiene advice should be provided to all patients. Many patients find the nocturnal episodes distressing, and this may cause anxiety, resulting in delay of bedtime that may in turn cause sleep deprivation and subsequently increase the risk of further episodes.

However, for people with severe or violent symptoms, medication may be indicated. The most commonly used drugs are clonazepam (long-acting benzodiazepine) or antidepressants. There is no licensed treatment, and there are to date no randomized clinical trials for treatment of NREM parasomnias. The efficacy of clonazepam has been reported in retrospective case series of patients with miscellaneous sleep disorders including NREM and REM parasomnias; around 85% achieved complete/nearly complete control of their sleep disorders (Schenck and Mahowald 1996). Importantly, in this study, there was little evidence of tolerance to clonazepam with long-term use.

The efficacy of antidepressants for NREM parasomnias has been illustrated in a case series of six patients using paroxetine where episodes were abolished in three of six patients, and in the remaining three patients, there was a reduction not further specified (Wilson et al. 1997). This forms the basis for the current clinical practice to use either clonazepam or antidepressant medication outside their usual licence to treat this sleep disorder. Side effects with daytime sedation often limit usage of clonazepam. There have also been case studies of NREM parasomnia episodes triggered by antidepressant medication such as bupropion and mirtazapine as well as paroxetine (see Kierlin and Littner 2011 for review). Randomized controlled studies are needed to establish the most appropriate treatment for patients with NREM parasomnias.

Clonazepam is the main treatment for RBD, although a host of other drugs have been tried with varying results (Table 14.2). The main alternative is usually melatonin. In a small placebo crossover study with 3 mg melatonin (Kunz and Mahlberg 2010), 7/8 improved with half having no dream enactment, and there was some improvement in the REM sleep atonia. A small randomized study of clonazepam

Table 14.2 Drugs used in the treatment of RBD (after Aurora et al. 2010)

Drug	Number of patients	Number of responders
Clonazepam	339	306
Melatonin	38	31
Pramipexole	29	13
Anticholinesterase inhibitors	28	23
Paroxetine	21	17
Zopiclone	12	9
Benzodiazepines (others)	12	9
Desipramine	3	1
Clozapine	3	3
Carbamazepine	5	5
Sodium oxybate	1	1

versus melatonin demonstrated no significant difference in efficacy in RBD (McCarter et al. 2013), but melatonin tended to be better tolerated.

Safety aspects are an important part of management of patients with parasomnias, in particular for patients with NREM parasomnias who may get out of bed and perform complex tasks that put themselves or others in danger. It is important that doors and windows are properly locked to reduce the risk of patients walking out of the house or falling out of windows. Sharp objects or other objects that could cause injury should be hidden or locked away. In more severe NREM parasomnias, it may be necessary to sleep in a separate room to reduce the risk of injuries as well as to reduce triggers—a bed partner moving may trigger an episode. Although people with RBD do not leave the bed, lashing out may injure the bed partner or themselves, necessitating separate beds.

Conclusion

Parasomnias, in particular NREM parasomnias, are common and can pose a differential diagnostic dilemma for the clinician. Clinical features can facilitate the differential diagnosis, but polysomnography is often needed. However, even with polysomnography, it may be difficult to diagnose these events with certainty. Medical treatment is often not needed, but clonazepam can be used for both NREM parasomnias and RBD in more severe cases, with antidepressants being an alternative treatment option for NREM parasomnias and melatonin for RBD. Randomized controlled trials are needed to clarify the best treatment options. Safety aspects and avoiding trigger factors are important for both disorders.

References

American Academy of Sleep Medicine. International classification of sleep disorders. Darien, IL: American Academy of Sleep Medicine; 2014. https://doi.org/10.1111/febs.12678.

Aurora RN, Zak RS, Maganti RK, et al. Best practice guide for the treatment of REM sleep behavior disorder (RBD). J Clin Sleep Med. 2010;6:85–95.

Bassetti C, Vella S, Donati F, et al. SPECT during sleepwalking. Lancet. 2000;356:484–5. https://doi.org/10.1016/S0140-6736(00)02561-7.

Ben-Hamou M, Marshall NS, Grunstein RR, et al. Spontaneous adverse event reports associated with zolpidem in Australia 2001-2008. J Sleep Res. 2011;20:559–68. https://doi.org/10.1111/j.1365-2869.2011.00919.x.

Boeve BF, Silber MH, Saper CB, et al. Pathophysiology of REM sleep behaviour disorder and relevance to neurodegenerative disease. Brain. 2007;130:2770–88. https://doi.org/10.1093/brain/awm056.

Bonakis A, Howard RS, Ebrahim IO, et al. REM sleep behaviour disorder (RBD) and its associations in young patients. Sleep Med. 2009;10:641–5. https://doi.org/10.1016/j.sleep.2008.07.008.

Chesson AL, Ferber RA, Fry JM, et al. The indications for polysomnography and related procedures. Sleep. 1997;20:423–87.

Derry CP, Davey M, Johns M, et al. Distinguishing sleep disorders from seizures: diagnosing bumps in the night. Arch Neurol. 2006;63:705–9. https://doi.org/10.1001/archneur.63.5.705.

Derry CP, Harvey AS, Walker MC, et al. NREM arousal parasomnias and their distinction from nocturnal frontal lobe epilepsy: a video EEG analysis. Sleep. 2009;32:1637–44.

Dolder CR, Nelson MH. Hypnosedative-induced complex behaviours : incidence, mechanisms and management. CNS Drugs. 2008;22:1021–36.

Fantini ML, Corona A, Clerici S, Ferini-Strambi L. Aggressive dream content without daytime aggressiveness in REM sleep behavior disorder. Neurology. 2005;65:1010–5. https://doi.org/10.1212/01.wnl.0000179346.39655.e0.

Fois C, Wright M-AS, Sechi G, et al. The utility of polysomnography for the diagnosis of NREM parasomnias: an observational study over 4 years of clinical practice. J Neurol. 2015;262:385–93. https://doi.org/10.1007/s00415-014-7578-2.

Hublin C, Kaprio J, Partinen M, et al. Prevalence and genetics of sleepwalking: a population-based twin study. Neurology. 1997;48:177–81.

Ju Y-ES. Rapid eye movement sleep behavior disorder in adults younger than 50 years of age. Sleep Med. 2013;14:768–74. https://doi.org/10.1016/j.sleep.2012.09.026.

Khalil A, Wright M-A, Walker MC, Eriksson SH. Loss of rapid eye movement sleep atonia in patients with REM sleep behavioral disorder, narcolepsy, and isolated loss of REM atonia. J Clin Sleep Med. 2013;9:1039–48. https://doi.org/10.5664/jcsm.3078.

Kierlin L, Littner MR. Parasomnias and antidepressant therapy: a review of the literature. Front Psych. 2011;2:71. https://doi.org/10.3389/fpsyt.2011.00071.

Kunz D, Mahlberg R. A two-part, double-blind, placebo-controlled trial of exogenous melatonin in REM sleep behaviour disorder. J Sleep Res. 2010;19:591–6. https://doi.org/10.1111/j.1365-2869.2010.00848.x.

Kushida CA, Littner MR, Morgenthaler T, et al. Practice parameters for the indications for polysomnography and related procedures: an update for 2005. Sleep. 2005;28:499–521.

Lam SP, Fong SYY, Ho CKW, Wing YK. Parasomnia among psychiatric outpatients: A clinical, epidemiologic, cross-sectional study. J Clin Psychiatry. 2008;69:1374–82.

Licis AK, Desruisseau DM, Yamada KA, et al. Novel genetic findings in an extended family pedigree with sleepwalking. Neurology. 2011;76:49–52. https://doi.org/10.1212/WNL.0b013e318203e964.

Lopez R, Jaussent I, Scholz S, et al. Functional impairment in adult sleepwalkers: a case-control study. Sleep. 2013;36:345–51. https://doi.org/10.5665/sleep.2446.

Manni R, Terzaghi M, Repetto A. The FLEP scale in diagnosing nocturnal frontal lobe epilepsy, NREM and REM parasomnias: data from a tertiary sleep and epilepsy unit. Epilepsia. 2008;49:1581–5. https://doi.org/10.1111/j.1528-1167.2008.01602.x.

Mayer G, Bitterlich M, Kuwert T, et al. Ictal SPECT in patients with rapid eye movement sleep behaviour disorder. Brain. 2015;138:1263–70. https://doi.org/10.1093/brain/awv042.

McCarter SJ, Boswell CL, St Louis EK, et al. Treatment outcomes in REM sleep behavior disorder. Sleep Med. 2013;14:237–42. https://doi.org/10.1016/j.sleep.2012.09.018.

McCarter SJ, St Louis EK, Duwell EJ, et al. Diagnostic thresholds for quantitative REM sleep phasic burst duration, phasic and tonic muscle activity, and REM atonia index in REM sleep behavior disorder with and without comorbid obstructive sleep apnea. Sleep. 2014;37:1649–62. https://doi.org/10.5665/sleep.4074.

Morrison I, Rumbold JMM, Riha RL. Medicolegal aspects of complex behaviours arising from the sleep period: a review and guide for the practising sleep physician. Sleep Med Rev. 2014;18:249–60. https://doi.org/10.1016/j.smrv.2013.07.004.

Ohayon MM, Caulet M, Priest RG. Violent behavior during sleep. J Clin Psychiatry. 1997;58:369–76. quiz 377.

Ohayon MM, Mahowald MW, Dauvilliers Y, et al. Prevalence and comorbidity of nocturnal wandering in the U.S. adult general population. Neurology. 2012;78:1583–9. https://doi.org/10.1212/WNL.0b013e3182563be5.

Oudiette D, De Cock VC, Lavault S, et al. Nonviolent elaborate behaviors may also occur in REM sleep behavior disorder. Neurology. 2009a;72:551–7. https://doi.org/10.1212/01.wnl.0000341936.78678.3a.

Oudiette D, Leu S, Pottier M, et al. Dreamlike mentations during sleepwalking and sleep terrors in adults. Sleep. 2009b;32:1621–7.

Pilon M, Montplaisir J, Zadra A. Precipitating factors of somnambulism: impact of sleep deprivation and forced arousals. Neurology. 2008;70:2284–90. https://doi.org/10.1212/01.wnl.0000304082.49839.86.

Postuma RB, Gagnon J-F, Montplaisir J. Rapid eye movement sleep behavior disorder as a biomarker for neurodegeneration: the past 10 years. Sleep Med. 2013a;14:763–7. https://doi.org/10.1016/j.sleep.2012.09.001.

Postuma RB, Gagnon J-F, Tuineaig M, et al. Antidepressants and REM sleep behavior disorder: isolated side effect or neurodegenerative signal? Sleep. 2013b;36:1579–85. https://doi.org/10.5665/sleep.3102.

Schenck CH, Mahowald MW. Long-term, nightly benzodiazepine treatment of injurious parasomnias and other disorders of disrupted nocturnal sleep in 170 adults. Am J Med. 1996;100:333–7. https://doi.org/10.1016/S0002-9343(97)89493-4.

Schenck CH, Bundlie SR, Ettinger MG, Mahowald MW. Chronic behavioral disorders of human REM sleep: a new category of parasomnia. Sleep. 1986;9:293–308.

Schenck CH, Boyd JL, Mahowald TW. A parasomnia overlap disorder involving sleepwalking, sleep terrors, and REM sleep behavior disorder in 33 polysomnographically confirmed cases. Sleep. 1997;20:972–81.

Schenck CH, Boeve BF, Mahowald MW. Delayed emergence of a parkinsonian disorder or dementia in 81% of older men initially diagnosed with idiopathic rapid eye movement sleep behavior disorder: a 16-year update on a previously reported series. Sleep Med. 2013;14(8):744. https://doi.org/10.1016/j.sleep.2012.10.009.

Shapiro CM, Trajanovic NN, Fedoroff JP. Sexsomnia--a new parasomnia? Can J Psychiatry. 2003;48:311–7.

Vignatelli L, Bisulli F, Provini F, et al. Interobserver reliability of video recording in the diagnosis of nocturnal frontal lobe seizures. Epilepsia. 2007;48:1506–11. https://doi.org/10.1111/j.1528-1167.2007.01121.x.

Wilson SJ, Lillywhite AR, Potokar JP, et al. Adult night terrors and paroxetine. Lancet. 1997;350:185.

Zadra A, Desautels A, Petit D, Montplaisir J. Somnambulism: clinical aspects and pathophysiological hypotheses. Lancet Neurol. 2013;12:285–94. https://doi.org/10.1016/S1474-4422(12)70322-8.

Nightmare Disorders

15

Ivana Rosenzweig

15.1 Introduction

Nightmares are a relatively prevalent parasomnia, associated with a range of psychiatric conditions and pathological symptoms (Nielsen and Levin 2007). They also occur at times of overall heightened arousal in otherwise healthy individuals. Nightmares are more frequent during childhood where they, not unlike other childhood parasomnias, probably represent a benign disorder caused by immaturity of neural circuits (Nevsimalova et al. 2013). Current knowledge about how nightmares are produced is still influenced by neo-psychoanalytic speculations, as well as by more recent personality, evolutionary and neurobiological models (Nielsen and Levin 2007). A majority of these models stipulate some type of emotionally adaptive function for dreaming, including image contextualization, affect desomatization, mood regulation or fear extinction (Nielsen and Levin 2007). It is generally accepted that dreams likely represent a state of consciousness, characterized by internally generated sensory, cognitive and emotional experiences occurring during sleep (Desseilles et al. 2011). Even normal dream reports tend to be abundant, with complex, emotional and perceptually vivid experiences after awakening from rapid eye movement (REM) sleep (Desseilles et al. 2011) or less often also during the non-REM (nREM) sleep. Emotional experiences in most dreams, not just nightmares, are frequent, intense and possibly biased towards negative emotions. Nightmares, on the other hand, can represent an intensified expression of an emotionally adaptive function, or, conversely, they can be taken as evidence of its breakdown (Nielsen and Levin 2007). One such example is highly emotionally loaded

I. Rosenzweig
Department of Neuroimaging, Sleep Disorders Centre, Guy's Hospital and Sleep and Brain Plasticity Centre, Institute of Psychiatry, Psychology and Neuroscience (IOPPN), King's College London, London, UK
e-mail: ivana.1.rosenzweig@kcl.ac.uk

© Springer-Verlag GmbH Germany, part of Springer Nature 2018
H. Selsick (ed.), *Sleep Disorders in Psychiatric Patients*,
https://doi.org/10.1007/978-3-642-54836-9_15

dreams and nightmares in post-traumatic stress disorder (PTSD) which can disrupt the maintenance of REM sleep (Nielsen and Levin 2007).

Various risk factors and pharmacological agents have, over the years, been implicated in the incidence and genesis of nightmares. The true aetiology and neuropathology of this sleep disorder remain yet to be fully understood, although the aetiology is likely best explained by an interaction between disposition and current stressors (Kushida 2013). Fortunately, the majority of nightmares do not require active treatment, and of those that do, a vast majority can be treated effectively with a brief and simple intervention method called imagery rehearsal therapy (Kushida 2013). Only severe, co-morbid and/or treatment-resistant nightmares may require further pharmacological treatment.

15.2 Description of Nightmare Disorder

Frequent nightmares can occur in many different psychopathological contexts, with wide variability in their relationship to, and implications for, overall functioning. Some nightmares are also seen in healthy individuals under conditions of internal stress and creative crisis. However, when nightmares form a primary feature of a presenting sleep disorder, the *International Classification of Sleep Disorders, 3rd Edition* (ICSD-3), definition refers to them as 'disturbing mental experiences that generally occur during REM sleep and that often result in awakening' (American Academy of Sleep Medicine 2015).

Nightmares are currently defined in two major nosologies (American Academy of Sleep Medicine 2015; American Psychiatric Association. DSM-5 Task Force 2013). They are characterized by awakenings, predominantly from REM sleep, with clear recall of disturbing mentation. The emotional component of nightmares is characteristically fear-related, although other less frequent emotions such as anger or disgust have also been documented (Zadra et al. 2006; Nielsen and Levin 2007). Traditionally, two major sub-classifications are recognized: idiopathic nightmares, for which the cause is unknown, and post-traumatic nightmares, which are more severe and distressing. The latter are frequently, although not exclusively, associated with PTSD (American Academy of Sleep Medicine 2015; American Psychiatric Association. DSM-5 Task Force 2013). Both types of nightmares are further distinguished from sleep terrors, which also involve fear-based arousals. Moreover, sleep terrors characteristically arise from nREM sleep and typically are not accompanied by vivid and extensive dreams. Also, they do not result in awakenings with clear recall of mentation.

Nightmare disorder is the only diagnosis in the ICSD-3 in which abnormal dreaming is the primary feature. The ICSD-3 states that 'Emotions usually involve anxiety, fear, or terror and frequently also anger, rage, embarrassment, disgust, and other negative feelings' (American Academy of Sleep Medicine 2015). The ICSD-3 also notes 'imminent physical danger to the individual' as particularly common content. Full consciousness is quickly attained with arousal, and there is often detailed recall of the preceding dream (Montagna and Chokroverty 2011).

Commonly, little or no movement accompanies arousal from nightmares. Difficulty falling back to sleep is also frequently reported, and, given that REM sleep is more present in the latter part of the night, most nightmares occur in that time period (American Psychiatric Association. DSM-5 Task Force 2013). Nightmares may, however, also occur during nREM sleep and may not always awaken the sleeper (American Psychiatric Association. DSM-5 Task Force 2013).

The following criteria need to be satisfied in order for the diagnosis of 'nightmare disorder' to be made according to the ICSD-3 (American Academy of Sleep Medicine 2015):

(a) Recurrent episodes of awakenings from sleep with recall of intensely disturbing dream mentation, usually involving fear or anxiety, but also anger, sadness, disgust and other dysphoric emotions.
(b) Full alertness on awakening, with little confusion or disorientation; recall of sleep mentation is immediate and clear.
(c) At least one of the following associated features is present: delayed return to sleep after the episodes and/or occurrence of episodes in the latter half of the habitual sleep period.

In children, the content of nightmares are age related, with imaginary creatures most common in 7–9-year-old children and being kidnapped common in 10–12-year-old children (American Psychiatric Association 2013). Other common themes are loss of control and fear of injury. Vocalizations may occur, but movement and autonomic symptoms are minimal. When awakened, the child becomes oriented, can be calmed and usually recalls details of the dream (Nevsimalova et al. 2013).

Developmental, genetic, psychological and organic factors can contribute to occurrence of nightmares. In early childhood, high prevalence of parasomnias has been associated with separation anxiety, and multiple studies have demonstrated that a child's general level of anxiety is related to nightmare severity and frequency (Petit et al. 2007; American Psychiatric Association. DSM-5 Task Force 2013).

15.3 Risk Factors

There are inconsistent reports of the prevalence of nightmare disorders in the literature. This is further complicated by the variable criteria and approaches to assessment used in various studies to date. It is, however, generally accepted that its prevalence in the adult population ranges somewhere between 2% and 8% (American Academy of Sleep Medicine 2015). Approximately 7% of individuals who have frequent nightmares also have a family history of nightmares. Nightmares occur in all races and cultures, with no reported differences in prevalence (American Academy of Sleep Medicine 2015). Young age and female gender appear to be amongst the risk factors. Up to 30% of children report having nightmares 'always' or 'often' (Partinen 1994). Several neuropsychiatric and neurological disorders have increased risk of abnormal mentation and nightmares. Of those, PTSD, depressive disorder, adjustment and anxiety disorder, borderline personality disorder, obstructive sleep apnoea (OSA), narcolepsy and migraine are just some that have, over the years, been associated with an increased risk for co-morbid nightmares. Several groups of medications, including sedative/hypnotics, dopamine agonists, beta-blockers and amphetamines, are the therapeutic modalities most frequently associated with nightmares (Thompson and Pierce 1999). These drug classes have a plausible pharmacologic mechanism to explain this effect; however, some other medications with less obvious mechanisms have also been implicated in causing nightmares in case studies, e.g. galantamine, mirtazapine and ciprofloxacin (Dang et al. 2008, 2009; Corbo et al. 2013).

15.3.1 Paediatric Nightmares

Nightmares often begin in childhood, at ages 3–5, and may persist through adulthood (Nevsimalova et al. 2013). Nightmares are more common in children with mental retardation, depression and central nervous system (CNS) diseases; an association has also been reported with febrile illnesses (Petit et al. 2007). The prevalence of nightmares and other parasomnias declines in school age and adolescence. This is thought to be due to progressive neurological maturation and reduction in separation anxiety (Kotagal 2009).

Daytime emotional conflicts and psychological stress often contaminate sleep and predispose children to nightmares (American Psychiatric Association. DSM-5 Task Force 2013). Nightmares are associated with anxiety disorders, particularly in adolescents (Bloomfield and Shatkin 2009).

Nightmares may result from a severe traumatic event in children, as well as in adults, and may indicate PTSD. Medications may also induce frightening dreams, either during treatment or following withdrawal. Withdrawal of medications that suppress REM sleep, including tricyclic antidepressants and selective serotonin reuptake inhibitors (SSRIs), can lead to an REM rebound effect that is accompanied by nightmares.

15.3.2 Psychopathology of Adult Age Nightmares

Amongst adults, nightmares are more frequently reported in women. Two main factors likely mediate the gender difference in nightmare frequency: neuroticism and overall dream recall frequency (Schredl 2014b). However, the gender difference in nightmare reporting is seen even when controlling for gender difference in dream recall. Also, in a Finnish twin cohort, a genetic predisposition to nightmares which continues into adulthood was reported (Hublin et al. 1999). Conversely, nightmares appear to be less frequent in elderly populations (Nielsen and Levin 2007; Salvio et al. 1992).

Many studies have investigated the relationship between the nightmare disorder and psychopathology and found an association in most instances, but not all (Zadra and Donderi 2000; Hublin et al. 1999). Nonetheless, it is widely acknowledged that nightmares are more frequent and more prevalent in psychiatric populations. Nightmares are frequently reported associated with anxiety and neuroticism, as well as with schizophrenia-spectrum symptoms. Patients with nightmares have heightened risk for suicide and dissociative phenomena. Frequent nightmares have been reported to increase the risk of suicidal thoughts by a factor of 1.5–3 and to increase the risk for suicide attempts by a factor of 3–4 (McCall and Black 2013; Susanszky et al. 2011). Moreover, nightmares are the single sleep pathology most consistently shown to be an independent risk factor for suicide and are seen as one of the modifiable risks for sui- cidality (McCall and Black 2013). Nightmares, especially when persistent over time, suggest high risk of repeated suicide attempts amongst those who had attempted sui- cide within the preceding 2 years (McCall and Black 2013; Sjostrom et al. 2007). The duration and intensity of nightmares are also predictive of suicide (McCall and Black 2013). It has been shown that the overall duration of insomnia and nightmares increases suicide risk independently of the severity of sleep disturbance and depres- sion (Nadorff et al. 2013b; McCall and Black 2013). This is of particular note, and any practicing sleep clinician should make it a crucial part of their clinical interview and history-taking to ask about the presence of suicidal ideation in these patients. However, the correlation between nightmares and suicide may not hold true in old age (Nadorff et al. 2013a), and this is thought to be due to the sleep changes that occur with increased age, such as altered REM sleep patterns and decreased number of reported nightmares (Nadorff et al. 2013a; McCall and Black 2013).

Nightmares are also associated with health behavioural problems, other sleep disturbances and PTSD. Numerous studies indicate that nightmares are reactive to intense stress. It has been proposed that all conditions which increase sleep frag- mentation, such as obstructive sleep apnoea (OSA) (Rosenzweig et al. 2014, 2015), can lead to more frequent nightmares (Youakim et al. 1998; Krakow et al. 2000). For example, in one study of veterans with PTSD and OSA, continuous positive airway pressure (CPAP) therapy was shown to reduce PTSD-associated nightmares and to improve overall PTSD symptoms (Tamanna et al. 2014). In the same manner, poor sleep hygiene, insufficient sleep and circadian rhythm disturbances are thought to increase the risk of nightmares. Also, nightmares themselves can lead to second- ary difficulties with sleep avoidance and insomnia (Krakow et al. 1995).

Of note is that two recent studies reported that up to 40% of narcolepsy patients might also suffer from nightmares (Pisko et al. 2014; Schredl 2014a). Here it has been suggested that the overactive REM sleep system itself is responsible for the increased nightmare frequency. Additionally, increased daytime stress in narcolepsy patients may contribute to increased nightmares. In yet another study, fear and anguish during dreaming were more frequently reported by migraine patients com- pared to controls, independent of anxiety and depression scores (De Angeli et al. 2014). The dreams in sufferers of migraine are reported to be abundant with nega- tive connotation, as well as fear and anguish. It was argued that this may be due to the recorded negative sensations induced by recurrent migraine pain. Alternatively, this may reflect a distinct activation of the mesolimbic structures in both dreaming and migraine attacks (De Angeli et al. 2014).

Some clinicians argue that nightmares are rarely truly idiopathic and primary and that nightmares should be always assessed as a symptom of an underlying psychiatric syndrome, for example, an anxiety disorder. Indeed, some studies suggest that approximately half of the sufferers with chronic nightmares have a co-morbid psychiatric disorder. Amongst psychiatric disorders, PTSD and severe depression are the most widely recognized risk factors for nightmares (Hartmann 1984; Ross et al. 1989). Recurrent nightmares are one of the recognized major symptoms of PTSD (Hartmann 1984). Of note is that in depression, nightmares were also associated with increased risk for suicidality (Marinova et al. 2014). So far this risk has only been conclusively shown for unipolar depression, whilst the results concerning bipolar depression are inconclusive (Marinova et al. 2014).

Moreover, an association between nightmare disorder and varied psychopathology has also been suggested by a number of studies (Hublin et al. 1999; Zadra and Donderi 2000). For example, the higher incidence of distressing nightmares and the association of nightmares with alexithymia suggest that an affect regulation disturbance may be common to the two sets of symptoms (Godin et al. 2013). Hartmann (1998) delineated a dimension of personality he refers to as thick versus thin boundaries and related it to the vulnerability to nightmares (Hartmann 1998). According to this division, people with thick boundaries tend to be solid, well-organized, logical and linear in thought. On the other hand, those with thin boundaries tend to be open, creative, sensitive and vulnerable. Hartmann reported that thin boundaries are associated with greater frequency of dream recall, more vivid, emotional and dream-like dream reports, and with nightmares (Hartmann 1998).

15.3.3 Iatrogenic Nightmares

Over the years, a large number of medications have been reported in association with nightmares. The highest frequency of complaints appears in association with dopamine agonists, beta-blockers and SSRIs. Hence a special consideration should be made when using some antiparkinsonian medications, as well as with several antihypertensives and antidepressants.

It should be noted that the early phase of antidepressant therapy may independently lead to temporary increased suicidal ideation (Isacsson and Ahlner 2014; Khan and Bernadt 2011). In those patients who additionally develop iatrogenic nightmares, this can be a contributory or additive risk factor, and careful monitoring during the first 2–3 weeks following the initiation may be required. The mechanism by which antidepressant drugs may increase suicidal thinking, suicidal behaviour and suicide is not yet established. Several mechanisms have been proposed over the years, one of which suggests that emergent anxiety and akathisia on starting treatment could play the role (Khan and Bernadt 2011). Also, some authors consider that some types of antidepressants (e.g. fluoxetine, SSRIs) promote suicidal thoughts per se and can initiate a painful round of pervasive suicidal thoughts in patients (Khan and Bernadt 2011). Whatever the underlying mechanism, it has been shown that the risk for nonfatal suicidal behaviour for the first 9 days of a new antidepressant prescription was raised fourfold in comparison with the risk for 90 days and beyond (Khan and Bernadt 2011).

Apart from antidepressants, many of above-listed medications may, in susceptible patients, cause disturbed dreams and in some cases lead to development of frank nightmares (Thompson and Pierce 1999; Pagel and Helfter 2003). Several hypnotics were also reported as associated with nightmares (Pagel and Helfter 2003). Of other groups of medications, those that affect the immunological response to infectious disease were reported as associated with nightmares in some patients. Some antibiotics (i.e. fluoroquinolones) are also associated with patient reports of insomnia and nightmares (Pagel and Helfter 2003). Additionally, several antiretrovirals were implicated in nightmares. Of those, the non-nucleoside reverse transcriptase inhibitor efavirenz is most commonly associated with central nervous system toxicity, causing insomnia, irritability and vivid dreams (Abers et al. 2014). Recent studies have suggested that the risk of developing these adverse effects is increased in patients with various cytochrome P450 2B6 alleles (Abers et al. 2014). Of all those listed, the individual medication most clearly associated with nightmares is the SSRI paroxetine (Voss et al. 2014).

Nightmares may also occur as a result of withdrawal from REM-suppressant agents such as alcohol, barbiturates as well as some antidepressants (Thompson and Pierce 1999). A possible association was also suggested to exist with agents affecting the neurotransmitters acetylcholine, GABA and histamine, as well as for some anaesthetics, antipsychotics and antiepileptic agents (Pagel and Helfter 2003). The proposed neuromechanisms behind the increased risk for nightmares appear to include the modulation of intrinsic neurotransmitters noradrenaline, serotonin and dopamine (Pagel and Helfter 2003) which in turn may lead to increases in qualities such as the intensity and vividness of dreaming, as well as genuine nightmares. For example, according to the noradrenergic mechanistic model, in some patients, an increased central nervous system noradrenergic state may lead to the disruption of normal REM sleep, in turn contributing to nightmares (Kung et al. 2012). Interestingly, it has been shown that REM sleep reduces, and thus likely restores, concentrations of noradrenaline to baseline, allowing for optimal wakeful functioning (Rosenzweig et al. 2015). It is possible that in some cases, a vicious cycle could be set when co-morbid disorders, such as PTSD or OSA, further disrupt REM's noradrenergic 'housekeeping' function (Rosenzweig et al. 2015). In such severe co-morbid cases, clinicians should perhaps consider pharmacological, along with psychological, treatment of nightmares as first-line treatment. Of note, prazosin (also see under Sect. 15.6), a lipid-soluble 1-adrenergic receptor antagonist that crosses the blood-brain barrier and decreases the sympathetic outflow in the brain, has been shown to be particularly effective in treatment of PTSD-associated nightmares (Kung et al. 2012).

Finally, to date, it is not clear whether nightmares induced by medications have long-term sequelae, i.e. continuing even after removing the offending agent (Aurora et al. 2010). Moreover, it is still far from clear if different types of nightmares share a common underlying pathophysiology (Zadra et al. 2006).

15.4 History

History-taking from someone presenting with a sleep disturbance is described in some detail in a previous chapter. When assessing the likelihood of nightmare disorder as a primary or secondary diagnosis, one should follow a similar approach as for other sleep disorders whilst paying particular attention to co-morbidities and known risk factors.

Good history-taking allows the clinician to rule out other sleep disorders that may mimic the diagnosis, may present concurrently (OSA, periodic limb movements, insomnia, etc.) and/or constitute plausible differential diagnosis for nightmares, such as night terrors. It is also important to distinguish whether the complaint is that of a primary sleep disorder or if nightmares arise co-morbid and secondary to other physical, neurological, neuropsychiatric or iatrogenic causes (also see under Sect. 15.3). Any suicidal risk should also be carefully explored, especially if nightmares present co-morbid to a psychiatric disorder, or following an initiation of a new antidepressant. However, at times, determining the causality might be difficult.

A differentiation is often made between so-called idiopathic nightmares and the nightmares that occur as a characteristic feature of PTSD. The latter are described as distinguished by the repetitive replay of scenes from a traumatic event and are the most consistently present symptom of PTSD. However, they may also involve emotions or sense of threat related to the experienced trauma without necessarily repeating the index event itself. Whether post-traumatic nightmares are based upon a different mechanism than ordinary nightmares has not been clearly established. PTSD can entail a broad range of disturbance, including mood disorder, and biological alterations may come into play in some cases. Patients with PTSD also suffer from insomnia due to a cognitive hyperarousal at sleep onset, which may reflect an abnormal activation of attentional networks in these patients during sleep (Pillar et al. 2000).

The most likely differential diagnosis for nightmare disorders is that of night terrors, post-traumatic re-enactments (flashbacks) or nocturnal panic attacks. Episodes of extreme panic and confusion associated with vocalization, movement and autonomic discharge suggest the diagnosis of sleep terrors as more likely. Equally, finding out when these episodes characteristically occur, from the patient or their bed partner, might be helpful. Unlike nightmares that are predominantly REM-associated, night terrors typically occur during nREM sleep. Also, children with night terrors are difficult to arouse and console and do not recall a dream or nightmare.

Finally, a more traditional psychoanalytical approach also advocates that nightmares should be assessed as psychologically meaningful mental products, arising from interactions amongst ongoing life circumstances, internal conflicts and personality structure, with links to childhood roots and to unresolved disturbing and traumatic experiences.

15.5   Investigations

Nightmares are not commonly associated with specific physical findings (American Psychiatric Association. DSM-5 Task Force 2013). Heart rate and respiratory rate may increase or show increased variability before the person awakens from a nightmare. Mild autonomic arousal, including tachycardia, tachypnoea and sweating, may also occur transiently upon awakening (Pollak et al. 2010). Movement is uncommon owing to REM sleep-induced atonia (American Psychiatric Association. DSM-5 Task Force 2013). Psychological evaluation is commonly indicated for patients whose nightmares occur more than twice a week over a period of several months or when the nightmares are of great severity (Neuspiel 2013).

The polysomnographic (PSG) investigations of nightmares have proven somewhat elusive in that they are rarely observed in the sleep laboratory. Also, the degree of autonomic arousal, when present at all, seems small in proportion to the intensity of the affects experienced (Fisher et al. 1970). However, in some clinical cases, the PSG is used to ascertain the presence of other co-morbid sleep disorders (e.g. OSA, periodic limb movements), which may lead to sleep fragmentation and in that way contribute to increased nightmare frequency.

Some authors propose that PTSD-induced nightmares and nocturnal post-traumatic re-enactments (Kushida 2013) should be seen as a form of memory intrusion and not dreams (Hartmann 1998). Several PSG studies suggest that PTSD nightmares may indeed differ somewhat from idiopathic ones in that some occur out of nREM sleep, particularly stage 2 (Kramer et al. 1984). They are also noted in a context of greater sleep disruption (Woodward et al. 2000) and, on average, earlier in the night (Woodward et al. 2000). They also appear to be more often associated with body movement (van der Kolk et al. 1984). However, the clinical implication of this putative theoretical difference is yet to be clarified.

15.6   Treatment

Approaches to the treatment of nightmare disorder can vary considerably, depending in part on the theoretical perspective. Some suggest that treatments may be classified in terms of whether they target the symptom of nightmares in relative isolation or whether they aim at working out underlying psychological issues viewed as causing nightmares and other interconnected symptoms and problems. Of importance from a clinical viewpoint is also to address an ongoing debate amongst some authors where the very benefits of treating the nightmare disorder are raised. However, in support of treatment, one should state that by definition nightmares disrupt sleep and that research indicates that nightmares are linked to impaired sleep quality even if daytime stress levels are statistically controlled (Schredl 2003). Also, daytime functioning is severely impaired after nights with nightmares (Köthe and Pietrowsky 2001). Moreover, as already mentioned, nightmares can be associated with suicidal ideation (Sjostrom et al. 2007). These findings indicate that nightmare treatment might be beneficial for patients suffering from frequent and chronic nightmares (Krakow and Zadra 2006; Krakow et al. 2001; Aurora et al. 2010; Cranston et al. 2011).

Currently the best level A evidence only exists for two respective treatments of nightmare disorders: imagery rehearsal therapy (IRT) and the antihypertensive medication prazosin (Aurora et al. 2010). IRT is recommended for treatment of both primary/idiopathic nightmare disorders and PTSD-associated nightmares, whilst prazosin is recommended for treatment of severe and PTSD-associated nightmares.

IRT is a psychological treatment approach that targets trauma-related nightmares (Cranston et al. 2011). In this approach, persistent nightmares are viewed as a learnt habit. Patients are taught positive imaging techniques and then work on changing some of their nightmares and practising the altered nightmare scenarios. Significant improvement has been reported with utilization of this technique in a number of patient groups (Krakow and Zadra 2006). The mechanism of change is thought to reside in recalling, scripting, changing (theme, storyline, ending or other parts) to be more positive and rehearsing the rewritten dream in an effort to displace the disturbing content of the actual dream (Cranston et al. 2011). Some authors have argued that although empirical results supporting the efficacy of IRT are impressive, the conceptual framework they provide for understanding nightmares and their resolution seems limited. However, overall, there is sufficient evidence for the use of IRT as a first-line psychological treatment for nightmares.

Prazosin is an α1-adrenergic receptor antagonist whose anti-nightmare effect likely includes reduction of noradrenergic activity in the brain of the individuals diagnosed with PTSD (Thompson et al. 2008). Several studies indicated that prazosin was superior to placebo in improving nightmares, sleep, overall PTSD symptom severity and moderate improvement in trauma-related nightmares and non-nightmare distressed awakenings (Cranston et al. 2011; Aurora et al. 2010). Length of treatment ranged from 3 to 20 weeks, with average dosages ranging from 9.5 to 9.6 mg/day (Cranston et al. 2011). In addition, prazosin is reported as well tolerated by participants with few reports of adverse effects (e.g. mild orthostatic hypotension and/or dizziness) (Cranston et al. 2011).

Although there are no current uniform guidelines, nightmares are generally considered treatment-resistant if no improvement is observed after treatment with first-line treatments (e.g. IRT) and/or antidepressants and hypnotics.

15.6.1 Other Second-Line Pharmacological Treatments

The use of clonidine in the treatment of PTSD-associated nightmares has been reported (level C). Similarly, there is some support in the literature for the treatment of PTSD-associated nightmares with these medications: trazodone, atypical antipsychotic medications, topiramate, low-dose cortisol, fluvoxamine, triazolam, nitrazepam, phenelzine, gabapentin, cyproheptadine and tricyclic antidepressants (Aurora et al. 2010).

Also, levomepromazine, an antipsychotic, can be used in severe cases of PTSD in combat veterans and for treatment-resistant nightmares (Cranston et al. 2011). Aukst-Margetić and colleagues reported a reduction in nightmares using levomepromazine in combat veterans with severe PTSD (Aukst-Margetic et al. 2004). The dose of levomepromazine used ranged from 25 to 100 mg ($M = 47.05$ mg, $SD = 27.78$ mg) (Aukst-Margetic et al. 2004). No adverse effects were reported, and statistically significant improvements were shown for recurrent distressing dreams, arousal, total sleep hours, sleep latency and subjective sleepiness after waking (Aukst-Margetic et al. 2004). More recently, a clinical potential for use of nabilone as a treatment in chronic and treatment-resistant PTSD patients was also suggested (Fraser 2009). This synthetic endocannabinoid receptor is purported to work via reducing arousal and stress response in the brain and by acting on the central nervous system to regulate the amygdala, hypothalamic-pituitary-adrenocortical and hippocampal activity. However, due to considerable adverse effects, this treatment is currently not recommended, and further empirical investigations through larger double-blind, placebo-controlled trials are needed (Cranston et al. 2011).

15.6.2 Other Psychological Treatments

Exposure, relaxation and rescripting therapy (ERRT) is a psychological treatment based on the amalgamation of IRT, exposure therapies for PTSD and insomnia treatments. The mechanism of ERRT-induced change is currently unknown but thought to be related to exposure to the feared content of the nightmare, mastery through rescripting the nightmare and modifying maladaptive sleep habits (Cranston et al. 2011).

Several other level B evidence treatments also exist; systematic desensitization and progressive deep muscle relaxation training are amongst the more widely used treatments of idiopathic nightmares (Aurora et al. 2010).

Moreover, some level C evidence supports the use of different behavioural therapies and several novel techniques. For example, sleep dynamic therapy, hypnosis, eye movement desensitization and reprocessing (EMDR) and the testimony method were suggested to be of use in some groups of patients for the treatment of PTSD-associated nightmares based on low-grade evidence (Aurora et al. 2010). Similarly, some authors suggest lucid dreaming therapy and self-exposure therapy (Aurora et al. 2010).

15.6.3 Not Recommended and/or Showing Some Future Promise

There is level B and level C evidence against use of venlafaxine (for PTSD-nightmares) and nefazodone (risk of hepatotoxicity), respectively, as a first-line therapy for nightmare disorder (Aurora et al. 2010). Also, the use of clonazepam and individual psychotherapy is currently not recommended as a first- or second-line treatment because of sparse data (Aurora et al. 2010).

However, even though individual exploratory or psychodynamic psychotherapy use is not supported by published evidence, it has to be taken into account that this is a very different kind of treatment approach from IRT or the use of medications. It aims to work out underlying conflicts and traumatic influences that are relevant not only to a specific symptom, such as nightmares, but to other interrelated symptoms, difficulties and impairments in overall functioning and capacities for satisfaction. It is also often more long term and intensive in scope. Hence this approach might be particularly useful in the treatment of chronic and treatment-resistant idiopathic nightmares or for those presenting with some other prominent psychiatric co-morbidities (e.g. anxiety or personality disorders).

Finally, one of the exciting novel experimental therapeutic modalities, non-invasive neurostimulation, shows potential promise for the treatment of nightmares. Recent experimental studies indicate that in the near future, we may indeed be able to enable an active change of dream content via artificial triggering of sleep-state lucid dreaming. During lucid dreams, sleeping individuals enter a state of consciousness in which they are aware that they are dreaming and can be theoretically taught to control dream events (Bray 2014). The modulation of sleep structure and induction of lucid dreaming have been shown to be possible in one study by non-invasive neuromodulation, e.g. with transcranial alternating current and by increasing prefrontal REM gamma oscillations (Voss et al. 2014). Given the current dearth of effective therapies for severe and refractory cases, psychotherapies based on inducing lucid dreaming could be a valuable, if alternative, addition to the clinician's armamentarium for treating patients with recurrent nightmares (Voss et al. 2014).

15.6.4 Special Considerations in Paediatric Population

Reassurance and conservative management are commonly the only treatment required for sporadic nightmares in children (American Psychiatric Association 2013; Nevsimalova et al. 2013). However, daytime stressors should be identified and resolution attempted. Bedtime should become a safe and comfortable time when parents read to and talk with the child (Neuspiel 2013). It has been suggested that parents should monitor media exposure as this influences dream content (Moore 2012). Television viewing should be avoided for about 2 h prior to bedtime (Sadeh 2005).

Although IRT is a treatment modality used successfully in adults, it is not well studied in children. Several different cognitive-behavioural methods have been reported to be effective in treating nightmares in children (Sadeh 2005). Hypnosis has also been reported to be effective in treating nightmares and other parasomnias in children and adults (Hauri et al. 2007). If the nightmare is recurrent, discussing dream content and rescripting may help.

Conclusion

Nightmares are a prevalent parasomnia with clinically significant frequencies of once a week or more, occurring in 2–8% of the population. Higher frequency of nightmares are reported amongst children, women and a wide range of patients with psychiatric, neurological and personality issues. Several models of nightmare production suggest that nightmares may be implicated in an emotional adaptation function (Kushida 2013; Desseilles et al. 2011). In dealing with complaints of nightmares, clinicians should optimize their treatment recommendations by collecting a variety of information about common precipitating risk factors (Kushida 2013; Nielsen and Levin 2007; Neuspiel 2013). Also, it should be ascertained whether the nightmares are idiopathic or secondary (e.g. PTSD-related), as this may further influence treatment decisions. In addition, a careful assessment of a patient's neuropsychiatric and neurological risks, as well as their personality traits and vulnerability to adjustment and distress reactions, is of importance.

In the majority of sporadic cases of nightmares, where significant neuropsychiatric or neurological co-morbidity is excluded, formal pharmacological or psychological treatment will not be necessary. However, the assessment of day-to-day levels of stress and an affect load that lead to a temporary period of bad dreams or nightmares is considered beneficial. This considerate approach will additionally strengthen the rapport between the clinician and the patient and offer a good basis for further reassurance and psychoeducation of the patient.

Acknowledgements Supported by the Wellcome Trust [103952/Z/14/Z]

References

Abers MS, Shandera WX, Kass JS. Neurological and psychiatric adverse effects of antiretroviral drugs. CNS Drugs. 2014;28(2):131–45. https://doi.org/10.1007/s40263-013-0132-4.

American Academy of Sleep Medicine. The international classification of sleep disorders: diagnostic and coding manual. 3rd ed. Westchester, IL: American Academy of Sleep Medicine; 2015.

American Psychiatric Association. Desk reference to the diagnostic criteria from DSM-5. Washington, DC: American Psychiatric Publishing; 2013.

American Psychiatric Association. DSM-5 Task Force. Diagnostic and statistical manual of mental disorders: DSM-5. 5th ed. Washington, DC: American Psychiatric Association; 2013.

Aukst-Margetic B, Margetic B, Tosic G, Bilic-Prcic A. Levomepromazine helps to reduce sleep problems in patients with PTSD. Eur Psychiatry. 2004;19(4):235–6. https://doi.org/10.1016/j.eurpsy.2003.12.007.

Aurora RN, Zak RS, Auerbach SH, Casey KR, Chowdhuri S, Karippot A, Maganti RK, Ramar K, Kristo DA, Bista SR, Lamm CI, Morgenthaler TI, Standards of Practice C, American Academy of Sleep Medicine. Best practice guide for the treatment of nightmare disorder in adults. J Clin Sleep Med. 2010;6(4):389–401.

Bloomfield ER, Shatkin JP. Parasomnias and movement disorders in children and adolescents. Child Adolesc Psychiatr Clin N Am. 2009;18(4):947–65. https://doi.org/10.1016/j.chc.2009.04.010.

Bray N. Sleep: Inducing lucid dreams. Nat Rev Neurosci. 2014;15(7):428. https://doi.org/10.1038/nrn3769.

Corbo JM, Brown JN, Moss JM. Galantamine-associated nightmares and anxiety. Consult Pharm. 2013;28(4):243–6. https://doi.org/10.4140/TCP.n.2013.243.

Cranston CC, Davis JL, Rhudy JL, Favorite TK. Replication and expansion of "Best Practice Guide for the Treatment of Nightmare Disorder in Adults". J Clin Sleep Med. 2011;7(5):549–53; . discussion 554–546. https://doi.org/10.5664/JCSM.1330.

Dang A, Kamat R, Padmanabh RV. Ciprofloxacin induced nightmares in an adult patient. Indian J Psychiatry. 2008;50(4):305–6. https://doi.org/10.4103/0019-5545.44757.

Dang A, Garg G, Rataboli PV. Mirtazapine induced nightmares in an adult male. Br J Clin Pharmacol. 2009;67(1):135–6. https://doi.org/10.1111/j.1365-2125.2008.03305.x.

De Angeli F, Lovati C, Giani L, D'Alessandro M, Raimondi E, Scaglione V, Castoldi D, Capiluppi E, Mariani C. Negative emotions in migraineurs dreams: the increased prevalence of oneiric fear and anguish, unrelated to mood disorders. Behav Neurol. 2014;2014:919627. https://doi.org/10.1155/2014/919627.

Desseilles M, Dang-Vu TT, Sterpenich V, Schwartz S. Cognitive and emotional processes during dreaming: a neuroimaging view. Conscious Cogn. 2011;20(4):998–1008. https://doi.org/10.1016/j.concog.2010.10.005.

Fisher C, Byrne JV, Edwards A, Kahn E. REM and NREM nightmares. Int Psychiatry Clin. 1970;7(2):183–7.

Fraser GA. The use of a synthetic cannabinoid in the management of treatment-resistant nightmares in posttraumatic stress disorder (PTSD). CNS Neurosci Ther. 2009;15(1):84–8. https://doi.org/10.1111/j.1755-5949.2008.00071.x.

Godin I, Montplaisir J, Gagnon JF, Nielsen T. Alexithymia associated with nightmare distress in idiopathic REM sleep behavior disorder. Sleep. 2013;36(12):1957–62. https://doi.org/10.5665/sleep.3238.

Hartmann E. The nightmare: the psychology and biology of terrifying dreams. New York, NY: Basic Books; 1984.

Hartmann E. Nightmare after trauma as paradigm for all dreams: a new approach to the nature and functions of dreaming. Psychiatry. 1998;61(3):223–38.

Hauri PJ, Silber MH, Boeve BF. The treatment of parasomnias with hypnosis: a 5-year follow-up study. J Clin Sleep Med. 2007;3(4):369–73.

Hublin C, Kaprio J, Partinen M, Koskenvuo M. Nightmares: familial aggregation and association with psychiatric disorders in a nationwide twin cohort. Am J Med Genet. 1999;88(4):329–36.

Isacsson G, Ahlner J. Antidepressants and the risk of suicide in young persons--prescription trends and toxicological analyses. Acta Psychiatr Scand. 2014;129(4):296–302. https://doi.org/10.1111/acps.12160.

Khan F, Bernadt M. Intense suicidal thoughts and self-harm following escitalopram treatment. Indian J Psychol Med. 2011;33(1):74–6. https://doi.org/10.4103/0253-7176.85400.

van der Kolk B, Blitz R, Burr W, Sherry S, Hartmann E. Nightmares and trauma: a comparison of nightmares after combat with lifelong nightmares in veterans. Am J Psychiatry. 1984;141(2):187–90.

Kotagal S. Parasomnias in childhood. Sleep Med Rev. 2009;13(2):157–68. https://doi.org/10.1016/j.smrv.2008.09.005.

Köthe M, Pietrowsky R. Behavioral effects of nightmares and their correlations to personality patterns. Dreaming. 2001;11:43–52.

Krakow B, Zadra A. Clinical management of chronic nightmares: imagery rehearsal therapy. Behav Sleep Med. 2006;4(1):45–70. https://doi.org/10.1207/s15402010bsm0401_4.

Krakow B, Tandberg D, Scriggins L, Barey M. A controlled comparison of self-rated sleep complaints in acute and chronic nightmare sufferers. J Nerv Ment Dis. 1995;183(10):623–7.

Krakow B, Lowry C, Germain A, Gaddy L, Hollifield M, Koss M, Tandberg D, Johnston L, Melendrez D. A retrospective study on improvements in nightmares and post-traumatic stress disorder following treatment for co-morbid sleep-disordered breathing. J Psychosom Res. 2000;49(5):291–8.

Krakow B, Hollifield M, Johnston L, Koss M, Schrader R, Warner TD, Tandberg D, Lauriello J, McBride L, Cutchen L, Cheng D, Emmons S, Germain A, Melendrez D, Sandoval D, Prince H. Imagery rehearsal therapy for chronic nightmares in sexual assault survivors with posttraumatic stress disorder: a randomized controlled trial. JAMA. 2001;286(5):537–45.

Kramer M, Schoen LS, Kinney L. Psychological and behavioral features of disturbed dreamers. Psychiatr J Univ Ott. 1984;9(3):102–6.

Kung S, Espinel Z, Lapid MI. Treatment of nightmares with prazosin: a systematic review. Mayo Clin Proc. 2012;87(9):890–900. https://doi.org/10.1016/j.mayocp.2012.05.015.

Kushida CE. Encyclopedia of sleep. Waltham, MA: Academic Press; 2013. p. 219–24. https://doi.org/10.1016/B978-0-12-378610-4.00429-0.

Marinova P, Koychev I, Laleva L, Kancheva L, Tsvetkov M, Bilyukov R, Vandeva D, Felthouse A, Koychev G. Nightmares and suicide: predicting risk in depression. Psychiatr Danub. 2014;26(2):159–64.

McCall WV, Black CG. The link between suicide and insomnia: theoretical mechanisms. Curr Psychiatry Rep. 2013;15(9):389. https://doi.org/10.1007/s11920-013-0389-9.

Montagna P, Chokroverty S. Sleep disorders. In: Handbook of clinical neurology, vol. 3. New York, NY: Elsevier, Edinburgh; 2011. p. 98–9.

Moore M. Behavioral sleep problems in children and adolescents. J Clin Psychol Med Settings. 2012;19(1):77–83. https://doi.org/10.1007/s10880-011-9282-z.

Nadorff MR, Fiske A, Sperry JA, Petts R, Gregg JJ. Insomnia symptoms, nightmares, and suicidal ideation in older adults. J Gerontol B Psychol Sci Soc Sci. 2013a;68(2):145–52. https://doi.org/10.1093/geronb/gbs061.

Nadorff MR, Nazem S, Fiske A. Insomnia symptoms, nightmares, and suicide risk: duration of sleep disturbance matters. Suicide Life Threat Behav. 2013b;43(2):139–49. https://doi.org/10.1111/sltb.12003.

Neuspiel DR. Nightmare disorder treatment & management. 2015. https://emedicine.medscape.com/article/914428-treatment

Nevsimalova S, Prihodova I, Kemlink D, Skibova J. Childhood parasomnia--a disorder of sleep maturation? Eur J Paediatr Neurol. 2013;17(6):615–9. https://doi.org/10.1016/j.ejpn.2013.05.004.

Nielsen T, Levin R. Nightmares: a new neurocognitive model. Sleep Med Rev. 2007;11(4):295–310. https://doi.org/10.1016/j.smrv.2007.03.004.

Pagel JF, Helfter P. Drug induced nightmares--an etiology based review. Hum Psychopharmacol. 2003;18(1):59–67. https://doi.org/10.1002/hup.465.

Partinen M. Epidemiology of sleep disorders. In: Kryger MH, Roth T, Dement WC, editors. Principles and practice of sleep medicine. 2nd ed. Philadelphia: Saunders; 1994. p. 437–52.

Petit D, Touchette E, Tremblay RE, Boivin M, Montplaisir J. Dyssomnias and parasomnias in early childhood. Pediatrics. 2007;119(5):e1016–25. https://doi.org/10.1542/peds.2006-2132.

Pillar G, Malhotra A, Lavie P. Post-traumatic stress disorder and sleep-what a nightmare! Sleep Med Rev. 2000;4(2):183–200. https://doi.org/10.1053/smrv.1999.0095.

Pisko J, Pastorek L, Buskova J, Sonka K, Nevsimalova S. Nightmares in narcolepsy: underinvestigated symptom? Sleep Med. 2014;15(8):967–72. https://doi.org/10.1016/j.sleep.2014.03.006.

Pollak C, Thorpy MJ, Yager J. The encyclopedia of sleep and sleep disorders. 3rd ed. New York, NY: Facts on File; 2010. Updated and revised edn.

Rosenzweig I, Williams SC, Morrell MJ. The impact of sleep and hypoxia on the brain: potential mechanisms for the effects of obstructive sleep apnea. Curr Opin Pulm Med. 2014;20(6):565–71. https://doi.org/10.1097/MCP.0000000000000099.

Rosenzweig I, Glasser M, Polsek D, Leschziner GD, Williams SCR, Morrell MJ. Sleep apnoea and the brain: a complex relationship. Lancet Respir Med. 2015;3:404. https://doi.org/10.1016/S2213-2600(15)00090-9.

Ross RJ, Ball WA, Sullivan KA, Caroff SN. Sleep disturbance as the hallmark of posttraumatic stress disorder. Am J Psychiatry. 1989;146(6):697–707.

Sadeh A. Cognitive-behavioral treatment for childhood sleep disorders. Clin Psychol Rev. 2005;25(5):612–28. https://doi.org/10.1016/j.cpr.2005.04.006.

Salvio MA, Wood JM, Schwartz J, Eichling PS. Nightmare prevalence in the healthy elderly. Psychol Aging. 1992;7(2):324–5.

Schredl M. Effects of state and trait factors on nightmare frequency. Eur Arch Psychiatry Clin Neurosci. 2003;253(5):241–7. https://doi.org/10.1007/s00406-003-0438-1.

Schredl M. Editorial for "Nightmares in narcolepsy - under-investigated symptom?" (SLEEP-D-13-00591) Understanding and treating nightmares in patients with narcolepsy. Sleep Med. 2014a;15(8):851–2. https://doi.org/10.1016/j.sleep.2014.05.003.

Schredl M. Explaining the gender difference in nightmare frequency. Am J Psychol. 2014b;127(2):205–13.

Sjostrom N, Waern M, Hetta J. Nightmares and sleep disturbances in relation to suicidality in suicide attempters. Sleep. 2007;30(1):91–5.

Susanszky E, Hajnal A, Kopp M. Sleep disturbances and nightmares as risk factors for suicidal behavior among men and women. Psychiatr Hung. 2011;26(4):250–7.

Tamanna S, Parker JD, Lyons J, Ullah MI. The effect of continuous positive air pressure (CPAP) on nightmares in patients with posttraumatic stress disorder (PTSD) and obstructive sleep apnea (OSA). J Clin Sleep Med. 2014;10(6):631–6. https://doi.org/10.5664/jcsm.3786.

Thompson DF, Pierce DR. Drug-induced nightmares. Ann Pharmacother. 1999;33(1):93–8.

Thompson CE, Taylor FB, McFall ME, Barnes RF, Raskind MA. Nonnightmare distressed awakenings in veterans with posttraumatic stress disorder: response to prazosin. J Trauma Stress. 2008;21(4):417–20. https://doi.org/10.1002/jts.20351.

Voss U, Holzmann R, Hobson A, Paulus W, Koppehele-Gossel J, Klimke A, Nitsche MA. Induction of self awareness in dreams through frontal low current stimulation of gamma activity. Nat Neurosci. 2014;17(6):810–2. https://doi.org/10.1038/nn.3719.

Woodward SH, Arsenault NJ, Murray C, Bliwise DL. Laboratory sleep correlates of nightmare complaint in PTSD inpatients. Biol Psychiatry. 2000;48(11):1081–7.

Youakim JM, Doghramji K, Schutte SL. Posttraumatic stress disorder and obstructive sleep apnea syndrome. Psychosomatics. 1998;39(2):168–71. https://doi.org/10.1016/S0033-3182(98)71365-9.

Zadra A, Donderi DC. Nightmares and bad dreams: their prevalence and relationship to well-being. J Abnorm Psychol. 2000;109(2):273–81.

Zadra A, Pilon M, Donderi DC. Variety and intensity of emotions in nightmares and bad dreams. J Nerv Ment Dis. 2006;194(4):249–54. https://doi.org/10.1097/01.nmd.0000207359.46223.dc.

Appendix A

1.1   Epworth Sleepiness Scale (ESS)

Name: _____ Today's date: _____

Your age (Yrs): _____ Your sex (Male = M, Female = F): _____

How likely are you to doze off or fall asleep in the following situations, in comparison to feeling just tired?

This refers to your usual way of life in recent times.

Even if you have not done some of these things recently try to work out how they would have affected you.

Use the following scale to choose the **most appropriate number** for each situation:

0 = would **never** doze
1 = **slight chance** of dozing
2 = **moderate chance** of dozing
3 = **high chance** of dozing

It is important that you answer each question as best as you can

Situation	Chance of Dozing (0–3)
Sitting and reading _____	___
Watching TV _____	___
Sitting still in a public place (e.g., a theatre, a cinema or a meeting) _____	___
As a passenger in a car for an hour without a break _____	___
Lying down to rest in the afternoon when circumstances allow _____	___
Sitting and talking to someone _____	___
Sitting quietly after a lunch without having drunk alcohol _____	___
In a car or a bus while stopped for a few minutes in traffic _____	___

THANK YOU FOR YOUR CO-OPERATION

ESS © MW Johns 1990-1997. Used under License

© Springer-Verlag GmbH Germany, part of Springer Nature 2018
H. Selsick (ed.), *Sleep Disorders in Psychiatric Patients*,
https://doi.org/10.1007/978-3-642-54836-9

Appendix B

Morningness-Eveningess Questionnaire

Instructions:
1. Please read each question very carefully before answering.
2. Answer ALL questions
3. Answer questions in numerical order.
4. Each question should be answered independently of others. Do NOT go back and check your answers.
5. All questions have a selection of answers. For each question place a cross alongside ONE answer only. Some questions have a scale instead of a selection of answers. Place a cross at the appropriate point along the scale.
6. Please answer each question as honestly as possible. Both your answers and the results will be kept, in strict confidence.
7. Please feel free to make any comments in the section provided below each question.

The Questionnaire with scores for each choice

1. Considering only your own "feeling best" rhythm, at what time would you get up if you were entirely free to plan your day?

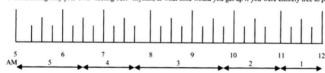

2. Considering only your own "feeling best" rhythm, at what time would you go to bed if you were entirely free to plan your evening?

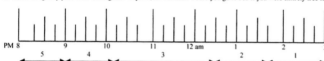

3. If there is a specific time at which you have to get up in the morning, to what extent are you dependent on being woken up by an alarm clock?

Not at all dependent	☐ 4
Slightly dependent	☐ 3
Fairly dependent	☐ 2
Very dependent	☐ 1

4. Assuming adequate environmental conditions, how easy do you find getting up in the mornings?

Not at all easy	☐ 1
Not very easy	☐ 2
Fairly easy	☐ 3
Very easy	☐ 4

5. How alert do you feel during the first half hour after having woken in the mornings?

Not at all alert	☐ 1
Slightly alert	☐ 2
Fairly alert	☐ 3
Very alert	☐ 4

6. How is your appetite during the first half-hour after having woken in the mornings?

Very poor	☐ 1
Fairly poor	☐ 2
Fairly good	☐ 3
Very good	☐ 4

15. You have to do two hours of hard physical work. You are entirely free to plan your day and considering only your own "feeling best" rhythm which ONE of the following times would you choose?

8:00-10:00 a.m.   □ 4
11:00 a.m.-1:00 p.m.   □ 3
3:00-5:00 p.m.   □ 2
7:00-9:00 p.m.   □ 1

16. You have decide to engage in hard physical exercise. A friend suggests that you do this for one hour twice a week and the best time for him is between 10-11 p.m. Bearing in mind nothing else but your own "feeling best" rhythm how well do you think you would perform?

Would be on good form   □ 1
Would be on reasonable form   □ 2
Would find it difficult   □ 3
Would find if very difficult   □ 4

17. Suppose that you can choose your own work hours. Assume that you worked a FIVE hour day (including breaks) and that your job was interesting and paid by results. Which FIVE CONSECUTIVE HOURS would you select?

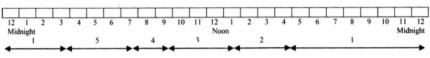

18. At what time of the day do you think that you reach your "feeling best" peak?

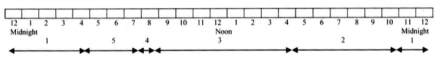

19. One hears about "morning" and "evening" types of people. Which ONE of these types do you consider yourself to be?

Definitely a "morning" type   □ 6
Rather more a "morning" than an evening type   □ 4
Rather more an "evening" than a "morning" type   □ 2
Definitely an "evening" type   □ 0

Scoring Instructions

For questions 3, 4, 5, 6, 7, 8, 9, 11, 12, 13, 14, 15, 16 and 19, the appropriate score for each response is displayed beside the answer box.

For questions 1, 2, 10 and 18, the cross made along each scale is referred to the appropriate score value range below the scale.

For question 17, the most extreme cross on the right-hand side is taken as the reference point and the appropriate score value range below this point is taken.

The scores are added together and the sum converted into a five-point morningness-eveningness scale:

Score

Definitely morning type 70–86
Moderately morning type 59–69
Neither type 42–58
Moderately evening type 31–41
Definitely evening type 16–30

(Horne and Ostberg 1976)

7. During the first half-hour after having woken in the morning, how tired do you feel?

Very tired ☐ 1
Fairly tired ☐ 2
Fairly refreshed ☐ 3
Very refreshed ☐ 4

8. When you have no commitments the next day, at what time do you go to bed compared to your usual bedtime?

Seldom or never later ☐ 4
Less than one hour later ☐ 3
1-2 hours later ☐ 2
More than two hours later ☐ 1

9. You have decided to engage in some physical exercise. A friend suggests that you do this one hour twice a week and the best time for him is between 7:00-8:00 a.m. Bearing in mind nothing else but your own "feeling best" rhythm, how do you think you would perform?

Would be on good form ☐ 4
Would be on reasonable form ☐ 3
Would find it difficult ☐ 2
Would find it very difficult ☐ 1

10. At what time in the evening do you feel tired and as a result in need of sleep?

11. You wish to be at your peak performance for a test which you know is going to be mentally exhausting and lasting for two hours. You are entirely free to plan your day and considering only your own "feeling best" rhythm which ONE of the four testing times would you choose?

8:00-10:00 a.m. ☐ 6
11:00 a.m.-1:00 p.m. ☐ 4
3:00-5:00 p.m. ☐ 2
7:00-9:00 p.m. ☐ 0

12. If you went to bed at 11 p.m. at what level of tiredness would you be?

Not at all tired ☐ 0
A little tired ☐ 2
Fairly tired ☐ 3
Very tired ☐ 5

13. For some reason you have gone to bed several hours later than usual, but there is no need to get up at any particular time the next morning. Which ONE of the following events are you most likely to experience?

Will wake up at usual time and will NOT fall asleep ☐ 4
Will wake up at usual time and will doze thereafter ☐ 3
Will wake up at usual time but will fall asleep again ☐ 2
Will NOT wake up until later than usual ☐ 1

14. One night you have to remain awake between 4-6 a.m. in order to carry out a night watch. You have no commitments the next day. Which ONE of the following alternatives will suit you best?

Would NOT go to bed until watch was over ☐ 1
Would take a nap before and sleep after ☐ 2
Would take a good sleep before and nap after ☐ 3
Would take ALL sleep before watch ☐ 4

Reference

Horne JA, Ostberg O. A self-assessment questionnaire to determine morningness-eveningness in human circadian rhythms. Int J Chronobiol. 1976;4(2):97–110.

Appendix C

Sleep Diary

Week starting	Last night I went to bed at	This morning I got up at	So I was in bed for (minutes)	It took me ? minutes to fall asleep	I woke ? number of times	During the night I was awake for (minutes)	In total I think I slept for (minutes)	Other info
Night 1								
Night 2								
Night 3								
Night 4								
Night 5								
Night 6								
Night 7								
Total			B					
Average in minutes							A	
Average in hours and minutes								

A divided by B × 100 = sleep efficiency A _____ /B _____ × 100 = _____

Printed by Printforce, the Netherlands